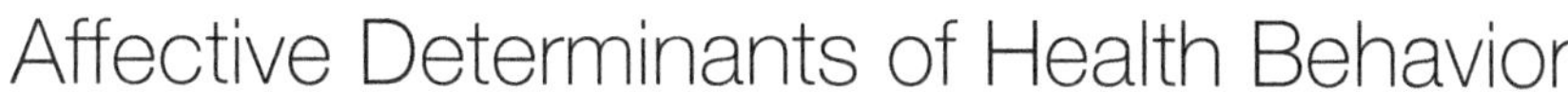

Affective Determinants of Health Behavior

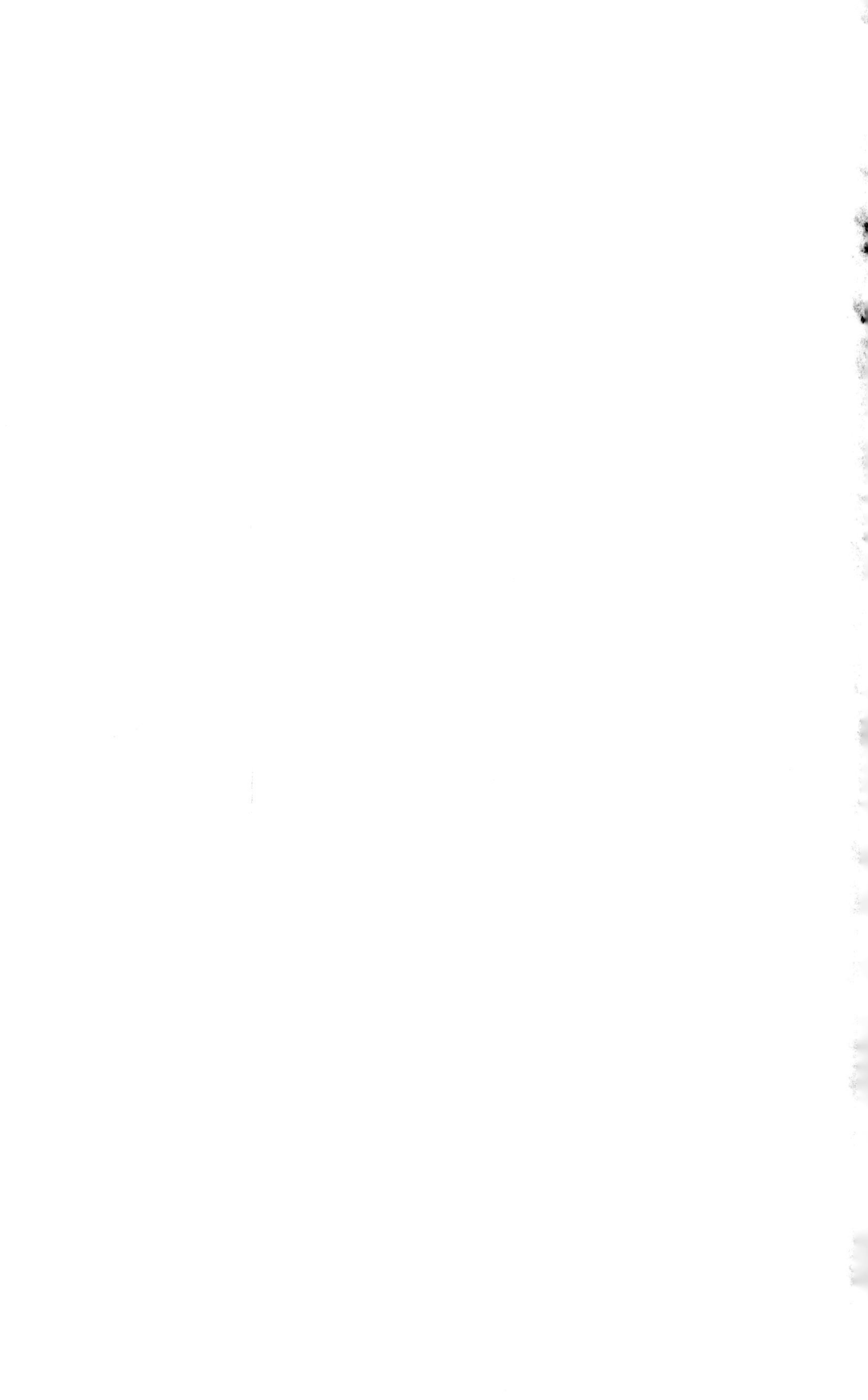

Affective Determinants of Health Behavior

EDITED BY

DAVID M. WILLIAMS

RYAN E. RHODES

MARK T. CONNER

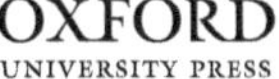

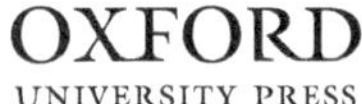

Oxford University Press is a department of the University of Oxford. It furthers the University's objective of excellence in research, scholarship, and education by publishing worldwide. Oxford is a registered trade mark of Oxford University Press in the UK and certain other countries.

Published in the United States of America by Oxford University Press
198 Madison Avenue, New York, NY 10016, United States of America.

Library of Congress Cataloging-in-Publication Data
Names: Williams, David M. (David Michael), 1976- editor. |
Rhodes, Ryan E., 1973- editor. | Conner, Mark T., 1962- editor.
Title: Affective determinants of health behavior / edited by
David M. Williams, Ryan E. Rhodes, Mark T. Conner.
Description: New York, NY : Oxford University Press, [2018] |
Includes bibliographical references and index.
Identifiers: LCCN 2017046501 | ISBN 9780190499037 (hardcover : alk. paper)
Subjects: | MESH: Health Behavior | Patient Acceptance of Health Care
Classification: LCC RA427.8 | NLM W 85 | DDC 613—dc23
LC record available at https://lccn.loc.gov/2017046501

9 8 7 6 5 4 3 2 1

Printed by Sheridan Books, Inc., United States of America

CONTENTS

PREFACE

Health behaviors such as poor diet, physical inactivity, smoking, risky sexual behavior, and alcohol and drug abuse are responsible for an ever-growing proportion of death and disease in developed and developing nations. Improving our understanding and ability to facilitate change in these health behaviors is thus a defining problem for 21st-century behavioral science and public health.

Behavioral and social scientists who study health behaviors have, until recently, placed heavy emphasis on cognitive factors—for example, beliefs, expectancies, intentions—in their theories of the determinants of health behavior. These theories include social cognitive theory, the health belief model, the theory of reasoned action, and the theory of planned behavior; they are based on the expectancy-value models that emerged at the time of the cognitive revolution in psychology in the 1950s. Such theories remain the dominant and most referenced accounts of the determinants of health behavior.

In the last couple of decades, however, health behavior scientists working in diverse disciplines have begun to place greater emphasis on affective factors—pleasure, displeasure, emotion—as determinants of why people engage in or do not engage in health behaviors. To be sure, these affective factors overlap in many ways with the cognitive factors that have been a focus of health behavior research for over 60 years: for example, research on anticipated affective response to exercise or drug use. It is only recently though that affective factors have become—in their own right—a major focus of research in health behavior science.

The burgeoning research on affective determinants of health behavior published in the last 20 years or so is characterized by two features. First, it has largely been domain- or behavior-specific, with separate literatures emerging in the context of addictive behaviors, food/eating, and physical activity research. Second, perhaps in part because of the aforementioned domain specificity, affective concepts have not been incorporated into the most-often used theories of health behavior; such theories remain cognitively focused.

The purpose of this book is to present in a single volume state-of-the-science theory and research on affective determinants of health behaviors across multiple behavioral domains. The book is divided into two parts. In the first part (chapters 2–10), theories of affect and behavior are presented in a way that is accessible and potentially applicable across multiple health behaviors. In part 2 (chapters 11–20), authors summarize research on one or more affective determinants within specific behavioral domains, including eating, smoking, sex, physical activity, alcohol and drug use, suntanning, blood donation, cancer screening, other cancer-related behaviors, and clinical decision-making. The precise structure of these chapters was left up to the authors with the one caveat that the focus be on health behavior as the dependent variable and affect as the putative determinant.

The intended audience for the book is graduate and advanced undergraduate students in psychology and other behavioral and social science fields, as well as applied fields such as behavioral medicine, nursing, public health, and medicine. We also expect the book to be useful to scientists currently conducting research for which the goal is to better understand and/or facilitate change in health behaviors, as well as those who are new to this burgeoning area of research.

We would like to thank the chapter authors for providing concise and informative summaries of work in their area. We would also like to thank Courtney McCarroll and Abby Gross at Oxford University Press for their help and enthusiasm in putting this book together.

CONTRIBUTORS

Kristen G. Anderson
Department of Psychology
Reed College
Portland, OR, USA

Austin S. Baldwin
Department of Psychology
Southern Methodist University
Dallas, TX, USA

Ryan P. Bell
Department of Psychology and Neuroscience
University of North Carolina—Chapel Hill
Chapel Hill, NC, USA

Krysten W. Bold
Department of Psychiatry
Yale University
New Haven, CT, USA

Charmaine Borg
Department of Clinical Psychology and Experimental Psychopathology
University of Groningen
Groningen, the Netherlands

Angela D. Bryan
Department of Psychology and Neuroscience
University of Colorado Boulder
Boulder, CO, USA

Mark T. Conner
School of Psychology
University of Leeds
Leeds, England, UK

Nathan S. Consedine
Department of Psychological Medicine
University of Auckland
Auckland, New Zealand

Jessica W. Cook
Department of Medicine
University of Wisconsin School of Medicine and Public Health
Madison, WI, USA

Elliot J. Coups
Rutgers Cancer Institute of New Jersey
Department of Medicine
Rutgers University
New Brunswick, NJ, USA

Stacey B. Daughters
Department of Psychology and Neuroscience
University of North Carolina—Chapel Hill
Chapel Hill, NC, USA

Ashley K. Day
Rutgers Cancer Institute of New Jersey
Rutgers University
New Brunswick, NJ, USA;
School of Psychology
University of Adelaide
Adelaide, Australia

Denise de Ridder
Department of Psychology
Utrecht University
Utrecht, the Netherlands

Panteleimon Ekkekakis
Department of Kinesiology
Iowa State University
Ames, IA, USA

Erin M. Ellis
Behavioral Research Program
National Cancer Institute
Rockville, MD, USA

Catharine Evers
Department of Psychology
Utrecht University
Utrecht, the Netherlands

Sarah W. Feldstein Ewing
Department of Child and Adolescent Psychiatry
Oregon Health & Science University
Portland, OR, USA

Eamonn Ferguson
School of Psychology
University of Nottingham
Nottingham, England, UK

Rebecca A. Ferrer
Behavioral Research Program
National Cancer Institute
Rockville, MD, USA

Geoffrey T. Fong
Department of Psychology
University of Waterloo
Waterloo, Ontario, Canada

Arielle S. Gillman
Department of Psychology and Neuroscience
University of Colorado Boulder
Boulder, CO, USA

Peter M. Gollwitzer
Department of Psychology
New York University
New York, NY, USA;
Department of Psychology
University of Konstanz
Konstanz, Germany

Samantha M. Gray
School of Exercise Science, Physical & Health Education
University of Victoria
Victoria, British Columbia, Canada

Martin S. Hagger
School of Psychology
Curtin University
Perth, Australia;
Faculty of Sport and Health Sciences
University of Jyväskylä
Jyväskylä, Finland

Peter A. Hall
School of Public Health and Health Systems
University of Waterloo
Waterloo, Ontario, Canada

Natasha S. Hansen
Department of Psychology and Neuroscience
University of Colorado Boulder
Boulder, CO, USA

Mark E. Hartman
Department of Kinesiology
Iowa State University
Ames, IA, USA

Jane Heyhoe
Bradford Institute for Health Research
Bradford, England, UK

Bernhard Hommel
Department of Psychology
Leiden University
Leiden, the Netherlands

Marc T. Kiviniemi
Department of Community Health and Health Behavior
University at Buffalo, SUNY
Buffalo, NY, USA

Lynne B. Klasko-Foster
Department of Community Health and Health Behavior
University at Buffalo, SUNY
Buffalo, NY, USA

Matthew A. Ladwig
Department of Kinesiology
Iowa State University
Ames, IA, USA

Rebecca Lawton
School of Psychology
University of Leeds
Leeds, England, UK;
Bradford Institute for Health Research
Bradford, England, UK

Teresa M. Leyro
Department of Psychology
Rutgers University
New Brunswick, NJ, USA

Cassandra J. Lowe
School of Public Health and Health Systems
University of Waterloo
Waterloo, Ontario, Canada

Barbara Masser
School of Psychology
The University of Queensland
Brisbane, Australia

Danielle E. McCarthy
Department of Medicine
University of Wisconsin School of Medicine and Public Health
Madison, WI, USA

Haruka Minami
Department of Psychology
Fordham University
Bronx, NY, USA

Gabriele Oettingen
Department of Psychology
New York University
New York, NY, USA;
Department of Psychology
University of Hamburg
Hamburg, Germany

Cleo Protogerou
School of Psychology
Curtin University
Perth, Australia;
Department of Psychology
University of Cape Town
Cape Town, South Africa

Elizabeth D. Reese
Department of Psychology and Neuroscience
University of North Carolina—Chapel Hill
Chapel Hill, NC, USA

Lisa M. Reynolds
Department of Psychological Medicine
University of Auckland
Auckland, New Zealand

Ryan E. Rhodes
School of Exercise Science, Physical & Health Education
University of Victoria
Victoria, British Columbia, Canada

Margarita Sala
Department of Psychology
Southern Methodist University
Dallas, TX, USA

Elske Salemink
Department of Psychology
University of Amsterdam
Amsterdam, the Netherlands

Paschal Sheeran
Gillings School of Global Public Health
University of North Carolina—Chapel Hill
Chapel Hill, NC, USA

Bram Van Bockstaele
Department of Psychology
University of Amsterdam
Amsterdam, the Netherlands

Thomas L. Webb
Department of Psychology
University of Sheffield
Sheffield, England, UK

Reinout W. Wiers
Department of Psychology
University of Amsterdam
Amsterdam, the Netherlands

David M. Williams
Department of Behavioral and Social Sciences
School of Public Health
Brown University
Providence, RI, USA

Jennifer Y. Yi
Department of Psychology and Neuroscience
University of North Carolina—Chapel Hill
Chapel Hill, NC, USA

Zachary Zenko
Center for Advanced Hindsight
Duke University
Durham, NC, USA

1

Overview of Affective Determinants of Health Behavior

DAVID M. WILLIAMS, RYAN E. RHODES, AND MARK T. CONNER

INTRODUCTION

This chapter provides a brief introduction to the topic of affective determinants of health behavior. First, we outline what is meant by health behavior. Second, we consider traditional views of the key determinants of such behaviors and the value of integrating affective determinants within health behavior theories. Third, and finally, the main section of the chapter offers a conceptualization of affective determinants in relation to health behaviors and a brief discussion of measurement of affect in the context of health behavior research.

HEALTH BEHAVIORS

A widely used definition of health behaviors is "overt behavioral patterns, actions and habits that relate to health maintenance, to health restoration and to health improvement" (Gochman, 1997, p. 3). A wide variety of behaviors would be included within such a definition including, but not limited to, eating, smoking, sex, physical activity, alcohol and drug use, suntanning, blood donation, cancer screening, other cancer-related behaviors, and clinical decision-making (all of which are addressed in this book, with some behaviors considered in several chapters). Most such behaviors are performed by individuals in ways that impact on their own health, although the definition does not necessarily exclude behaviors performed as part of one's professional role (see Lawton & Heyhoe, this volume). The evidence supporting the health impacts of behaviors such as smoking, eating, sedentary behavior, physical inactivity, substance abuse, and sex is substantial, and together health behaviors account for a significant proportion of chronic disease and death worldwide and in high-income countries in particular (Danaei et al., 2009; GBD 2016 Risk Factors Collaborators, 2017; Mokdad, Marks, Stroup, & Gerberding, 2004). Informative reviews of the broad range of research on prominent health behaviors (healthy diet: de Ridder, Kroese, Evers, Adriaanse, & Gillebaart, 2017; physical activity: Rhodes, Janssen, Bredin, Warburton, & Bauman, 2017; binge drinking: Kuntsche, Kuntsche, Thrul, & Gmel, 2017; smoking: West, 2017) can be found in a recent themed issue of the journal *Psychology and Health* (Conner & Norman, 2017; see also Ferrer & Mendes, 2018, for a special issue devoted to affect and health behaviors).

A variety of distinctions between types of health behaviors have been made (see McEachan, Lawton, & Conner, 2010). For example, Rothman and Salovey (1997) highlight the distinction between preventive (those that aim to prevent onset of ill-health), detective (those that aim to detect potential problems), and curative (those that aim to cure or treat a health problem) health behaviors. Other distinctions have focused on distinguishing among health behaviors on the basis of frequency of occurrence (frequent versus infrequent) or whether the positive health outcomes are associated with performing more or less of the behavior. However, there does not appear to be any simple mapping between such distinctions among health behaviors and the relative importance of affective determinants. For example, the current volume considers various preventive (e.g., physical activity: Ekkekakis, Zenko, Ladwig, & Hartman, this volume; Hall, Fong, & Lowe, this volume; Hagger & Protogerou, this volume; Rhodes, Janssen, et al., this volume; Sheeran, Webb, Gollwitzer, & Oettinge, this volume; diet/eating: de Ridder & Evers, this volume; Hall et al., this volume; Rhodes, Janssen, et al., this volume; Sheeran et al., this volume; drinking alcohol: Reese, Yi, Bell, & Daughters, this volume; Wiers, Anderson, Van Bockstaele, Salemink, & Hommel, this volume; sexual behaviors: Hansen, Gillman, Feldstein Ewing, & Bryan, this volume; smoking: McCarthy, Cook, Leyro, Minami, & Bold, this volume; Wiers et al., this volume; suntanning: Day & Coups, this volume), detective, or curative (e.g., screening: Consedine, Reynolds, & Borg, this volume; cancer-related behaviors: Ellis & Ferrer, this volume) health behaviors. It also considers health behaviors that are more (e.g., smoking: McCarthy et al., this volume; Wiers et al., this volume; physical activity: Ekkekakis et al., this volume; Hall et al., this volume; Hagger & Protogerou, this volume; Rhodes, Janssen, et al., this volume; Sheeran et al., this volume; diet/eating: de Ridder et al., this volume; Hall et al., this volume; Rhodes, Janssen, et al., this volume; Sheeran et al., this volume) or less (e.g., blood donation: Ferguson & Masser, this volume; health screening: Consedine et al., this volume) frequently performed. In addition, health behaviors that can be classified as either approach (e.g., physical activity: Ekkekakis et al., this volume; Hall et al., this volume; Hagger & Protogerou, this volume; Rhodes, this volume; Sheeran et al., this volume) or avoidance (e.g., drinking alcohol: Reese et al., this volume; Wiers et al., this volume; smoking: McCarthy et al., this volume; Wiers et al., this volume; substance use: Reese et al., this volume; Wiers et al., this volume; suntanning: Day et al., this volume) behaviors are addressed. The role of affective determinants in relation to healthcare decision-making has also become an area of interest and is addressed in a chapter in this book (Heyhoe & Lawton, this volume).

KEY DETERMINANTS OF HEALTH BEHAVIORS

Understanding the determinants of health behaviors is important in order to predict future behavior and develop successful behavior-change interventions. The dominant health behavior theories (HBTs; see Conner & Norman, 2015a; Glanz & Bishop, 2010; Painter, Borba, Hynes, Mays, & Glanz, 2008) emphasize conscious behavior-specific cognitions as determinants of health behavior (Ajzen, 1991; Bandura, 1986; Fishbein, 1979; Prochaska & DiClemente, 1983; Rosenstock, 1966) consistent with the cognitive paradigm in psychology that came into favor in the 1950s (Edwards, 1954; Rotter, 1954; Tolman, 1955). Such theories account for substantial portions of the variance in health behaviors based on variables such as intentions, attitudes, norms, and self-efficacy (Conner & Norman, 2015b). Such theories place a heavy emphasis on the systematic processing of information usually following the weighted consideration of expectancies and values (Edwards, 1954) to inform plans or intentions to act. However, they have been criticized for not explaining more variance (Baranowski, Anderson, & Carmack, 1998; Webb & Sheeran, 2006) and having modest utility when used as the basis for behavior change interventions (Johnson, Scott-Sheldon, & Carey, 2010; Prestwich et al., 2013). In order to better understand the determinants of health behavior and develop novel targets for behavior-change interventions, the scope of HBTs might be expanded beyond their current emphasis on cognition.

Previous efforts to expand the scope of HBTs have mainly focused on environmental and policy factors (e.g., Sallis, Owen, & Fisher, 2008; Stokols, 1996) and, more recently, nonconscious psychological processes (e.g., Hofmann, Friese, & Wiers, 2008; Sheeran, Gollwitzer, & Bargh, 2013). The present volume is concerned, in part, with developing such theories by considering the role of affect-related concepts—including affect proper (i.e., core affect, emotion, and mood) as well as concepts that involve or refer to cognitively mediated affect (e.g., affective attitudes, anticipated affect, affective associations). Thus in addition to considering the importance of affective determinants of health behaviors in their own right, the present volume attempts to consider the impact of such determinants alongside those already identified in existing HBTs. Such an approach naturally leads to consideration of various relationships among cognitive and affective determinants of health behaviors, including direct and mediated effects and various moderation models. For example, Ekkekakis et al. (this volume) and McCarthy et al. (this volume) both focus on direct effects of core affect on behavior, while a variety of other chapters look at direct verses mediated effects of affect (Baldwin & Sala, this volume; Conner, this volume; Consedine et al., this volume; de Ridder et al., this volume; Ferguson et al., this volume; Ellis & Ferrer, this volume; Hagger & Protogerou, this volume; Kiviniemi & Klasko-Foster, this volume; Reese et al., this volume; Rhodes et al., this volume; Sheeran et al., this volume; Williams, this volume). For example, Conner (this volume) considers how affective attitudes and anticipated affective reactions might impact health behaviors directly (a less reasoned route) alongside other cognitive determinants or have mediated effects on behavior through intentions (a more reasoned route). Chapters also consider moderated relationships for affect. For example, Rhodes, Janssen, et al. (this volume) considers moderated relationships between affective and cognitive determinants of health behaviors such as intention.

Much of the evidence reported in this volume in relation to affective determinants of health behaviors is correlational. Many of these correlational studies employ prospective designs allowing us to assess causal direction. In addition, some of these correlational studies explore the effects of controlling for past behavior and/or nonaffective determinants as potential third variables that might account for affect–behavior relationships. A small but growing number of studies explore the experimental evidence in relation to manipulating the affective determinants of health behaviors. For example, Kiviniemi & Klasko-Foster (this volume) give examples of how affective associations can be manipulated without influencing cognitive factors, while Conner (this volume) reviews evidence relating to experimental manipulations of affective attitudes and anticipated affective reactions and their impacts on health behavior. Experimental manipulations of affective determinants are also reviewed in a number of other chapters (e.g., Consedine et al., this volume; Day & Coups, this volume; Hansen et al., this volume; Kiviniemi & Klasko-Foster, this volume; Reese et al., this volume; Rhodes, this volume; Sheeran et al., this volume; Wiers et al., this volume). Such work is likely to be particularly valuable where we wish to move beyond understanding of the affective determinants of health behaviors to changing such behaviors in order to promote positive health outcomes (see Prestwich, Kenworthy, & Conner, 2017, for a recent review of work on health behavior change). In addition, comparisons of correlational and experimental work should allow us to gauge whether correlational studies overestimate the magnitude of the causal effect of affect on behavior (as has been shown to be the case for intentions: Webb & Sheeran, 2006). Shedding light on the affective determinants of health behavior whether considered on their own or alongside other key determinants is a key focus of this book.

CONCEPTUALIZING AFFECT

One potential barrier to research on affective determinants of health behavior is the lack of consensus regarding the conceptualization of affect. Indeed, there are a multitude of unresolved questions in this area: What is affect? Where is the boundary between affect and cognition? Are there differences between affect, moods, and emotions? If so, what are they? Which among the cognitive, physiological, behavioral, and experiential components of affect are essential to, versus products of, affect? In what order does one experience the various components of affect and what are their causal interconnections? Is there a set of basic evolutionarily hardwired emotions experienced by all humans? If so, what are those emotions? Or, are specific emotions socially constructed? Are discrete emotions best viewed as categorical or as situated along one or more dimensions? If the former, how many emotion categories are there, and what constitutes a discrete emotion? If the latter, how many dimensions are there, and how are the dimensions best labeled and conceptualized? Finally, from what regions of the brain does affect emanate? And are there certain brain regions that merely encode, inhibit, or enhance affective states (the prefrontal cortex?) rather than cause them?

The goal here is not to provide a resolution of these issues or choose sides on each of these conceptual controversies. Instead, a broad conceptualization of affect is offered in order to provide the largest possible conceptual space for research on affect-related determinants of health behavior. Specifically, *affect* is defined herein as an evaluative neurobiological state that manifests in: (1) coordinated patterns of physiological (e.g., release of hormones, increased heart rate) and involuntary behavioral (e.g., facial expression, vocalization) changes, and (2) subjective experiential feelings (e.g., the phenomenal experience of pleasure, anger, embarrassment, etc.). This broad definition of affect is consistent with its use as an umbrella term encompassing a range of interrelated concepts, including core affect (e.g., hedonic response [pleasure/displeasure] and arousal), emotions (e.g., anger, fear, sorrow, joy), and moods (e.g., happy, contented, depressed, irritable) (Davidson, Scherer, & Goldsmith, 2009; Ekkekakis, 2013; Kahneman, Diener, & Schwarz, 1999; Lewis, Haviland-Jones, & Barrett, 2008; Manstead, Frijda, & Fischer, 2004).

Core Affect

According to multiple theorists, all affect includes a *core affect* component (Larsen, 2000; Russell, 1980; Thayer, 1978; Watson & Tellegen, 1985). In Russell's circumplex model, core affect is characterized by two orthogonal dimensions: a "valence" dimension ranging from positive to negative, and an "activation" dimension ranging from high to low (Russell, 1980). Alternatively, in Watson and Tellegen's (1985) "rotated" core affect circumplex the valence and activation dimensions are rotated 45 degrees, yielding (1) a "positive activation" dimension ranging from the union of positive valence and high activation (e.g., excited) to the union of negative valence and low activation (e.g., fatigued) and (2) a "negative activation" dimension ranging from the union of negative valence and high activation (e.g., anxious) to the union of positive valence and low activation (e.g., tranquil).

The differences between Russell's (1980) unrotated circumplex model and Watson and Tellegen's (1985) rotated circumplex model have led to considerable confusion in affective science regarding the terms *positive affect* and *negative affect* (Russell & Carroll, 1999a, 1999b; Watson & Tellegen, 1999). This confusion has spilled over into research on health behaviors (Ekkekakis, 2013, pp. 76–95). The problem stems from the original labeling of the dimensions of Watson and Tellegen's (1985) rotated circumplex model as "positive affect" and "negative affect." As a result of this labeling, the rotated core affect dimensions are often incorrectly interpreted as descriptors of pure positive and negative valence, as in Russell's (1980) "unrotated" valence dimension. Because of this confusion, Watson and Tellegen have renamed their rotated dimensions "positive activation" and "negative activation" to distinguish them from the opposite (positive and negative) poles of Russell's hedonic valence dimension (Watson, Wiese, Vaidya, & Tellegen, 1999). Unfortunately, this solution to the problem has often gone unrecognized in health behavior science and thus the confusion and misinterpretation of the literature persists.[1]

Regardless of the specific characterization and labeling of core affect dimensions, core affect is posited to be ever present when a person is conscious and awake, though it may not always be the focus of one's attention (Lambie & Marcel, 2002; Russell, 1980). Core affect may shift in direction or magnitude in response to transient stimuli that do not require cognitive appraisals, such as when stubbing one's toe. Alternatively, changes in core affect may underlie more complex appraisal-based emotions and moods (Russell & Barrett, 1999).

Emotions and Moods

Emotions (e.g., anger, fear, sorrow, joy) involve cognitive appraisals of a specific stimulus, which lead to a combination of coordinated and distinctive physiological and/or behavioral responses and experiential feelings with an underlying core affect component (Frijda, 2008). For example, the emotion of anger involves the appraisal that one has been wronged, accompanied by increased heart rate, flushed skin, a scowling facial expression, and an increase in negative activated affect, culminating in the distinctive phenomenal experience (i.e., feeling) of anger. *Moods* (e.g., happy, contented, anxious, depressed/sad, irritable) involve the same components as emotions (i.e., cognitive appraisal, change in core affect, physiological, behavioral, and experiential manifestations), but, relative to emotions are (1) more diffuse rather than focused on a specific stimulus; and (2) less time-limited (Morris, 1999). Thus, relative to the emotion of anger, an irritable mood may not be attributable to any specific stimulus and can last for days or weeks, with no distinct beginning and end.

Integral Versus Incidental Affect

Affect can be further organized into integral and incidental affect—categories that are orthogonal to the previous distinctions among core affect, emotions, and moods. *Integral affect* is one's *affective response* to the target behavior or the immediate consequences of the behavior, the latter including the taste of the food that one is eating, the sensation of vigorous exercise, or the feeling of alcohol or drug intoxication. *Incidental affect* is affect that is not experienced in the context of the behavior but may nonetheless influence the behavior (e.g., effects of job-related stress on smoking) or be influenced by the behavior (e.g., effects of regular exercise on general mood or well-being) (Bodenhausen, 1993).

Integral affect may be further characterized by whether it occurs during or immediately following the target behavior. This distinction may be particularly important for many health-related behaviors for which the during-behavior affective response has a valence that is opposite from the postbehavior affective response. For example, people often experience pleasure while eating calorie-dense foods, but afterward may feel guilty or disappointed in themselves. Conversely, many people experience pain or discomfort during vigorous exercise, but feel a sense of satisfaction or accomplishment once they are done.

Affect Processing, Affective Judgments, Cognitively Mediated Affect

"Affect processing," "affective judgments," and "cognitively mediated affect" are umbrella terms that encompass cognitive processing of previous or anticipated affective responses to the target behavior (Conner, McEachan, Taylor, O'Hara, & Lawton, 2015; Rhodes, Fiala, & Conner, 2009; Williams & Evans, 2014). (For ease of exposition, we hereafter use the term "affect processing," but the three terms are essentially synonymous.) Included in the category of affect processing are *anticipated affect, affective attitudes, implicit attitudes*, and *affective associations*. Although the concepts in this category are fundamentally cognitive in nature, they are considered within the purview of affective determinants of behavior because they either directly refer to affect (i.e., anticipated affective reaction) or include an affective component (i.e., affective associations, affective attitudes, and implicit attitudes). Conceptually, affect processing is posited to partially or completely mediate the effects of previous integral affect on future behavior (Figure 1.1).

Anticipated affect is an expectation of one's affective response to the target behavior, consistent with the broader notion of outcome expectancy in sociocognitive theories of behavior (Ajzen, 1991; Bandura, 1986; Fishbein, 1979; Prochaska & DiClemente, 1983; Rosenstock, 1966). *Affective attitudes* are evaluations of the target behavior based on aggregation of anticipated affective responses. Affective attitudes differ from *instrumental attitudes* in which the target behavior is evaluated (e.g., beneficial versus harmful) based on aggregation of expected instrumental outcomes

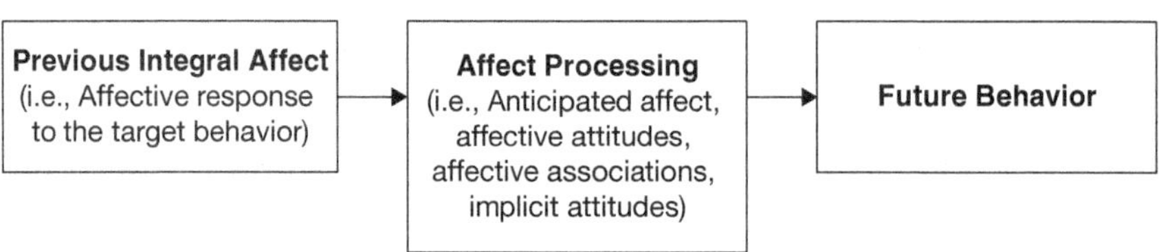

Figure 1.1. A model of the impact of integral affect on behavior.

(e.g., health-related outcomes) (Ajzen, 1991; Crites, Fabrigar, & Petty, 1994). Anticipated affect and affective attitudes are distinct from actual affective responses to the target behavior in that the former are *about the behavior* and thus can be experienced and reported at any time, whereas affective responses are how one feels *in response to performing* the behavior and thus is only relevant in the context of the target behavior.

Attitudes may be either explicit or implicit (Gawronski & Bodenhausen, 2006). Explicit attitudes, including both affective and instrumental subtypes, are based on an aggregation of thoughtful consideration of the affective or instrumental outcomes of the behavior (see above). *Implicit attitudes*, on the other hand, are automatically activated evaluations of the target behavior based on an aggregation of affective associations (Gawronski & Bodenhausen, 2006). *Affective associations*, in turn, are automatic associations between the target behavior and previously experienced affective responses to the target behavior (Kiviniemi, Voss-Humke, & Seifert, 2007). Thus, theoretically, anticipated affect is the deliberate and thoughtful consideration of potential affective consequences of behavior and underlies (explicit) affective attitudes, while affective associations are automatically triggered associations between the target behavior and an affective response and underlie implicit attitudes (Williams & Evans, 2014).

MEASURING AFFECT IN THE CONTEXT OF HEALTH BEHAVIOR

Affect can be assessed objectively via physiological, behavioral, or neuroimaging measures, or subjectively via self-report. Objective physiological measures include inference of affective arousal based on galvanic skin response or heart rate. Behavioral measures include inference of affective valence (i.e., pleasure versus displeasure) or discrete emotions (e.g., anger, fear, joy, sadness) based on facial expressions, which can be assessed through observation or electromyography. Neuroimaging can be used to infer emotions such as fear or anxiety based on activation of specific brain regions (e.g., amygdala), although such assessments are usually performed in conjunction with self-report.

Self-report of affect may, despite its subjectivity, be considered the "gold standard" method of assessment to the extent that affect is defined in terms of experiential feeling states. Indeed, none of the aforementioned objective measures of affect are necessary or sufficient indicators of affect. On the other hand, the experience of affect, assuming it is genuinely reported, is a sufficient, if not necessary (depending on one's definition of affect), indicator of affect. Moreover, generally speaking, relative to objective measures, self-report of affect is easier to obtain and thus more conducive to field-based applied research on health-related behaviors.

Self-report measures of affect can be categorized based on a number of orthogonal characteristics. Such measures may (1) be standardized versus created for specific use in an individual study; (2) be domain-specific (i.e., designed to assess affect in the context of a particular health-related behaviour) versus domain-general; and (3) assess retrospective versus real-time affective states. Regardless of the content of the affect assessment, self-reported affect may be assessed via interview, traditional questionnaire (paper or computer-based), or ecological momentary assessment (EMA).

Assessment of Affect Processing

Unlike affect proper, affect processing is not conceptualized in terms of any particular physiological or behavioral manifestation. Moreover, the neurobiology of affect processing is more diffuse and thus harder to distinguish from other cognitive processing. For these reasons, measures of affect processing are, with the exception of implicit attitudes, limited to self-report. Such measures are almost always domain-specific (i.e., about a specific behavior) consistent with the conceptualization of affect processing concepts. As with measures of affect proper, measures of anticipated affect, affective attitudes, and affective associations may be standardized based on use in prior studies, or created for the purposes of an individual study. Assessment of implicit attitudes is based on computer-based reaction-time measures, such as the implicit association test (Greenwald, Poehlmann, Uhlmann, & Banaji, 2009), thus increasing the likelihood that responses are based on automatic rather than controlled processing.

Despite the conceptual differences between different affect processing constructs, they may be difficult to disentangle empirically. Indeed, measures of anticipated affect (e.g., when I exercise I expect to feel good [or bad]), affective attitudes (e.g., exercise is pleasant versus unpleasant), and affective associations (e.g., when I think about exercise I feel excited [or bored]) may seem quite similar to typical questionnaire respondents who are not used to splitting hairs among these subtly different constructs. Moreover, such questionnaire-based assumptions are likely to be strongly associated with reaction-time measures of implicit attitudes (Ayres, Conner, Prestwich, & Smith, 2012; Conner, Prestwich, & Ayres, 2011).

CONCLUSION

Although this book focuses on affective determinants of health behaviors, many of the considerations are general to a broader set of social behaviors (e.g., voting, consumer choice, helping behavior, etc.). We would argue that the study of health behaviors provides a useful testbed for exploring the role of affective determinants of behavior as well as being an important and consequential area of study in its own right. The various chapters in this book show the important and exciting ways in which researchers are exploring the impacts of affective determinants of health behaviors.

NOTE

1. Most problematic, researchers often argue that positive affect and negative affect are orthogonal, which is theoretically true if use of these labels refers to Watson and Tellegen's rotated circumplex dimensions, but is erroneous when these labels are used (as they often are) to refer to the opposite (i.e., positive and negative) poles of Russell's hedonic valence dimension (e.g., Cheetham, Allen, Yucel, & Lubman,

2010). To further complicate the issue, there is empirical evidence that the positive and negative poles of Russell's hedonic valence dimension may be mediated by different neurological circuits (Cacioppo & Berntson, 1994; Cacioppo & Gardner, 1999), though likely integrated in experience, such that one cannot feel (pure) good and bad at the same time (Ekkekakis, 2013, pp. 88–89). This issue should not, however, be conflated with the erroneous interpretation of Watson and Tellegen's (1985) circumplex model as indicating that positive and negative *hedonic valence* are orthogonal.

REFERENCES

Ajzen, I. (1991). The theory of planned behavior. *Organizational Behavior and Human Decision Processes, 50*, 179–211. doi: 10.1016/0749-5978(91)90020

Ayres, K., Conner, M. T., Prestwich, A., & Smith, P. (2012). Do implicit measures of attitudes incrementally predict snacking behaviour over explicit affect-related measures? *Appetite, 58*, 835–841.

Bandura, A. (1986). *Social foundations of thought and action: A social cognitive theory*. Englewood Cliffs, NJ: Prentice-Hall.

Baranowski, T., Anderson, C., & Carmack, C. (1998). Mediating variable framework in physical activity interventions: How are we doing? How might we do better? *American Journal of Preventive Medicine, 15*, 266–297. doi: 10.1016/S0749-3797(98)00080-4

Bodenhausen, G. V. (1993). Emotions, arousal, and stereotype-based discrimination: A heuristic model of affect and stereotyping. In D. M. Mackie & D. L. Hamilton (Eds.), *Affect, cognition, and stereotyping: Interactive processes in group perception* (pp. 13–35). San Diego, CA: Academic.

Cacioppo, J. T., & Berntson, G. G. (1994). Relationship between attitudes and evaluative space: A critical review, with emphasis on the separability of positive and negative substrates. *Psychological Bulletin, 115*, 401–423. doi: 10.1037/0033-2909.115.3.401

Cacioppo, J. T., & Gardner, W. L. (1999). Emotion. *Annual Review of Psychology, 50*, 191–214. doi: 10.1146/annurev.psych.50.1.191

Cheetham, A., Allen, N. B., Yucel, M., & Lubman, D. I. (2010). The role of affective dysregulation in drug addiction. *Clinical Psychology Review, 30*, 621–634. doi: 10.1016/j.cpr.2010.04.005

Conner, M., McEachan, R., Taylor, N., O'Hara, J., & Lawton, J. (2015). Role of affective attitudes and anticipated affective reactions in predicting health behaviors. *Health Psychology, 34*, 642–652. doi: 10.1037/hea0000143

Conner, M., & Norman, P. (2015a). (Eds.). *Predicting and changing health behaviour: Research and practice with social cognition models* (3rd ed.). Maidenhead: Open University Press.

Conner, M., & Norman, P. (2015b). Predicting and changing health behaviour: A social cognition approach. In M. Conner & P. Norman (Eds.), *Predicting and changing health behaviour: Research and practice with social cognition models* (3rd ed., pp. 1–29). Maidenhead: Open University Press.

Conner, M., & Norman, P. (2017). Editorial: Health behaviour: Current issues and challenges. *Psychology and Health, 32*, 895–906.

Conner, M., Prestwich, A., & Ayres, K. (2011). Using explicit affective attitudes to tap impulsive influences on health behavior: A commentary on Hofmann et al. (2008). *Health Psychology Review, 5*, 145–149.

Crites, S. L., Fabrigar, L. R., & Petty, R. E. (1994). Measuring the affective and cognitive properties of attitudes: Conceptual and methodological issues. *Personality and Social Psychology Bulletin, 6*, 619–634. doi: 10.1177/0146167294206001

Danaei, G., Ding, E. L., Mozaffarian, D., Taylor, B., Rehm, J., Murray, C. J., & Ezzati, M. (2009). The preventable causes of death in the United States: Comparative risk assessment of dietary, lifestyle, and metabolic risk factors. *PLoS Med, 6*, e1000058. doi: 10.1371/journal.pmed.1000058

Davidson, R. J., Scherer, K. R., & Goldsmith, H. H. (Eds.). (2009). *Handbook of affective sciences*. New York, NY: Oxford University Press.

de Ridder, D., Kroese, F., Evers, C., Adriaanse, M., & Gillebaart, M. (2017). Healthy Diet: Health impact, prevalence, correlates, and interventions. *Psychology and Health, 32*, 907–941.

Edwards, W. (1954). The theory of decision making. *Psychological Bulletin, 51*, 380–417. doi: 10.1037/h0053870

Ekkekakis, P. (2013). *The measurement of affect, mood, and emotion: A guide for health-behavioral research*. New York, NY: Cambridge University Press.

Ferrer, R., & Mendes, W. (2018). Editorial: Emotion, health decision-making, and health Behaviour. *Psychology and Health, 33*, 1–16.

Fishbein, M. (1979). A theory of reasoned action: Some applications and implications. *Nebraska Symposium on Motivation, 27*, 65–116. doi: 1982-21194-001

Frijda, N. (2008). The psychologists point of view. In M. Lewis, J. M. Haviland-Jones, & L. F. Barrett (Eds.), *Handbook of emotions* (3rd ed., pp. 68–87). New York, NY: Guilford.

Gawronski, B., & Bodenhausen, G. V. (2006). Associative and propositional processes in evaluation: An integrative review of implicit and explicit attitude change. *Psychological Bulletin, 132*, 692–731. doi: 10.1037/0033-2909.132.5.692

GBD 2016 Risk Factors Collaborators (2017). Global, regional, and national comparative risk assessment of 84 behavioural, environmental and occupational, and metabolic risks or clusters of risks, 1990–2016: A systematic analysis for the Global Burden of Disease Study 2016. *Lancet, 390*, 1345–1422.

Glanz, K., & Bishop, D. B. (2010). The role of behavioral science theory in development and implementation of public health interventions. *Annual Review of Public Health, 31*, 399–418. doi: 10.1146/annurev.publhealth.012809.103604

Gochman, D. S. (Ed.). (1997). *Handbook of health behavior research* (Vols 1–4). New York, NY: Plenum.

Greenwald, A. G., Poehlmann, T. A., Uhlmann, E. L., & Banaji, M. R. (2009). Understanding and using the implicit association test: III. Meta-analysis of predictive validity. *Journal of Personality and Social Psychology, 97*, 17–41.

Hofmann, W., Friese, M., & Wiers, R. W. (2008). Impulsive versus reflective influences on health behavior: A theoretical framework and empirical review. *Health Psychology Review, 2*, 111–137. doi: 10.1080/17437190802617668

Johnson, B. T., Scott-Sheldon, L. A., & Carey, M. P. (2010). Meta-synthesis of health behavior change meta-analyses. *American Journal of Public Health, 100*, 2193–2198. doi: 10.2105/AJPH.2008.155200

Kahneman, D., Diener, E., & Schwarz, N. (Eds.). (1999). *Well-being: The foundations of hedonic psychology*. New York, NY: Russell Sage.

Kiviniemi, M. T., Voss-Humke, A. M., & Seifert, A. L. (2007). How do I feel about the behavior? The interplay of affective associations with behaviors and cognitive beliefs as influences on physical activity behavior. *Health Psychology, 26*, 152–158. doi: 10.1037/0278-6133.26.2.152

Kuntsche, E., Kuntsche, S., Thrul, J., & Gmel, G. (2017). Binge drinking: Health impact, prevalence, correlates, and interventions. *Psychology and Health, 32*, 976–1017.

Lambie, J. A., & Marcel, A. J. (2002). Consciousness and the varieties of emotion experience: A theoretical framework. *Psychological Review, 109*, 219–259. doi: 10.1037/0033-295X.109.2.219

Larsen, R. J. (2000). Toward a science of mood regulation. *Psychological Inquiry, 11*, 129–141. doi: 10.1207/S15327965PLI1103_01

Lewis, M., Haviland-Jones, J. M., & Barrett, L. F. (Eds.). (2008). *Handbook of emotions* (3rd ed.). New York, NY: Guilford.

Manstead, A. S. R., Frijda, N., & Fischer, A. (Eds.). (2004). *Feelings and emotions: The Amsterdam symposium*. New York, NY: Cambridge University Press.

McEachan, R. R. C., Lawton, R. J., & Conner, M. (2010). Classifying health-related behaviours: Exploring similarities and differences amongst behaviours. *British Journal of Health Psychology, 15*, 347–366. doi: 10.1348/135910709X466487

Mokdad, A. H., Marks, J. S., Stroup, D. F., & Gerberding, J. L. (2004). Actual causes of death in the United States, 2000. *Journal of the American Medical Association, 291*, 1238–1245. doi: 10.1001/jama.291.10.1238

Morris, W. N. (1999). The mood system. In D. Kahneman, E. Diener, & N. Schwarz (Eds.), *Well-being: The foundations of hedonic psychology* (pp. 169–189). New York, NY: Russell-Sage.

Painter, J. E., Borba, C. P., Hynes, M., Mays, D., & Glanz, K. (2008). The use of theory in health behavior research from 2000 to 2005: A systematic review. *Annals of Behavioral Medicine, 35*, 358–362. doi: 10.1007/s12160-008-9042-y

Prestwich, A., Kenworthy, J., & Conner, M. (2017). *Health behavior change: Theories, methods and interventions*. Abingdon, UK: Routledge.

Prestwich, A., Sniehotta, F. F., Whittington, C., Dombrowski, S. U., Rogers, L., & Michie, S. (2013). Does theory influence the effectiveness of health behavior interventions? Meta-analysis. *Health Psychology, 33*, 465–474. doi: 10.1037/a0032853

Prochaska, J. O., & DiClemente, C. C. (1983). Stages and processes of self-change of smoking: Toward an integrative model of change. *Journal of Consulting and Clinical Psychology, 51*, 390–395. doi: 10.1037/0022-006X.51.3.390

Rhodes, R. E., Fiala, B., & Conner, M. (2009). Affective judgments and physical activity: A review and meta-analysis. *Annals of Behavioral Medicine, 38*, 180–204.

Rhodes, R., Janssen, I., Bredin, S., Warburton, D., & Bauman, A. (2017). Physical activity: Health impact, prevalence, correlates and interventions. *Psychology and Health, 32*, 942–975.

Rosenstock, I. M. (1966). Why people use health services. *Milbank Memorial Fund Quarterly, 44* (Suppl): 94–127. doi: 10.1111/j.1468-0009.2005.00425.x

Rothman, A. J., & Salovey, P. (1997). Shaping perceptions to motivate healthy behaviour: The role of message framing. *Psychological Bulletin, 121*, 3–19.

Rotter, J. B. (1954). *Social learning and clinical psychology*. Englewood Cliffs, NJ: Prentice-Hall.

Russell, J. A. (1980). A circumplex model of affect. *Journal of Personality and Social Psychology, 39*, 1161–1178. doi: 10.1037/h0077714

Russell, J. A., & Barrett, L. F. (1999). Core affect, prototypical emotional episodes, and other things called emotion: Dissecting the elephant. *Journal of Personality and Social Psychology, 76*, 805–819. doi: 10.1037/0022-3514.76.5.805

Russell, J. A., & Carroll, J. M. (1999a). On the bipolarity of positive and negative affect. *Psychological Bulletin, 125*, 3–30. doi: 10.1037/0033-2909.125.1.3

Russell, J. A., & Carroll, J. M. (1999b). The phoenix of bipolarity: Reply to Watson & Tellegen. *Psychological Bulletin, 125*, 611–617. doi: 10.1037/0033-2909.125.5.611

Sallis, J. F., Owen, N., & Fisher, E. B. (2008). Ecological models of health behavior. In K. Glanz, B. K. Rimer, & K. Viswanath (Eds.), *Health behavior and health education: Theory, research and practice* (pp. 465–485). San Francisco, CA: Jossey-Bass.

Sheeran, P., Gollwitzer, P. M., & Bargh, J. A. (2013). Nonconscious processes and health. *Health Psychology, 32*, 460–473. doi: 10.1037/a0029203

Stokols, D. (1996). Translating social ecological theory into guidelines for community health promotion. *American Journal of Health Promotion, 10*, 282–298. doi: 10.4278/0890-1171-10.4.282

Thayer, R. E. (1978). Factor analytic and reliability studies on the Activation-Deactivation Adjective Check List. *Psychological Reports, 42*, 747–756. doi: 10.2466/pr0.1978.42.3.747

Tolman, E. C. (1955). Principles of performance. *Psychological Review, 62*, 315–326. doi: 10.1037/h0049079

Watson, D., & Tellegen, A. (1985). Toward a consensual structure of mood. *Psychological Bulletin, 98*, 219–235. doi: 10.1037/0033-2909.98.2.219

Watson, D., & Tellegen, A. (1999). Issues in the dimensional structure of affect—Effects of descriptors, measurement error, and response formats: Comment on Russell and Carroll. *Psychological Bulletin, 125*, 601–610. doi: 10.1037/0033-2909.125.5.601

Watson, D., Wiese, D., Vaidya, J., & Tellegen, A. (1999). The two general activation systems of affect: Structural findings, evolutionary considerations, and psychobiological evidence. *Journal of Personality and Social Psychology, 76*, 820–838. doi: 10.1037/0022-3514.76.5.820

Webb, T. L., & Sheeran, P. (2006). Does changing behavioral intentions engender behavior change? A meta-analysis of the experimental evidence. *Psychological Bulletin*, *132*, 249–268. doi: 10.1037/0033-2909.132.2.249

West, R. (2017). Tobacco smoking: Health impact, prevalence, correlates and interventions. *Psychology and Health*, *32*, 1018–1036.

Williams, D. M., & Evans, D. R. (2014). Current emotion research in health behavior science. *Emotion Review*, *6*, 277–287. doi: 10.1177/1754073914523052

PART 1

Theoretical Perspectives

2

Affect in the Process of Action Control of Health-Protective Behaviors

RYAN E. RHODES AND SAMANTHA M. GRAY

INTRODUCTION

Chronic diseases, such as heart disease and cancer, now constitute the leading causes of death in all industrialized countries (World Health Organization, 2014). Furthermore, the personal, social, and economic impacts of these diseases are enormous and involve low quality of life, workplace absenteeism, familial distress, and high costs for treatment (Mascie-Taylor & Karim, 2003; Walker, 2007). Thus, initiatives that can prevent the onset of chronic disease and improve rehabilitation outcomes are critical for all levels of society. Most chronic diseases have complex etiologies that involve environmental, genetic, and behavioral antecedents (Kujala, 2011; Mulle & Vaccarino, 2013). Behavioral factors, in particular, are responsible for considerable explanation of most chronic diseases (Warburton, Nicol, & Bredin, 2006). Unfortunately, very few people in most developed nations engage in protective health behaviors such as physical activity (PA), and healthy eating behavior (J. N. Hall, Moore, Harper, & Lynch, 2009; Hallal et al., 2012). Clearly, promotion efforts are needed.

Theoretical understanding of the determinants behind these health behaviors has been a line of research inquiry for over half a century (Rosenstock, 1974). The premise behind this research is that a sound understanding of health behavior determinants will aid in intervention success. Theories represent an organizing framework to provide structure, function, and common nomenclature to critical variables under study (Michie, West, Campbell, Brown, & Gainforth, 2014). While the breadth of theories applied to understand health-protective behaviors has been growing in diversity, the dominant approach has been through the social cognitive tradition (Conner & Norman, 2015). Theories from this tradition each have unique aspects, yet almost all suggest that expectations of the outcomes from behavioral action and the perception of one's capability to perform the behavior affect the formation of intentions. These intentions, in turn, impact behavior (Fishbein et al., 2001).

Action Control in Health Behavior

Social cognitive approaches to understanding health behavior have been useful, but are not without some limitations that have been a subject of recent debate (e.g., Sheeran, Gollwitzer, & Bargh, 2013; Sniehotta, Presseau, & Araújo-Soares, 2014). One of the most common criticisms is the modest association between intention and behavior, when these theoretical models tend to suggest that intention should be the critical proximal determinant of behavior. To be clear, the relationship between intention and health behaviors is substantial. For example, the most recent meta-analysis of the theory of planned behavior applied to PA and eating behavior showed $r = .48$ and $r = .44$ respectively (McEachan, Conner, Taylor, & Lawton, 2011). Still, the finding also suggests that 77%–81% of the variance in these behaviors is unexplained. The relationship is also further attenuated when examining change in PA and healthy eating (i.e., controlling for past behavior), which is arguably more accurate when attempting to understand intention and its role in behavior change (Weinstein, 2007); the relationship between PA and healthy eating with intention reduces to $r = .22$ and $r = .28$, respectively. While this is still suggestive of a meaningful effect (Cohen, 1992), the evidence is not as convincing that intentions are a strong predictor of behavior.

Examinations of the absolute, rather than relative, value of intention–behavior relations have also shown considerable discordance (Sheeran, 2002; Webb & Sheeran, 2006). For example, experimental manipulations that increase PA intention ($d = .45$ or $r = .22$) result in much lower and clinically less meaningful increases in PA ($d = .15$ or $r = .08$) (Rhodes & Dickau, 2012). Dichotomization of the intention and PA relationship around public health guidelines also showed that 48% of intenders failed to follow through with PA (Rhodes & de Bruijn, 2013a). Perhaps most important is the lowered practical value of theories that place intention as the proximal antecedent of health behavior. It is extremely common for participants in healthy eating and PA interventions to report to the trial with high intentions at baseline—often an almost circular reasoning for even volunteering in the first place—yet low participation in the behavior. The repeated and regular nature of these behaviors highlights how adherence may be more an ongoing process of navigating good intentions into behavior rather than a discrete and certain coupling.

One way to address these concerns is in theories that separate intention formation from intention translation, or what is sometimes referred to as action control (Kuhl, 1984). This line of thinking is not novel and traces back to the early 20th century (Ach, 1905), but most of our models in the social cognitive tradition have focused heavily on intention formation, with an assumption that the intention construct itself can account for translation. Bagozzi (1992) delineated the concerns of this approach well during the construction of his volitional model of goal-directed behavior, by indicating "It seems, however, that we ask too much of the concept of intentions when we expect it to capture directional, planning, and motivational elements in a single construct" (pp. 198–199). While the intention construct has enough evidence as a necessary process in the pursuit of health behaviors, research into intention–behavior discordance clearly shows that nearly all variability comes from intenders failing to act (Rhodes & de Bruijn, 2013a; Sheeran, 2002). Action control models that attempt to understand who translates intentions into behavior in order to foster effective interventions is a viable and important area of future health behavior research (Rhodes & Yao, 2015).

While volitional strategies, such as implementation intentions (Gollwitzer & Sheeran, 2006) or regulatory plans (Schwarzer, 2008), are clearly the hallmark of most action control models, affective aspects, defined as the experience of a feeling or emotion (Emerson & Williams, 2015), are likely crucial. The purpose of this chapter is to overview how affective factors may impact action control in protective health behaviors. Using action control approaches that include affective factors highlighted in a prior review (Rhodes & Yao, 2015), we propose several potential links (see Figure 2.1). These have been divided into sections representing reflective affect (i.e., affective judgments, anticipated affective reactions), affective factors in volitional self-regulation behaviors (e.g., planning,

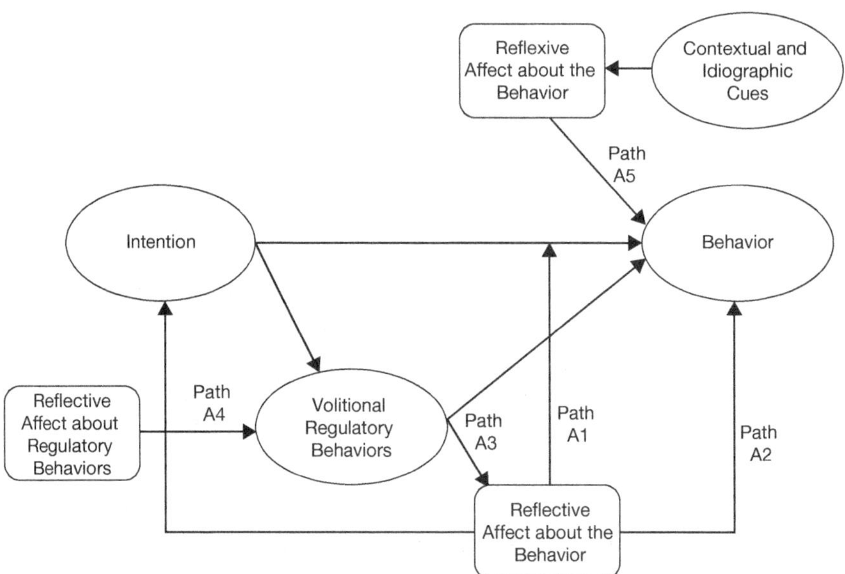

Figure 2.1. The possible pathways affect determines health-behavior action control.

self-monitoring), and reflexive affect (e.g., affective associations, peripheral affect) with an assessment of the current state of evidence for each in relation to repeated behaviors like healthy eating and regular PA. We conclude the chapter by discussing the testing of a conceptual frame for affect and action control relationships and proposing future research directions.

REFLECTIVE AFFECTIVE CONSTRUCTS AND ACTION CONTROL

Affect-related constructs in health behavior are clearly complex (Williams & Evans, 2014), and the sources and characteristics of the construct appear central to understanding how these can differ in meaningful ways for understanding and promoting behavior. Dual process approaches highlight the differences between reflective and reflexive sources of behavioral enactment (Deutsch & Strack, 2006; Evans & Stanovich, 2013). Reflective sources of motivation are marked by longer processing times, expectations of a given behavior made outside of the context of the behavior, and more judgmental processing of multiple lines of stimuli. By contrast, reflexive sources of motivation are abrupt, in-context "hot" reactions that are more often considered a function of context and associations. We believe these distinctions are very useful for understanding the role of affect in health behavior. In this section, we highlight two potentially powerful reflective affect constructs that have evidence for affecting action control.

Affective Judgments

"Affective judgments" is considered an umbrella term to encompass the expected feelings of pleasure/displeasure and enjoyment surrounding an experience of performing a given behavior (Rhodes, Fiala, & Conner, 2009). The term is meant to provide an overarching reach for concepts such as affective attitude (Ajzen, 2006), perceived enjoyment (Kendzierski & DeCarlo, 1991), and intrinsic regulation (Deci & Ryan, 1985). The construct is separate from affective states because affective judgments are expectations of an experience out of context and thus representative of reflective sources of motivation. Further, affective judgments are considered to use more cognitive processing than state or incidental affect (feelings in the moment) and can be based on many factors, from the expected affective state induced from performing the behavior to various aspects related to the expected context, which could include social and environmental factors (Rhodes, Fiala, et al., 2009). In the PA domain, this diversity of reasons for affective judgments has been validated (Riecken, Mark, & Rhodes, 2013), although past state affect from performing the behavior is a large source of affective judgments (Rhodes & Kates, 2015).

Affective judgments are most commonly positioned as antecedents of intention: if one expects a health behavior will be pleasant and satisfying, one is more likely to intend to act upon that behavior. Certainly, a strong relationship between affective judgments with intention has been substantiated in areas such as PA and eating. For example, in a meta-analysis of PA, Rhodes, Fiala, et al. (2009) showed that the relationship between intention and affective judgments was $r = .65$ across 42 samples. In a study of healthy eating behavior in casual dining settings, Jun and Arendt (2016) showed that affective attitudes and intention were correlated $r = 0.42$ in a sample of 744 adults. Clearly, there is good evidence that affective judgments are related to the intentions people form in health behavior.

We propose that there is also evidence that affective judgments may play a role in action control (see Figure 2.1). The role that affective judgments may take in action control is via two routes. First, affective judgments may represent moderators of intention–behavior relations primarily by creating more stable initial intentions over time (Figure 2.1 Path A1). While this is represented by a moderator arrow, we view this as an indicator of ostensibly stronger intentions than those formed for other potential reasons. Keer et al. (2013), for example, showed that intentions formed from affective judgments were more stable across time than intentions formed for other reasons. Thus, people who intend to engage in a behavior because they enjoy it are more likely to hold to their intentions and thus follow through with behavior.

Second, affective judgments about a behavior may augment health behavior performance after one makes an intention to perform the behavior (Figure 2.1 Path A2). This may happen naturally/incidentally or through active volitional regulation on the part of the individual in order to enhance the likelihood of action control (Figure 2.1 Path A2 via Path A3). For example, both Bagozzi (1992) and Kuhl (1984) suggest the importance of active regulation of affective judgments using volitional strategies in their models of action control. Other affect-related behavioral processes, such as building social interactions into the act (helping relationships) are also considered in the processes of change within the transtheoretical model (Prochaska & Velicer, 1997). In a related approach, Rhodes and colleagues (Rhodes & de Bruijn, 2013b; Rhodes & Yao, 2015) have suggested that higher levels of affective judgments are required to translate an intention into behavior than form the initial intention, in their model of multiprocess action control (M-PAC). In a series of observational studies used to validate M-PAC, seven of eight tests showed that unsuccessful intenders (those who had intention but did not act) held significantly lower affective judgments than successful intenders (those with intention who acted) (Rhodes & Yao, 2015).

The most convincing evidence for this effect of affective judgments on behavior independent of intention, however, comes from experimental manipulations of affective judgments. For example, Conner, Rhodes, Morris, McEachan, and Lawton (2011) examined the effect of affective-based persuasive material on subsequent performance of PA over 2 weeks and found that participants exposed to the material compared to controls (and to more instrumental material) significantly increased PA through an increase in affective judgments. Intention scores, however, were high at baseline and did not change during the intervention. Similarly, Rhodes, Warburton, et al. (2009) showed that exposure to exergame cycling activity increased affective judgments compared to a control stationary bike condition and this was linked to continued use of the bike over 6 weeks. Intention, on the other hand, was high at baseline and did not change as a result of exposure to the conditions.

The independent role of affective judgments on behavior from intention is also present within the eating domain. Lawton, Conner, and McEachan (2009) explored affective attitudes and their role in predicting behaviors such as healthy eating. A sample of 390 adults completed measures of affective and instrumental attitudes and intentions, and then 1 month later, they completed measures of their behaviors. After controlling for intention, analyses showed that affective attitudes remained a significant predictor of fruit and vegetable consumption as well as eating a low-fat diet after controlling for intention. This provides support for Figure 2.1 Path A2 and suggests that some reflective affect may guide healthy eating behavior regardless of intent.

Anticipated Affective Reactions

While affective judgments are reliable correlates of health behavior, there is also evidence that the anticipated affective experience from performing the behavior may be different from the anticipated affective reaction to not performing the behavior (Conner, McEachan, Taylor, O'Hara, & Lawton, 2015). These anticipated affective reactions to abstention are typically labeled anticipated regret (Abraham & Sheeran, 2003). Conner and colleagues (2015) propose the theoretical process for how anticipated regret affects health behaviors is via self-conscious emotions (e.g., guilt) (Giner-Sorolla, 2001), although (Rhodes & Mistry, 2016) have demonstrated that much of the regret stems from simple missed opportunities and not personal shame. In either case, however, negative emotions are anticipated preemptively and serve as motivation to avoid the outcome (Simonson, 1992). Given the anticipated nature of the construct, it is still considered a reflective affective process and not reflexive because the source of motivation is preemptive and not context- or situationally driven.

Like affective judgments, anticipated regret has typically been considered an antecedent of intention. This has strong support in the PA domain in observational studies, where anticipated regret has contributed to explaining intention independent of social cognitive factors in the theory of planned behavior (Abraham & Sheeran, 2004; Conner & Abraham, 2001; Sandberg & Conner, 2011; Wang, 2011). Nevertheless, the anticipated regret construct also has convincing evidence as a moderator of intention–behavior relations (Rhodes & Dickau, 2013; Rivis, Sheeran, & Armitage, 2009). Thus, we propose that anticipated regret may be a critical affective construct in translating intentions into health behavior (Figure 2.1).

Interestingly, the mechanisms for how anticipated regret works in PA action control are still rather unclear. Abraham and Sheeran (2003) showed that manipulating anticipated regret increased intentions, which subsequently also remained more stable over time (Figure 2.1 Path A1). By contrast, Sandberg and Conner have shown there is some evidence for a small indirect effect on behavior, independent of intention (Sandberg & Conner, 2008). Furthermore, these authors have shown that manipulations of anticipated regret to exercise may improve action control mainly under conditions of high initial intentions and do not modify intentions themselves (Sandberg & Conner, 2011). This suggests that considerations of anticipated regret help prime people about the importance of the reasons behind forming intentions in the first place and augment motivation beyond the initial intention (Figure 2.1 Path A2). It seems possible that, as with affective judgments, people could also use volitional strategies to enhance feelings of anticipated regret as a mechanism for ensuring action control through social commitments (Rhodes & Mistry, 2016) and various contracts or cues (Prochaska & Velicer, 1997), but this has not received much formal research examination. Thus, while anticipated regret has relatively convincing evidence that it interacts with intentions and behavior, its exact role in action control still requires exploration.

AFFECT AND VOLITIONAL REGULATION BEHAVIORS

The hallmark of many postintentional models is the inclusion of volitional regulatory behaviors used to maintain or augment intentions. Theorists suggest that people who form intentions need to then become strategic in order to implement their intentions across the backdrop of competing forces for their attention, motivation, and time (Heckhausen & Gollwitzer, 1987; Schwarzer, 2008). This is conceived either as a mediator and/or moderator of intention–behavior relations with evidence for both approaches (Carraro & Gaudreau, 2013). The number and type of volitional regulatory behaviors suggested also vary greatly from very specific concepts such as action plans or implementation intentions to a more general array of behaviors such as self-monitoring, scheduling, enlisting support, prioritizing, and problem-solving. Volitional behaviors used to maintain or hone intentions have sound empirical evidence in PA (Bélanger-Gravel, Godin, & Amireault, 2013; Carraro & Gaudreau, 2013; Conn, Hafdahl, & Mehr, 2011; Kwasnicka, Presseau, White, & Sniehotta, 2013) and eating behavior (Godinho, Alvarez, Lima, & Schwarzer, 2014; Richert et al., 2010; Stadler, Oettingen, & Gollwitzer, 2010) domains generally.

What has seen less attention, yet seems extremely relevant to the implementation of these approaches, however, is how affect may impact volitional strategy use. That is, while the use of volitional strategies has strong evidence for successfully closing the intention–behavior gap, these strategies are microbehaviors themselves and likely impacted by motivational factors independent of the motivation to perform the health behavior. Indeed, the adherence to self-regulatory strategies in interventions is very modest (Sniehotta, 2009). This is readily observed in the dietary domain with examples of self-monitoring applications. For example, Helander, Kaipainen, Korhonen, and Wansink (2014) examined adherence rates to a free mobile app designed to promote healthy eating via photography, peer feedback, and dietary self-monitoring (The Eatery). Adherence rates were extremely low, with regular use at 2.58% across a sample of 189,770 participants. Those who did continue using the app were already healthy eaters. Another example relates to MyFitnessPal, an app for dietary monitoring, calorie counting, and exercise journaling. One study in overweight primary care patients revealed that though intervention participants were satisfied with the app, usage decreased drastically within 1 month of initial download, and this low use was attributed to the null results of the trial (Laing et al., 2014). The researchers suggested that MyFitnessPal may only have utility for those that are motivated to self-monitor.

The exploration of motivation to use and adhere to volitional self-regulatory strategies is currently underdeveloped, but appears to be critical (Mistry, Sweet, Latimer, & Rhodes, 2015). While most attempts at improving volitional self-regulatory behaviors have catered to improving skills and abilities (Locke & Latham, 1990), the largest reason behind low use appears to be the hassle and boredom associated with constant self-regulation. For example, in a qualitative study of middle-aged men and healthy eating, the consensus across participants was that it took more time and effort than they were willing to give to organize the preparation of healthy meals, despite acknowledging a desire to ultimately eat healthy (Caperchione et al., 2012). Another qualitative study highlighted similar barriers among young men toward healthy eating, which is well summarized in the following statement:

> It certainly takes much more time to think about preparing a balanced diet for a week and hitting everything, all the food groups and a variety of foods and preparing that all and stuff which, I guess if you are busy, you're not going to prioritise it, there's always something else more urgent. (Ashton et al., 2015 p. 5)

We propose that affective judgments are likely a critical determinant of adherence to volitional self-regulation tactics (see Figure 2.1 Path A4), but this has been relatively unexplored. Some evidence is present in how serious games improve self-regulation strategies. Given their captivating properties and engaging storylines, a review was conducted on video games as means for health-related behavior change (Baranowski, Buday, Thompson, & Baranowski, 2008). The authors identified a subset of studies that aimed to change both diet and PA behaviors via self-regulation processes. There were four video games found that used a story as an overarching structure supported with minigames aimed at increasing self-regulation behaviors. Results subsequently showed some change in diet and PA behavior. Thus, making the experience of engaging in volitional regulation behaviors more captivating may improve self-regulation and subsequently increase protective health behavior.

REFLEXIVE AFFECTIVE CONSTRUCTS AND ACTION CONTROL

Reflective constructs, denoted by "cold" and reasoned processes, are a mainstay in the most popular social cognitive models used to understand health protective behaviors (Conner & Norman, 2015). By contrast, reflexive sources of motivation are abrupt, "hot" reactions that are a function of contextual stimuli and associations. These more implicit components to behavioral action or inaction have not received as much research attention as their reflective counterparts (Deutsch & Strack, 2006), but the area has seen enormous growth in recent years (Rebar et al., 2016). The affect domain may be a critical link in the functioning of implicit determinants of protective health behavior (Rhodes & Kates, 2015; Williams & Evans, 2014). In this section, we highlight three potentially powerful ways that reflexive affect may influence action control.

Automatic Affective Associations

Given our changing contextual environments, opportunities to perform health behaviors are likely impacted by very fast—in the moment—approach or avoidance processing. These automatic associations are the immediate affective responses a person has toward an event or stimulus, which go on to influence decisions and behaviors (Bargh, Chaiken, Raymond, & Hymes, 1996; Cunningham, Raye, & Johnson, 2004). These associations are generally thought to be from prior experiences that have linked the stimulus with a certain affective response and thus serve as a very fast warning system to engage or disengage from a course of action. Within the consideration of action control, we view these as either impacting protective health behaviors directly by thwarting or augmenting intention translation (Figure 2.1 Path A5). Another way to conceptualize these associations is by considering them impulses or cravings such as those specified in PRIME theory (West, 2009; West & Brown, 2013), where these associations can either facilitate or derail original intentions that were derived primarily from the reflective system.

While research evaluating affective associations and health-protective behaviors is still relatively new, there are early indicators to support these proposed pathways. For example, in the eating behavior domain, over 400 adults were surveyed regarding their affective associations and behavior for fruit and vegetable consumption. Those reporting more positive affective words for fruit and vegetable consumption, such as "joy," "delighted," and "happy," reported more daily consumption of fruit and vegetables (Kiviniemi & Duangdao, 2009). In the PA domain, people who automatically associate PA with the word "pleasantness" are more physically active than people who do not have these associations (Bluemke, Brand, Schweizer, & Kahlert, 2010) and the effect on behavior appears independent of intention (Rebar, Ram, & Conroy, 2015). Specifically, Rebar and colleagues found that participants who processed affective words about PA more efficiently were more likely to engage in behavior, objectively monitored over 14 days, independent of their intentions such as denoted in Figure 2.1 Path 5. More generally, the in-task affective response to a bout of PA has been reliably associated with the performance of future PA in a recent review of this literature (Rhodes & Kates, 2015) and this state-level affect has been shown to moderate future intention–PA relations (Kwan & Bryan, 2010). Commensurate with Figure 2.1 Path 4, those individuals reporting a positive affective experience were more likely to follow through with positive intentions than those who reported a less positive affect while engaging in a bout of PA. While it is entirely possible that much of this basic affective response to PA is mediated by future affective judgments in the more reflexive system of motivation, this basic affect and PA relationship may also provide the groundwork for affective associations (Rhodes & Kates, 2015). More research is needed to disentangle the two processes in action control.

Peripheral Affect

While affective judgments are focused on the feeling-states toward enactment of the behavior itself, and automatic associations are "tripwire" connections between a stimulus and affect, people also enter any situation with peripheral affect. Peripheral affect is either incidental (e.g., bad or good mood) to the target behavior or tangentially linked to its performance (e.g., accumulating feelings of distress due to incomplete goals in the day). Some of this peripheral affect is likely core affect, which is posited to be ever-present (Lambie & Marcel, 2002; Russell, 1980), while much of this affect may involve more complex appraisal-based emotions and moods from events throughout the day (Morris, 1999).

Peripheral affect and its relationship to health behavior is present in theories of general behavior (Morris & Reilly, 1987; Wegener & Petty, 1994), and also features prominently in theoretical models of more specific health behaviors (see Williams & Evans, 2014, for a review). Most of these approaches position negative peripheral affect as a mechanism for derailing health behaviors, yet the facilitating effect of positive affect has also been explored (Lyubomirsky, King, & Diener, 2005). Peripheral negative affect, however, has also been theorized as a motivator for PA under specific contexts where it is linked to identity (Stryker & Burke, 2000). Identity theory, for example, suggests that miss-matches between behavior and one's identity provide negative affect and dissonance that serve to motivate identity-consistent behavioral actions (Stets & Burke, 2000). We have made a simple adaptation of these prior approaches to an action control framework in Figure 2.1, with peripheral affect representing internal cues toward more reflexive affective motivation to either facilitate the behavior and augment or to derail intentions (Path A5).

Current evidence in the PA domain is available to support this path within Figure 2.1. Incidental positive and negative affective states have been associated with subsequent bouts of directly assessed PA among children (Dunton et al., 2013). More importantly adults reporting positive affect above their typical values, were over two times more likely to translate their positive PA intentions into behavior in a study using ecological momentary assessment (Maher et al., 2017). The same study showed that those reporting negative peripheral affect compared to typical daily values were 28% less likely to follow through on their good intentions.

Peripheral affect has been extensively studied with eating behavior. For instance, negative emotions have been shown to trigger emotional eating in which intention is overridden, often leading to overconsumption regardless of feelings of hunger (Kemp, Bui, & Grier, 2013; van Strien, Frijters, Bergers, & Defares, 1986). Peripheral affect, which is incidental or tangentially linked to a target behavior, is tied to emotional eating: a behavior in which one consumes food without regard for hunger but in response to emotional stimuli. Much research has focused on emotional eating in response to negative emotions such as anxiety and depression, however this behavior also occurs in response to boredom (Koball, Meers, Storfer-Isser, Domoff, & Musher-Eizenman, 2012). For example, Armitage (2015) showed that boredom was a more common trigger for emotional eating than depression and anxiety in an intervention setting where participants were asked to identify their most common peripheral affect that preempts eating behavior. Another study captured qualitative data in an effort to understand internal and external factors that contribute to emotional eating. One quote exemplifies the common struggle of emotional eaters:

> Everyday I get up with the intention of trying to eat better. I honestly do. I want to eat better. I want to be healthy . . .. But food is comfort to me. If I am sad, I want chips, fried food or gumbo. . . . I try not to eat these things, but I do. (Kemp et al., 2013, p. 204)

Food indulgence brings comfort to many and unfortunately, in several cases, can derail intentions to eat well. In an investigation of the stress-eating behavior relationship, O'Connor, Jones, Conner, McMillan, and Ferguson (2008) assessed its moderators in a naturalistic setting with 422 adult men and women. Findings indicated that daily stresses were associated with higher consumption of high-fat and high-sugar foods and decreased consumption of main meals and vegetables; the leading moderator was emotional eating.

Rhodes, Kaushal, and Quinlan, (2016) have also recently reviewed studies that manipulate hypothetical peripheral affect within the context of PA identity. Three studies by Strachan and colleagues (Strachan & Brawley, 2008; Strachan, Brawley, Spink, & Jung, 2009; Strachan, Flora, Brawley, & Spink, 2011) showed that a vignette asking people to imagine they are too busy to exercise resulted in much higher negative affect and lower positive affect for those with exercise identities than those who reported lower exercise identities. Strachan and Brawley (2008) also presented a similar vignette to people asking them to imagine they were too busy to eat healthily; those reporting high healthy-eater identity had higher negative affect and lower positive affect in response to the vignette than those reporting lower healthy-eater identity (Strachan & Brawley, 2008). This peripheral affect has not been field tested with intention and behavior, but Rhodes's review did show consistent evidence in seven of eight studies that those who have higher scores on measures of identity are significantly more likely to translate intention into behavior. According to theory, this peripheral negative affect is context-activated and reflexive (Stets & Burke, 2000), initiating the motivation to enact the behavior.

Affect and the Enablement of Habit

One of the most researched and integral implicit processes in health behavior is the formation of habits (Rebar et al., 2016; Sheeran et al., 2013). Habit has been defined as a process by which a stimulus cues a learned stimulus-response (Gardner, 2015). Habits are also directly related to action control as they are typically viewed as initially goal-directed automatic behavior (Bargh, 1989). They also feature prominently in several models of action control such as the motivation-ability-opportunity-behavior model (Olander & Thogersen, 1995), M-PAC (Rhodes & de Bruijn, 2013b), PRIME theory (West, 2009), theory of consumption (Baggozi, 2000), theory of interpersonal behavior (Triandis, 1977), and temporal self-regulation theory (P. A. Hall & Fong, 2007).

The antecedents of habit are still an area of considerable debate, although reinforcement and reward are often considered fundamental to habit development (Lally & Gardner, 2011; Lally, van Jaarsveld, Potts, & Wardle, 2009). Kaushal and Rhodes (2015) have suggested that, in terms of PA, the affective response to a behavior and affective judgments about the behavior are likely to have some impact on the development or facilitation of habit formation (in line with internal reinforcement or reward). Specifically, if PA affective judgments are strongly negative, then this may prompt rumination (e.g., dread) and thus heighten the awareness of performing the behavior, which should limit the extent to which it can be habituated. Relatedly, if the affective response to PA is construed as unpleasant, then pain-related awareness would likely thwart habituation. Initial evidence has supported this conjecture. Kaushal and Rhodes showed that affective judgments were a significant predictor of habit development of exercise behavior among new gym members, second only to the consistency of practice. Further, while a direct examination of the affective response to PA and habit has not yet been performed, Rhodes and de Bruijn (2010) did show that moderate intensity PA had a stronger relationship with habit than vigorous intensity PA. Vigorous intensity PA provides a less pleasant response than moderate PA (Ekkekakis, Hall, & Petruzzello, 2008) so the affect response was deemed the most likely reason for the lowered habituation of vigorous compared to moderate PA.

Eating behaviors are also often linked to strong habits, and this has supported theoretical conjecture based on how habits can form (Lally & Gardner, 2011). For example, if someone repeatedly eats confectionary snacks while watching television, the action of watching television becomes a cue to consume a sugary snack, resulting in a poor dietary habit (Kremers, van der Horst, & Brug, 2007). The role of affect on this type of habit formation seems to involve hedonic hunger. Hedonic hunger is consumption based on pleasure rather than internal hunger cues, which is thought to thwart intentional dietary control (Stroebe, Papies, & Aarts, 2008). Naughton, McCarthy, and McCarthy (2015) showed some support for this theorizing, as habit mediated the relationship between hedonic hunger and consumption of high-sugar foods. There is evidence that intended behavior and behavioral control are quieted by strong habits: factors such as self-monitoring and dietary planning are competing against unhealthy habits in a model of sugar consumption (where intention translation on sugar consumption is fully mediated by habits). Put simply, regardless of one's intended healthy eating behavior, the presence of a desirable confectionary food may lead to its consumption through a maladaptive habit of unhealthy eating.

FUTURE DIRECTIONS AND IMPLICATIONS FOR INTERVENTION

Guided by several action control frameworks, we have proposed pathways in which affect may determine action control in Figure 2.1 and three main affective processes. Clearly, some of these lines of research have more advanced evidence than others at present but all research on affect and action control is relatively new. In this section, we highlight how these may be tested and future directions to examine these various pathways.

Reflective affect in the form of affective judgments, followed by anticipated regret has the most advanced research in action control thus far due to its testing within the theory of planned behavior (Lawton et al., 2009; Rhodes, Fiala, et al., 2009; Sandberg & Conner, 2008). Nevertheless, as noted in this theory, much of these examinations have been designed merely to predict or raise intentions in experimental designs with the assumption that this will subsequently increase behavior. Action control experiments to test a moderation pathway of increased intention stability (Figure 2.1 Path A1) should be designed with nonintending populations of the target behavior and manipulations of reflective affect (either judgments or regret) compared to other sources of exposure (e.g., instrumental attitudes, perceived behavioral control) meant to promote intentions. If both approaches can relatively equally increase intentions, Path A1 will be supported by evidence that the reflective affect intervention did not result in more behavior over time and falsified if evidence is not supportive of a difference in behavior change.

In contrast to Path A1, examinations of Figure 2.1 Path A2 are likely best examined among randomized experimental designs with intenders of the target health behavior, who are in the initial phase of behavior change. Manipulations of reflective affect (either judgments or regret) should augment intention and result in better behavior change results compared to controls. By contrast, Path A2 would be falsified if these manipulations showed change in affective judgments compared to controls, but did not result in higher behavioral enactment.

As previously noted, volitional regulation behaviors have seen considerable empirical testing in many health behaviors, yet the role of affect has seen limited attention. Examinations of how volitional regulatory behaviors can improve behavioral enactment via increased reflective affect (Figure 2.1 Path A3) can be examined among randomized experimental designs with intenders of the target health behavior, who are in the initial phase of behavior change. Volitional strategies used to improve reflective affect (e.g., plans that involve enjoyable opportunities, tasty recipes, social outcomes) should augment intention and result in better behavior change results compared to controls.

The impact of reflective affect about regulatory behaviors on the repeated use of these volitional regulatory behaviors (Figure 2.1 Path A4) can also be tested using randomized experimental designs with intenders of the target health behavior, who are in the initial phase of behavior change. Manipulations to the affective judgments about using these volitional strategies (e.g., games, social contexts) can be compared to a control group with no such manipulation and instead just instructions to use the same strategies. Path A4 would be supported if volitional regulation behaviors were higher in the affect condition, and particularly telling if this followed to subsequently higher enactment of the target behavior.

Finally, examination of Figure 2.1 Path A5 is among the least tested pathways in current research and may still benefit from initial daily diary or ecological momentary assessment approaches used to examine the peripheral mood, habit, identity, and behavior among those with initially high intentions to enact the target health behavior. These observational designs may yield helpful initial support on whether there is enough basic evidence for Path A5 before conducting randomized experimental studies.

In summary, affect may have several routes to partially determine the action control of protective behaviors such as PA and healthy eating. At present there is good evidence that reflective affective factors such as affective judgments and anticipated regret can both moderate intention–behavior relations presumably from more stable original intentions and augment initial intentions with direct effects on behavior. There has been far less research on how affect may impact volitional regulation behaviors, yet prior theories suggest that many volitional tactics may involve constructing improved reflective affect in order to facilitate successful action control. Finally, reflexive affect has just begun to see research attention in health behavior and its role in action control may be through various means such as identity, habit, incidental affect, and affective associations. Carefully designed future studies should help justify or falsify several of the proposed pathways we have suggested in our model of affect and action control.

ACKNOWLEDGMENT

RER is supported by a Canadian Cancer Society Senior Scientist Award and the Right to Give Foundation with additional funds from the Canadian Cancer Society, the Social Sciences and Humanities Research Council of Canada and the Canadian Institutes for Health Research.

REFERENCES

Abraham, C., & Sheeran, P. (2003). Acting on intentions: The role of anticipated regret. *British Journal of Social Psychology*, 495–511.

Abraham, C., & Sheeran, P. (2004). Deciding to exercise: The role of anticipated regret. *British Journal of Health Psychology*, *9*, 269–278.

Ach, N. (1905). *Uber die Willenstatigkeit und das Denken*. Gottingen: Vandenhoeck & Ruprecht.

Ajzen, I. (2006). Constructing a theory of planned behavior questionnaire. http://people.umass.edu/aizen/pdf/tpb.measurement.pdf

Armitage, C. J. (2015). Randomized test of a brief psychological intervention to reduce and prevent emotional eating in a community sample. *Journal of Public Health*, 438–444.

Ashton, L. M., Hutchesson, M. J., Rollo, M. E., Morgan, P. J., Thompson, D. I., & Collins, C. E. (2015). Young adult males' motivators and perceived barriers towards eating healthily and being active: a qualitative study. *International Journal of Behavioral Nutrition and Physical Activity*, *12*, 1–10.

Baggozi, R. P. (2000). The poverty of economic explanations of consumption and an action theory alternative. *Managerial and Decision Economics*, *21*, 95–109.

Bagozzi, R. P. (1992). The self-regulation of attitudes, intentions, and behavior. *Social Psychology Quarterly*, *55*, 178–204.

Baranowski, T., Buday, R., Thompson, D. I., & Baranowski, J. (2008). Playing for real: Video games and stories for health-related behavior change. *American Journal of Preventive Medicine, 34*, 74–82.

Bargh, J. A. (1989). Conditional automaticity: Varieties of automatic influence in social perception and cognition. In J. S. Uleman & J. A. Bargh (Eds.), *Unintended thought* (pp. 3–51). New York, NY: Guilford Press.

Bargh, J. A., Chaiken, S., Raymond, P., & Hymes, C. (1996). The automatic evaluation effect: Unconditional automatic attitude activation with a pronunciation task. *Journal of Experimental Social Psychology, 32*, 104–128.

Bélanger-Gravel, A., Godin, G., & Amireault, S. (2013). A meta-analytic review of the effect of implementation intentions on physical activity. *Health Psychology Review, 7*(1), 1–32.

Bluemke, M., Brand, R., Schweizer, G., & Kahlert, D. (2010). Exercise might be good for me, but I don't feel good about it: Do automatic associations predict exercise behavior. *Journal of Sport and Exercise Psychology, 32*, 137–153.

Caperchione, C. M., Vandelanotte, C., Kolt, G. S., Duncan, M., Ellison, M., George, E., & Mummery, W. K. (2012). What a man wants: Understanding the challenges and motivations to physical activity participation and healthy eating in middle-aged Australian men. *American Journal of Men's Health, 6*, 453–461.

Carraro, N., & Gaudreau, P. (2013). Spontaneous and experimentally induced action planning and coping planning for physical activity: A meta-analysis. *Psychology of Sport and Exercise, 14*, 228–248.

Cohen, J. (1992). A power primer. *Psychological Bulletin, 112*, 155–159.

Conn, V. S., Hafdahl, A. R., & Mehr, D. R. (2011). Interventions to increase physical activity among healthy adults: Meta-analysis of outcomes. *American Journal of Public Health, 101*, 751–758.

Conner, M., & Abraham, C. (2001). Conscientiousness and the theory of planned behavior: Toward a more complete model of the antecedents of intentions and behavior. *Personality and Social Psychology Bulletin, 27*, 1547–1561.

Conner, M., McEachan, R., Taylor, N., O'Hara, J., & Lawton, R. (2015). Role of affective attitudes and anticipated affective reactions in predicting health behaviors. *Health Psychology, 34*, 642–652.

Conner, M., & Norman, P. (2015). *Predicting health behaviour: Research and practice with social cognition models*. Berkshire, UK: Open University Press.

Conner, M., Rhodes, R. E., Morris, B., McEachan, R., & Lawton, R. (2011). Changing exercise through targeting affective or cognitive attitudes. *Psychology and Health, 26*, 133–149.

Cunningham, W., Raye, C., & Johnson, M. (2004). Implicit and explicit evaluation: fMRI correlates of valence, emotional intensity, and control in the processing of attitudes. *Journal of Cognitive Neuroscience, 16*, 1717–1729.

Deci, E. L., & Ryan, R. M. (1985). *Intrinsic motivation and self-determination in human behavior*. New York, NY: Plenum Press.

Deutsch, R., & Strack, F. (2006). Duality models in social psychology: From dual processes to interacting systems. *Psychological Inquiry, 17*, 166–172.

Dunton, G. F., Huh, J., Leventhal, A. M., Riggs, N., Hedeker, D., Spruijt-Metz, D., & Pentz, M. (2013). Momentary assessment of affect, physical feeling states, and physical activity in children. *Health Psychology*. doi: 10.1037/a0032640

Ekkekakis, P., Hall, E. E., & Petruzzello, S. J. (2008). The relationship between exercise intensity and affective responses demystified: To crack the 40 year-old nut, replace the 40-year-old nutcracker! *Annals of Behavioral Medicine*, *35*, 136–149.

Emerson, J. A., & Williams, D. M. (2015). The multifaceted relationship between physical activity and affect. *Social and Personality Psychology Compass*, *9*, 419–433.

Evans, J. S. B. T., & Stanovich, K. E. (2013). Dual-process theories of higher cognition: Advancing the debate. *Perspectives on Psychological Science*, *8*, 223–241.

Fishbein, M., Triandis, H. C., Kanfer, F. H., Becker, M., Middlestadt, S. E., & Eichler, A. (2001). Factors influencing behavior and behavior change. In A. Baum & T. A. Revenson (Eds.), *Handbook of health psychology* (pp. 3–17). Mahwah, NJ: Erlbaum.

Gardner, B. (2015). A review and analysis of the use of "habit" in understanding, predicting and influencing health-related behaviour. *Health Psychology Review*, *9*, 277–295. doi: 10.1080/17437199.2013.876238

Giner-Sorolla, R. (2001). Guilty pleasures and grim necessities: Affective attitudes in dilemmas of self-control. *Journal of Personality and Social Psychology*, *80*, 206–221.

Godinho, C. A., Alvarez, M. J., Lima, M. L., & Schwarzer, R. (2014). Will is not enough: Coping planning and action control as mediators in the prediction of fruit and vegetable intake. *British Journal of Health Psychology*, *19*, 856–870.

Gollwitzer, P. M., & Sheeran, P. (2006). Implementation intentions and goal achievement: A meta-analysis of effects and processes. *Advances in Experimental Social Psychology*, *38*, 69–119.

Hall, J. N., Moore, S., Harper, S. B., & Lynch, J. W. (2009). Global variability in fruit and vegetable consumption. *American Journal of Preventive Medicine*, *36*, 402–409.

Hall, P. A., & Fong, G. T. (2007). Temporal self-regulation theory: A model for individual health behavior. *Health Psychology Review*, *1*, 6–52.

Hallal, P. C., Andersen, L. B., Bull, F. C., Guthold, R., Haskell, W., Ekelund, U., & Wells, J. C. (2012). Global physical activity levels: Surveillance progress, pitfalls, and prospects. *Lancet*, *380*, 247–257.

Heckhausen, H., & Gollwitzer, P. M. (1987). Thought contents and cognitive functioning in motivational and volitional states of mind. *Motivation and Emotion*, *11*, 101–120. doi: doi: 10.1007/BF00992338

Helander, E., Kaipainen, K., Korhonen, I., & Wansink, B. (2014). Factors related to sustained use of a free mobile app for dietary self-monitoring with photography and peer feedback: Retrospective cohort study. *Journal of Medical Internet Research*, *16*, e109.

Jun, J., & Arendt, S. W. (2016). Understanding healthy eating behaviors at casual dining restaurants using the extended theory of planned behavior. *International Journal of Hospitality Management*, *53*, 106–115.

Kaushal, N., & Rhodes, R. E. (2015). Exercise habit in new gym members: A longitudinal study. *Journal of Behavioral Medicine*, *38*, 652–663.

Keer, M., Conner, M., Van den Putte, B., & Neijens, P. (2013). The temporal stability and predictive validity of affect-based and cognition-based intentions. *British Journal of Social Psychology*, 1–13.

Kemp, E., Bui, M., & Grier, S. (2013). When food is more than nutrition: Understanding emotional eating and overconsumption. *Journal of Consumer Behavior, 12*, 204–213.

Kendzierski, D., & DeCarlo, K. J. (1991). Physical activity enjoyment scale: Two validation studies. *Journal of Sport and Exercise Psychology, 13*, 50–64.

Kiviniemi, M. T., & Duangdao, K. M. (2009). Affective associations mediate the influence of cost-benefit beliefs on fruit and vegetable consumption. *Appetite, 52*, 771–775.

Koball, A. M., Meers, M. R., Storfer-Isser, A., Domoff, S. E., & Musher-Eizenman, D. R. (2012). Eating when bored: Revision of the Emotional Eating Scale with a focus on boredom. *Health Psychology, 31*, 521–524.

Kremers, S. P. J., van der Horst, K., & Brug, J. (2007). Adolescent screen-viewing behaviour is associated with consumption of sugar-sweetened beverages: The role of habit strength and perceived parental norms. *Appetite, 48*, 345–350.

Kuhl, J. (1984). Motivational aspects of achievement motivation and learned helplessness: Towards a comprehensive theory of action control. In B. A. Maher & W. B. Maher (Eds.), *Progress in experimental personality research* (Vol. 13, pp. 99–171). New York, NY: Academic Press.

Kujala, U. M. (2011). Physical activity, genes, and lifetime predisposition to chronic disease. *European Review of Aging and Physical Activity, 8*, 31–36.

Kwan, B., & Bryan, A. D. (2010). In-task and post-task affective response to exercise: Translating exercise intentions into behaviour. *British Journal of Health Psychology, 15*, 115–131.

Kwasnicka, D., Presseau, J., White, M., & Sniehotta, F. F. (2013). Does planning how to cope with anticipated barriers facilitate health-related behaviour change? A systematic review. *Health Psychology Review*. doi:10.1080/17437199.2013.766832

Laing, B. Y., Mangione, C. M., Tseng, C. H., Leng, M., Vaisberg, E., Mahida, M., & Bell, D. S. (2014). Effectiveness of a smartphone application for weight loss compared with usual care in overweight primary care patients. *Annals of Internal Medicine, 161*, S5–S12.

Lally, P., & Gardner, B. (2011). Promoting habit formation. *Health Psychology Review*, 1–22.

Lally, P., van Jaarsveld, C. H. M., Potts, H. W. W., & Wardle, J. (2009). How are habits formed: Modelling habit formation in the real world. *European Journal of Social Psychology, 40*, 998–1009.

Lambie, J. A., & Marcel, A. J. (2002). Consciousness and the varieties of emotion experience: A theoretical framework. *Psychological Review, 109*, 219–259.

Lawton, R., Conner, M., & McEachan, R. (2009). Desire or reason: Predicting health behaviors from affective and cognitive attitudes. *Health Psychology, 28*, 56–65.

Locke, E. A., & Latham, G. P. (1990). *A theory of goal setting performance*. Englewood Cliffs, NJ: Prentice Hall.

Lyubomirsky, S., King, L., & Diener, E. (2005). The benefits of frequent positive affect: Does happiness lead to success?. *Psychological Bulletin, 131*, 803–855.

Maher, J. P., Rhodes, R. E., Dzubur, E., Huh, J., Intille, S., & Dunton, G. F. (2017). Momentary assessment of physical activity intention-behavior coupling in adults. *Translational Behavioral Medicine, 7*(4), 709–718.

Mascie-Taylor, C. G. N., & Karim, E. (2003). The burden of chronic disease. *Science, 302*, 1921–1922.

McEachan, R., Conner, M., Taylor, N. J., & Lawton, R. J. (2011). Prospective prediction of health-related behaviors with the theory of planned behavior: A meta-analysis. *Health Psychology Review, 5*, 97–144.

Michie, S., West, R., Campbell, R., Brown, J., & Gainforth, H. (2014). *ABC of theories of behaviour change*. Great Britain, London: Silverback Publishing.

Mistry, C., Sweet, S., Latimer, A., & Rhodes, R. E. (2015). Predicting changes in planning behaviour and physical activity among adults. *Psychology of Sport and Exercise, 17*, 1–6.

Morris, W. N. (1999). The mood system. In D. Kahneman, E. Diener, & N. Schwarz (Eds.), *Well-being: The foundations of hedonic psychology* (pp. 169–189). New York, NY: Russell-Sage.

Morris, W. N., & Reilly, N. P. (1987). Toward the self-regulation of mood: Theory and research. *Motivation and Emotion, 11*, 215–249.

Mulle, J. G., & Vaccarino, V. (2013). Cardiovascular disease, psychosocial factors, and genetics: The case of depression. *Progress in Cardiovascular Diseases, 55*, 557–562.

Naughton, P., McCarthy, M., & McCarthy, S. (2015). Acting to self-regulate unhealthy eating habits: An investigation into the effects of habit, hedonic hunger and self-regulation on sugar consumption from confectionery foods. *Food Quality and Preference, 46*, 173–183.

O'Connor, D. B., Jones, F., Conner, M., McMillan, B., & Ferguson, E. (2008). Effects of daily hassles and eating style on eating behavior. *Health Psychology, 27*, 20–31.

Olander, F., & Thogersen, J. (1995). Understanding of consumer behaviour as a prerequisite for environmental protection. *Journal of consumer Policy, 18*, 345–385.

Prochaska, J. O., & Velicer, W. F. (1997). The transtheoretical model of health behavior change. *American Journal of Health Promotion, 12*, 38–48.

Rebar, A., Ram, N., & Conroy, D. E. (2015). Using the EZ-diffusion model to score a Single-Category Implicit Association Test of physical activity. *Psychology of Sport and Exercise, 16*, 96–105.

Rebar, A. L., Dimmock, J. A., Jackson, B., Rhodes, R. E., Kates, A., Starling, J., & Vandelanotte, C. (2016). A systematic review of the effects of non-conscious regulatory processes in physical activity. *Health Psychology Review, 10*, 395–407.

Rhodes, R. E., & de Bruijn, G. J. (2010). Automatic and motivational correlates of physical activity: Does intensity moderate the relationship? *Behavioral Medicine, 26*, 44–52.

Rhodes, R. E., & de Bruijn, G. J. (2013a). How big is the physical activity intention-behaviour gap? A meta-analysis using the action control framework. *British Journal of Health Psychology, 18*, 296–309.

Rhodes, R. E., & de Bruijn, G. J. (2013b). What predicts intention-behavior discordance? A review of the action control framework. *Exercise and Sports Sciences Reviews, 41*, 201–207.

Rhodes, R. E., & Dickau, L. (2012). Meta-analysis of experimental evidence for the intention-behavior relationship in the physical activity domain. *Health Psychology, 31*, 724–727.

Rhodes, R. E., & Dickau, L. (2013). Moderators of the intention-behavior relationship in physical activity: A systematic review. *British Journal of Sports Medicine, 47*, 215–225. doi: doi:10.1136 bjsports-2011-090411

Rhodes, R. E., Fiala, B., & Conner, M. (2009). Affective judgments and physical activity: A review and meta-analysis. *Annals of Behavioral Medicine, 38*, 180–204.

Rhodes, R. E., & Kates, A. (2015). Can the affective response to exercise predict future motives and physical activity behavior? A systematic review of published evidence. *Annals of Behavioral Medicine, 49*, 715–731.

Rhodes, R. E., Kaushal, N., & Quinlan, A. (2016). Is physical activity a part of who I am? A review and meta-analysis of identity, schema and physical activity. *Health Psychology Review, 10*, 204–225.

Rhodes, R. E., & Mistry, C. D. (2016). Understanding the reasons behind anticipated regret for missing regular physical activity. *Frontiers in Psychology, 7*, 1–6.

Rhodes, R. E., Warburton, D. E. R., & Bredin, S. S. (2009). Predicting the effect of interactive video bikes on exercise adherence: An efficacy trial. *Psychology, Health and Medicine, 14*, 631–641.

Rhodes, R. E., & Yao, C. (2015). Models accounting for intention-behavior discordance in the physical activity domain: A user's guide, content overview, and review of current evidence. *International Journal of Behavioral Nutrition and Physical Activity, 12*(9), 1–15.

Richert, J., Reuter, T., Wiedemann, A. U., Lippke, S., Ziegelmann, J., & Schwarzer, R. (2010). Differential effects of planning and self-efficacy on fruit and vegetable consumption. *Appetite, 54*, 611–614.

Riecken, K. H. B., Mark, R., & Rhodes, R. E. (2013). Qualitative elicitation of affective beliefs related to physical activity. *Psychology of Sport and Exercise, 14*, 786–792.

Rivis, A., Sheeran, P., & Armitage, C. J. (2009). Expanding the affective and normative components of the theory of planned behavior: A meta-analysis of anticipated affect and moral norms. *Journal of Applied Social Psychology, 39*, 2985–3019.

Rosenstock, I. M. (1974). Historical origins of the health belief model. *Health Education Monographs, 2*, 1–9.

Russell, J. A. (1980). A circumplex model of affect. *Journal of Personality and Social Psychology, 39*, 1161–1178.

Sandberg, T., & Conner, M. (2008). Anticipated regret as an additional predictor in the theory of planned behaviour: A meta-analysis. *British Journal of Social Psychology, 47*, 589–606.

Sandberg, T., & Conner, M. (2011). Understanding self-generated validity to promote exercise behavior. *British Journal of Social Psychology, 50*, 769–783.

Schwarzer, R. (2008). Modeling health behavior change: How to predict and modify the adoption and maintenance of health behaviors. *Applied Psychology, 57*, 1–29.

Sheeran, P. (2002). Intention-behaviour relations: A conceptual and empirical review. In M. Hewstone & W. Stroebe (Eds.), *European review of social psychology* (Vol. 12, pp. 1–36). Chichester, UK: Wiley.

Sheeran, P., Gollwitzer, P. M., & Bargh, J. A. (2013). Nonconscious processes and health. *Health Psychology, 32*, 460–473.

Simonson, I. (1992). The influence of anticipated regret and responsibility on purchase decision. *Journal of Consumer Research, 19*, 105–118.

Sniehotta, F. F. (2009). Towards a theory of intentional behaviour change: Plans, planning, and self-regulation. *British Journal of Health Psychology, 14*, 261–273.

Sniehotta, F. F., Presseau, J., & Araújo-Soares, V. (2014). Time to retire the theory of planned behavior. *Health Psychology Review, 8*, 1–7.

Stadler, G., Oettingen, G., & Gollwitzer, P. M. (2010). Intervention effects of information and self-regulation on eating fruits and vegetables over two years. *Health Psychology, 29*, 274–283.

Stets, J. E., & Burke, P. J. (2000). Identity theory and social identity theory. *Social Psychology Quarterly, 63*, 224–237.

Strachan, S. M., & Brawley, L. R. (2008). Reactions to a perceived challenge to identity: A focus on exercise and healthy eating. *Journal of Health Psychology, 13*, 575–588.

Strachan, S. M., Brawley, L. R., Spink, K. S., & Jung, M. (2009). Strength of exercise identity and identity-exercise consistency: Affective and cognitive relationships. *Journal of Health Psychology, 14*, 1196–1206.

Strachan, S. M., Flora, P. K., Brawley, L. R., & Spink, K. S. (2011). Varying the cause of a challenge to exercise identity behaviour: Reactions of individuals of differing identity strength. *Journal of Health Psychology, 16*, 572–583.

Stroebe, W., Papies, E. K., & Aarts, H. (2008). From homeostatic to hedonic theories of eating: Self-regulatory failure in food-rich environments. *Applied Psychology, 57*, 172–193.

Stryker, S., & Burke, P. J. (2000). The past, present and future of an identity theory. *Social Psychology Quarterly, 63*, 284–297.

Triandis, H. C. (1977). *Interpersonal behavior*. Monterey, CA: Brooks/Cole.

van Strien, T., Frijters, J. E. R., Bergers, G. P. A., & Defares, P. B. (1986). The Dutch Eating Behavior Questionnaire (DEBQ) for assessment of restrained, emotional, and external eating behavior. *International Journal of Eating Disorders, 5*, 295–315.

Walker, A. E. (2007). Multiple chronic diseases and quality of life: Patterns emerging from a large national sample, Australia. *Chronic Illness, 3*, 202–218.

Wang, X. (2011). The role of anticipated negative emotions and past behavior in individuals' physical activity intentions and behaviors. *Psychology of Sport and Exercise, 12*, 300–305.

Warburton, D. E. R., Nicol, C. W., & Bredin, S. S. (2006). Health benefits of physical activity: The evidence. *Canadian Medical Association Journal, 174*, 801–809.

Webb, T. L., & Sheeran, P. (2006). Does changing behavioral intentions engender behavior change? A meta-analysis of the experimental evidence. *Psychological Bulletin, 132*, 249–268.

Wegener, D. T., & Petty, R. E. (1994). Mood management across affective states: The hedonic contingency hypothesis. *Journal of Personality and Social Psychology, 66*, 1034–1048.

Weinstein, N. D. (2007). Misleading tests of health behavior theories. *Annals of Behavioral Medicine, 33*(1), 1–10.

West, R. (2009). The multiple facets of cigarette addiction and what the mean for encouraging and helping smokers to stop. *Journal of Chronic Obstructive Pulmonary Disease*, 6, 277–283.

West, R., & Brown, J. (2013). *Theory of addiction* (2nd ed.). Oxford: Wiley-Blackwell.

Williams, D. M., & Evans, D. R. (2014). Current emotion research in health behavior science. *Emotion Review*, 6, 282–292.

World Health Organization. (2014). Fact Sheet No. 310—The top ten causes of death. http://www.who.int/mediacentre/factsheets/fs310/en/

3

Experiential Attitude and Anticipated Affect

MARK T. CONNER

INTRODUCTION

The psychological determinants of health behaviors have been an important focus of health psychology for over 30 years. Health behavior–specific thoughts and feelings, or health cognitions, have received particular attention (Conner & Norman, 1995, 2005, 2015). This has been justified as a search for modifiable determinants of health behavior that can be targeted in interventions to change health behaviors and subsequently improve health outcomes. Models such as the theory of planned behavior (TPB), social cognitive theory, health belief model, and protection motivation theory have been widely used in this way (Conner & Norman, 2015). They suggest that the thoughts and feelings I have now about a behavior will predict whether I perform that behavior in the future (partly because they inform my current decision or intention to perform that behavior and partly because that decision plus those thoughts and feelings impact on performance of the behavior when the opportunity to act presents itself). For example, the TPB (Ajzen, 1991) suggests behavior is determined by intention, which in turn is determined by attitude, subjective norm, and perceived behavioral control. Intention here taps the plans or decision to act. Attitude taps the overall evaluation of the behavior, while subjective norm assesses perceptions of the reactions and the behavior of important others. Perceived behavioral control measures the perceived degree of control or confidence the individual has over performing the behavior. Prospective tests of the TPB have shown it to predict a wide range of health behaviors, with meta-analyses indicating that it explains 44.3% of the variance in intention and 19.3% of the variance in action across health behaviors (McEachan, Conner, Taylor, & Lawton, 2011).

However, models like the TPB are firmly grounded in the cognitive tradition and focus on cognitive influences at the expense of affective influences. In addition, given the focus on predicting behavior, attempts to integrate affect within such models have mainly focused on cognitively mediated affect rather than experienced affect (see Sheeran, Webb, Gollwitzer, and Oettingen, this volume, for discussion of this issue). Research has long highlighted the failure of models like the TPB to adequately account for the role of affect (e.g., Manstead & Parker, 1995; van der Pligt, Zeelenberg, van Dijk, de Vries, & Richard, 1998). Yet, despite there being a long established distinction between, for example, instrumental/cognitive and experiential/affective attitudes (e.g., Abelson, Kinder, Peters, & Fiske, 1982; Trafimow & Sheeran, 1998), it is only recently that there have been moves to reflect such distinctions in theories. For example, Fishbein and Ajzen (2010) in their reasoned action approach (RAA), developed out of the TPB and earlier theory of reasoned action, noted that attitude measures should tap both components (also see Ajzen & Fishbein, 2005) labeled experiential and instrumental attitudes. Considerable research has also shown distinctions between types of norms and types of perceived behavioral control. For example, the RAA approach splits norms into injunctive (what others perceived to want) and descriptive (what others perceived to do) norms and perceived behavioral control into capacity (similar to self-efficacy) and autonomy (or perceived control).

A distinct body of predictive research has conceptualized the role of affect in a different way. The measures used in such research are usually labeled anticipated affect to distinguish them from the experiential attitudes described previously. These two types of affective evaluations can be distinguished in three important ways. First, work on anticipated affect tends to focus on the affect that is expected to follow after performance or nonperformance of a behavior rather than that expected to occur while the behavior is being performed. Second, anticipated affect measures tend to focus on what Giner-Sorolla (2001) describes as self-conscious emotions (e.g., regret, guilt), whereas experiential attitudes tend to focus on hedonic emotions (e.g., enjoyment, excitement). Third, research on anticipated affect has tended to examine the negative affect (particularly associated with nonperformance of the behavior) while experiential attitudes tend to focus on positive affect.

The present chapter reviews the role of experiential attitudes and anticipated affect on health behaviors in the context of models such as the TPB/RAA that include other established determinants of behavior. The effects of experiential attitudes and anticipated affect are considered individually before considering their combined effects. Both correlational and experimental findings are presented along with meta-analytic summaries. Where possible the focus is on prospective and experimental studies that employ objective measures of health behavior and explore the effects of controlling for other health cognitions and past behavior. The main focus is on health behaviors in general although the power of affective influences for different types of health behavior such as risk behaviors (e.g., smoking), protection behaviors (e.g., physical activity), and detection behaviors (e.g., cervical screening) is noted where evidence is available.

Lawton, Conner, and McEachan (2009) used Russell's (2003) theory of emotion to argue that the influence of experiential attitude will be strongest for those behaviors that have a more immediate impact on the senses or physiological state and weakest among behaviors where the impact is less immediate. Russell (2003) proposes that affective qualities are attributed to behaviors as a result of experiencing the emotion when enacting the behavior and that this guides intention and action. In modulating our general mood state we may engage in behaviors to which we attribute changes in affect. So when we engage in exercise we do so to make ourselves feel energized or when we smoke we do so to feel relaxed. These affective qualities attributed to the behaviors may then motivate further enactment of the behavior, particularly in circumstances where core affect is off-balance, for example, when we feel tired or anxious. Conner, McEachan, Taylor, O'Hara, and Lawton (2015) argue that various health risk (e.g., drinking alcohol) and health protection (e.g., exercise) behaviors are likely to have more immediate impact on the senses or physiological state, while various detection behaviors (e.g., self-examination) are likely to have less immediate impact. On this basis we might expect experiential attitude to have a stronger impact on intention and behavior for risk and protection compared to detection behaviors. Although less clear cut, anticipated affect might be expected to have a stronger effect on detection compared to protection or risk behaviors because it is the less immediate anticipated affect such as regret or guilt that are likely to dominate here in the absence of experiential attitude effects.

Experiential Attitudes

In this section correlational and then experimental studies on experiential attitudes are reviewed.

Correlational Studies

The relative importance of experiential and instrumental attitudes in predicting the performance of health behavior is usefully illustrated in a study by Lawton et al. (2009). In this study a sample of members of the general public completed questionnaires tapping components of attitudes in relation to a range of different health behaviors and two months later self-reported their intention to perform these behaviors and actual performance of the behaviors over the past two months. Importantly, respondents completed single item semantic differential measures of both experiential and instrumental attitudes. Experiential attitude was tapped by how "not enjoyable–enjoyable" the behavior might be and instrumental attitude was tapped by how "harmful-beneficial" the behavior might be expected to be. Comparisons of the simple correlations showed that compared to instrumental attitude, experiential attitude was a stronger predictor of intention (10 out of 14 behaviors) and behavior (13 out of 14 behaviors). Importantly when both types of attitude were simultaneously entered, the beta weight for experiential attitude was significantly stronger than the beta weight for instrumental attitude when predicting intention (7 out of 14 behaviors) and behavior (9 out of 14 behaviors). This pattern was replicated by Lawton, Conner, and Parker (2007) using multiple-item measures of experiential and instrumental attitude (based on sets of behavioral beliefs) and objective measures of behavior and controlling for other TPB components for exceeding the posted speed limit in an adult sample of drivers and smoking initiation in an adolescent sample. Relatedly, Rhodes and Conner (2010) argue that such behavioral beliefs vary along the dimensions of cognitive-affective, proximal-distal and positive-negative. It is notable that for many health behaviors the affective outcomes also tend to be more proximal than the cognitive outcomes.

A number of other studies have also reported stronger effects for experiential/affective compared to instrumental/cognitive attitudes and beliefs (see Glasman & Albarracin, 2006 for a general review). For example, Conner et al. (2008) reported that in three studies, experiential compared to instrumental attitudes were stronger predictors of intention to have unprotected sex in women (effects reversed in men) and their impact was significantly increased by intoxication with alcohol. Lawton, Ashley, Dawson, Waiblinger, and Conner (2012) reported experiential attitude compared to instrumental attitude to be significantly stronger predictors of intention to breastfeed and breastfeeding behavior when controlling for variables from the RAA plus moral norm. Research has indicated the importance of experiential attitude as a correlate of intention and behavior for a range of health behaviors (e.g., Elliott, Thomson, Robertson, Stephenson, & Wicks, 2013; Godin, 1987; Kiviniemi, Jandorf, & Erwin, 2014; Kiviniemi, Voss-Humke, & Seifert, 2007; Lowe, Eves, & Carroll, 2002; Rhodes, Blanchard, & Matheson, 2006; Trafimow et al., 2004; Van den Berg, Manstead, van der Pligt, & Wigboldus, 2005). Relatedly, it has been shown that intentions based on experiential compared to instrumental attitudes are more predictive of behavior. For example, Keer, Conner, Van den Putte, and Neijens (2014) across two studies showed that intention based on experiential attitude was a stronger predictor of health behaviors compared to intention based on instrumental attitude.

More recent research has suggested that experiential attitude may be a stronger predictor for health risk compared to health protection behaviors. For example, Conner, McEachan, Lawton, and Gardner (2017) in a test of the RAA showed both instrumental and experiential attitudes to be predictors of intention to engage in a range of health behaviors including risk and protection health behaviors (when controlling for other RAA predictors plus past behavior). For predictions of behavior, both types of attitude were significant when controlling for other RAA predictors, although experiential attitude was a stronger predictor for risk compared to protection health behaviors. When past behavior was also controlled for, only experiential attitude was significant and was again significantly stronger in risk compared to protection behaviors. This work suggests that experiential attitude has both an indirect (via intentions) and direct "impulsive" impact on health behaviors and their effect is particularly strong for risk compared to protection health behaviors (see Rhodes & Gray, this volume for further discussion of different pathways).

Meta-analyses of correlational studies have confirmed the importance of experiential attitudes in predicting intention and behavior. For example, reviews of studies of physical activity have shown experiential attitudes to have medium-sized effects on behavior in both adult ($r_+ = .39$, $k = 83$: Rhodes, Fiala, & Conner, 2010) and adolescent ($r_+ = .26$, $k = 56$: Nasuti & Rhodes, 2013) samples. A more recent review (McEachan et al., 2016) reported the more relevant comparison of studies that included both instrumental and experiential attitude measures across a range of health behaviors. Again experiential attitude was found to be significantly more strongly related to intention (experiential attitude: $r_+ = .55$, $k = 48$; instrumental attitude: $r_+ = .38$, $k = 48$) and behavior (experiential attitude: $r_+ = .30$, $k = 47$; instrumental attitude: $r_+ = .20$, $k = 47$). Both types of attitude were significantly stronger predictors of intention and behavior for risk compared to protection behaviors. In regressions controlling for other RAA predictors, experiential compared to instrumental attitudes were stronger predictors of intention and significant direct predictors of behavior, while instrumental attitude was not directly predictive of behavior. There were too few studies in the review to permit separate regressions for risk compared to protection behaviors.

In general, the correlational data to date appears to be strongly supportive of the importance of experiential attitude in determining both intention and action for various health behaviors. The data would appear to suggest that experiential attitude is generally at least as strong as instrumental attitude and in some cases a considerably stronger correlate of intention and behavior. More recent data would suggest that this pattern is particularly strong for risk compared to protection behaviors. It may be that experiential attitude better taps the more hedonic and impulsive influences often considered to predict risk behaviors (Ayres, Conner, Prestwich, & Smith, 2012; Gibbons & Gerrard, 1995; Strack & Deutsch, 2004; see Conner, Prestwich, & Ayres, 2011, for a commentary on this issue). However, to be considered useful targets in interventions designed to change health behaviors we need experimental studies that show experiential attitude can be readily changed and that such changes impact on behavior.

Experimental Studies

There have been a number of experimental studies showing the value of targeting experiential attitude. For example, Sirriyeh, Lawton, and Ward (2010) showed that receiving a daily affective text (SMS) messages (i.e., physical activity is enjoyable) over a 2-week period compared to a cognitive (i.e., physical activity is beneficial) or a combined message was sufficient to significantly increase self-reported physical activity. Parrott, Tennant, Olejnik, and Poudevigne (2008) also reported that a positively framed e-mail message partly targeting experiential attitude was effective in changing experiential attitude and increasing exercise behavior over a 3-week period. Conner, Rhodes, Morris, McEachan, and Lawton (2011) also looked at physical activity in two studies testing a written message presented as a leaflet targeting affective outcomes with a more traditional message targeting cognitive outcomes and a no message control. In both studies, self-reported physical activity was highest in the affective message condition at follow-up (3 weeks post-baseline) and this difference remained significant after controlling for baseline physical activity (see also Morris, Lawton, McEachan, Hurling, & Conner, 2015). Importantly changes in experiential attitude were shown to partially mediate the changes in physical activity supporting a causal role of experiential attitude change. The second study also showed the affective intervention to be more effective for particular groups of individuals, that is, those high in need for affect. Carfora, Caso, and Conner (2016) showed that daily affective text messages also significantly increased self-reported fruit and vegetable consumption in a sample of adolescents. Mediation analyses again indicated the effects to be explained by changes in experiential attitude. In addition, the affective text messages were more effective than similar cognitive text messages. It would be useful if future studies in this area could demonstrate these effects on objectively measured behavior. For example, Walsh and Kiviniemi (2014) manipulated affective reactions to fruit using an implicit priming task and showed it resulted in significantly more choices of fruit in an objective task (see also Smith & De Houwer, 2015, on affective antismoking messages and implicit evaluations; Helfer, Elhai, & Geers, 2015, on affective expectation and exercise intention).

Meta-analyses of experimental studies would also appear to support the idea that changing experiential attitude can be a useful way to change health behavior, although the reported effect sizes tend to be small. In relation to physical activity, reviews by Rhodes and colleagues (Rhodes et al., 2010; Nasuti & Rhodes, 2013) showed interventions targeting experiential attitude were associated with small- to medium-sized effects on behavior ($d_+ = .35$, $k = 25$; 95%CI .23 to .48). These are comparable effect sizes to those reported for a broader range of health behaviors where interventions have changed overall attitudes. For example, Sheeran et al. (2016) reported that studies changing overall attitudes about health behaviors were associated with small to medium effects on intentions

($d_+ = .48$, $k = 59$) and behavior ($d_+ = .38$, $k = 67$). Although there is no published meta-analysis of studies that change experiential attitudes there is a meta-analysis of studies that changed anticipatory (hedonic) emotions such as fear and worry that could be considered similar to experiential attitudes. Sheeran, Harris, and Epton (2014) reported that studies that had changed anticipatory emotion ($d_+ = .72$, $k = 107$) were associated with a small change in intention ($d_+ = .31$, $k = 97$) and behavior ($d_+ = .21$, $k = 46$). Further studies that examine the individual and combined effects of manipulating experiential and instrumental attitudes might provide further insights into their relative importance in determining intention and behavior. However, the difficulty of separately manipulating experiential and instrumental attitudes or indeed attitudes separately from norms should not be underestimated.

Anticipated Affect

In this section correlational and then experimental studies on anticipated affect are reviewed.

Correlational Studies

Anticipated affect (or self-conscious affect) has also received attention as a determinant of intention and behavior in relation to health behaviors. A particular focus of attention has been anticipated negative affect such as *regret* and to a lesser extent *guilt*. Anticipated positive affect such as pride or satisfaction has received less attention (but see Amireault, Godin, Vohl, & Pérusse, 2008; Conner, Godin, Sheeran, & Germain, 2013; Dunton & Vaughan, 2008; see Baldwin, this volume, for further consideration of satisfaction in particular). In one correlational study, Ferrer et al. (2014) showed anticipated affect to predict intentions to receive self-threatening genetic risk information, while Liao, Wong, and Fielding (2013) showed anticipated regret to directly predict influenza vaccination uptake in Chinese adults. Brewer, DeFrank, and Gilkey (2016) provide the most comprehensive review to date of the impact of anticipated regret on health behaviors in correlational studies. Across 81 studies, anticipated regret was a significant predictor of intention ($r = .50$, $k = 80$) and behavior ($r = .29$, $k = 48$). Anticipated regret was also a significantly stronger predictor than other anticipated emotions (i.e., worry) for both intention and behavior.

Other studies have examined the effects of anticipated affect while controlling for other known predictors of intention and behavior. One example of a correlational study in this area is that by Conner, Sandberg, McMillan, and Higgins (2006). This study looked at the role of anticipated regret (e.g., I would feel depressed if I smoked this term) in the context of the TPB on smoking intentions and objectively assessed smoking initiation in a sample of adolescents. Anticipated regret showed a strong correlation with intentions ($r = .55$) and a small to medium correlation with behavior ($r = .23$). In regressions to predict intention, anticipated regret remained significant when controlling for other TPB variables (attitudes, norms, perceived behavioral control). However, in regressions to predict behavior, anticipated regret did not remain significant when controlling for other TPB variables (intention, attitude, subjective norm, perceived behavioral control). The meta-analysis of Sandberg and Conner (2008) explored the effect of anticipated regret when controlling for other predictors of intention and behavior from the TPB (see also Rivis, Sheeran, & Armitage, 2009). Overall, anticipated regret showed a strong effect on intention ($r_+ = .47$, $k = 25$) and a small to medium effect on behavior ($r_+ = .28$, $k = 8$). Regressions of the meta-analytic correlations indicated anticipated regret was a significant predictor of both intention and behavior when controlling for TPB variables, however, only the impact on intention remained significant when also controlling for past behavior. Overall the correlation findings for anticipated affect and anticipated regret in particular suggest that it has a small to medium effect on behavior and that this effect may be partially mediated by intention. However, to consider it a useful target for interventions to change health behaviors, we need experimental studies to show that anticipated affect can be readily changed and that such changes impact on behavior.

Experimental Studies

Experimental studies targeting anticipated affect have been less commonly reported. In part this may be attributable to the difficulty of changing how much regret or guilt an individual anticipates experiencing. One way round this problem is to manipulate how much the individual's attention is drawn to potential anticipated affect. For example, we can compare groups who receive and complete versus are not exposed to anticipated affect questions. A number of studies have shown this "question-behavior effect" for anticipated regret for behaviors such as condom use (Richard, van der Pligt, & de Vries, 1996) and blood donation (Godin, Sheeran, Conner, & Germain, 2008). Sandberg and Conner (2009) specifically looked at the effect of including such anticipated regret questions in relation to a sample of women invited for cervical screening. Women were randomly allocated to receive a normal invitation for screening, to receive a normal invitation plus complete a TPB questionnaire about screening, or to receive a normal invitation plus complete a TPB questionnaire about screening that included anticipated regret questions. Intention to treat analyses indicated that screening attendance as measured by medical records showed significantly higher attendance in the two TPB conditions (26%) compared to the no questionnaire condition (21%). Among those who completed and returned the questionnaire (and were therefore definitely exposed to the regret questions), attendance was considerably higher in the TPB plus regret condition (65%) compared to the TPB only condition (44%). Further analyses showed this was mainly due to changes in attendance among those with a strong intention to attend for screening. A similar set of findings was reported for objectively assessed exercise (sports center use) by Sandberg and Conner (2011). Importantly this study showed that this effect of measuring regret on behavior was probably mediated by intention. Only when the anticipated regret questions preceded the intention question was a significant effect on behavior observed. More recently, Cox, Sturm, and Cox (2014) showed that anticipated regret questions increase mothers' intentions to vaccinate their daughters with the HPV shot, while Conner, Sandberg, Nekitsing, Hutter, Wood, Jackson, Godin, and Sheeran (2017) showed that measuring anticipated regret questions increased influenza vaccination compared to a no questionnaire control condition. Nevertheless, a recent meta-analysis of the question-behavior effect (Wood et al., 2016) reported that studies including anticipated regret items had significantly smaller effect sizes ($d_+ = 0.08$, $k = 10$) than studies that did not include such items ($d_+ = 0.26$, $k = 106$). This might reflect the idea that a question-behavior effect for anticipated affect is dependent on first measuring anticipated affect and then intention.

Sheeran, Harris, and Epton (2014) in a meta-analysis of studies that changed anticipated affective reactions like regret and guilt ($d_+ = .39$, $k = 10$), reported that where changes in anticipated affect were observed a small but significant change in intention ($d_+ = .27$, $k = 10$) and behavior ($d_+ = .30$, $k = 3$) was also observed. The authors note that the observed effects were stronger for studies focusing on anticipated guilt than for studies focusing on anticipated regret, although the limited number of studies means such findings should be treated with caution. In an unpublished review of anticipated affect studies, Conner (2013) reported a small but significant effect of changing anticipated affect on health behavior ($d_+ = .29$, $k = 6$; Cho & Salmon, 2006; Kellar & Abraham, 2005; Richard et al., 1996; Sandberg & Conner, 2009, 2011; Wardle et al., 2003). Further studies that identify effective means to change anticipated affect are required to provide better estimates of the causal effects of anticipated affect on behavior. Exploration of interventions that change different types of negative (e.g., regret, guilt) and positive (satisfaction, pride) anticipated affect would be particularly valuable.

Experiential Attitude Plus Anticipatory Affect

The research presented previously supports a small but significant role for both experiential attitude and anticipated affect on intention and behavior for various health behaviors. However, it leaves open the question of what their combined effect on intention and behavior are. This is a question of discriminant and predictive validity of the two affect constructs. Earlier it was argued that there are a number of reasons to distinguish the two. Here a number of studies that have tested their discriminant validity and independent power to predict intention and behavior for health behaviors are discussed.

Correlational Studies

Among the correlational studies available to assess this issue was a study testing the power of instrumental and experiential attitudes alongside positive and negative anticipated affect in predicting intention and behavior for blood donation in a large sample of blood donors (Conner et al., 2013). Confirmatory factor analysis showed that measures of experiential attitude, instrumental attitude, negative anticipated affect, and positive anticipated affect could be distinguished. This supports the discriminant validity of the different constructs. Experiential attitude and (positive and negative) anticipated affect showed only moderate intercorrelation ($r = .42–.43$). Predictive validity was examined by regression. Regressions indicated that it was instrumental attitude and both positive and negative anticipated affect that were predictive of intention (along with perceived behavioral control from the TPB); while it was just negative anticipated affect that was predictive of donation behavior (along with intention and perceived behavioral control from the TPB). However, a weakness of this study was that the focal behavior, blood donation, may not be representative of other health behaviors. For example, affective attitudes may be considerably less important for behaviors like blood donation compared to health protection behaviors like physical activity or health risk behaviors like drinking alcohol.

Sandberg, Hutter, Richetin, and Conner (2016) in a study of a range of health and social behaviors across two studies found both that experiential attitude and anticipated regret were independent significant predictors of intention controlling for instrumental attitude, subjective norm, perceived behavioral control and past behavior. However, in Study 1, which focused on "protection" behaviors, neither construct was predictive of behavior when controlling for intention, instrumental attitude, subjective norm, perceived behavioral control and past behavior. In Study 2, which focused on "protection" and "risk" behaviors, both experiential attitude and anticipated regret were significant predictors of behavior when controlling for intention, instrumental attitude, subjective norm, capacity (similar to self-efficacy) and autonomy. When also controlling for past behavior, anticipated regret remained significant although experiential attitude became nonsignificant. Moderation and simple slopes analyses also indicated that both experiential attitude and anticipated regret were significantly stronger predictors for risk compared to protection behaviors.

Conner et al. (2015, Study 2) report a similar multibehavior study but focusing on health behaviors. Across behaviors, both experiential attitude and anticipated affect were significant independent predictors of intention when controlling for instrumental attitude, subjective norm, perceived behavioral control, and past behavior. Anticipated affect was the stronger predictor of intention. Moderation analyses indicated that the power of anticipated affect but not experiential attitude varied across behavior types. Simple slopes analyses indicated that anticipated affect was most strongly related to intention for detection, then protection, and then risk health behaviors. In relation to predictions of behavior, experiential attitude was a significant independent predictor of behavior but anticipated affect was not when also controlling for intention, instrumental attitude, subjective norm, perceived behavioral control, and past behavior. Moderation and simple slopes analyses indicated that experiential attitude was a significantly stronger predictor of behavior for protection compared to risk or detection behaviors, while anticipated affect was only a significant predictor for detection behaviors.

Relatedly, Conner, McEachan, Lawton, and Gardner (2016) reported that when simultaneously comparing intention based on various other constructs including cognitive and affective attitude and anticipated affective reactions it was only the latter that was a significant moderator of the intention–behavior relationship across a range of health behaviors. They suggest that anticipated affective reactions may be particularly effective in binding individuals to their intention.

Conner et al. (2015, Study 1) report a meta-analytic review of the limited number of available studies that have measured both experiential attitude and anticipated affect (k = 16). Only a small to medium sized relationship between experiential attitude and anticipated affect was observed (r_+ = .29, k = 16) supporting their discriminant validity. Both affective constructs showed similar sized relationships with intention (r_+ = .40 vs. .47, for experiential attitude and anticipated affect respectively) and behavior (r_+ = .27 vs. .23, for experiential attitude and anticipated affect respectively). Regressions of the meta-analytic correlations indicated that only experiential attitude was an independent significant predictor of intention when controlling for instrumental attitude, subjective norm, and perceived behavioral control. Regressions of the meta-analytic correlations also indicated that both experiential attitude and anticipated affect were independent significant predictors of behavior when controlling for intention, instrumental attitude, subjective norm, and perceived behavioral control.

The available correlational data support the discriminant validity of experiential attitude and anticipated affect in relation to health behaviors. However, the predictive validity data are somewhat mixed, with different studies showing only one of the two constructs (and not always the same one) or both the constructs to be independent predictors of intention and behavior when controlling for other predictors. Similarly, the available work on different types of health behavior suggests a variable impact on the power of experiential attitude and anticipated affect to predict intention and behavior.

Experimental Studies

Experimental studies that have attempted to manipulate both experiential attitude and anticipated affect and observed effects on intention and behavior for health behaviors are extremely limited and represent an important gap in the literature. Indeed, only Wardle et al. (2003) appear to have designed an intervention to change both experiential attitudes and anticipated affect simultaneously. This study focused on colorectal screening using flexible sigmoidoscopy and compared a standard leaflet with one that targeted barriers and positive expectations in a large sample of adults (and designed to change both experiential attitude and anticipated regret).

The study produced small- to medium-sized changes in both experiential attitude ($d_+ = .38$) and anticipated affect ($d_+ = .36$) but only small effects on intention ($d_+ = .18$) and very small effects on behavior ($d_+ = .07$). These values are smaller than those we noted earlier when reporting reviews of experimental studies changing just experiential attitude ($d_+ = .31$ to .37 for intentions; $d_+ = .20$ to .35 for behavior) or just anticipated affect ($d_+ = .27$ for intention; $d_+ = .29$ to .30 for behavior). Although the available evidence is not supportive, further experimental studies are clearly required before we can draw any definitive conclusions about the value of targeting both experiential attitudes and anticipated affect as a means to produce change in intention and behavior.

CONCLUSIONS

The existing literature would suggest that when trying to change intention and behavior there is value in focusing on affective influences on health behavior probably in conjunction with other more widely studied influences (e.g., capacity/self-efficacy, instrumental attitudes, norms). Affective influences probably have both direct effects on behavior, effects mediated by intention, and also effects on the intention–behavior relationship (e.g., Conner et al., 2016; Keer et al., 2014). There is good evidence from both correlational and experimental studies to support a focus on either experiential attitude or anticipated affect, although the effect sizes on behavior change may only be in the small to medium range. The impact on long-term behavior change is a further focus that could benefit research examining different types of affective influence. The overlap between experiential attitude and anticipated affect would be another useful area on which to focus. Current evidence would suggest the two are only modestly correlated perhaps because they are based on different influences. In addition, the evidence concerning the value of jointly targeting experiential attitude and anticipated affect in order to change health behavior is weak. Further experimental studies in this area would be particularly valuable. We need to know more about whether one construct can be changed without changing the other and the impact of changing one or both on observed behavior change. A final useful area for research is potential moderators. A range of moderators might be usefully explored, including differences between behavior (e.g., risk versus protection versus detection behaviors) and individual factors (e.g., need for affect, need for cognition).

REFERENCES

Abelson, R. P., Kinder, D. R., Peters, M. D., & Fiske, S. T. (1982). Affective and semantic components in political person perception. *Journal of Personality and Social Psychology, 42,* 619–630.

Ajzen, I. (1991). The theory of planned behavior. *Organizational Behavior and Human Decision Processes, 50,* 179–211. doi:10.1016/0749-5978(91)90020-t

Ajzen, I., & Fishbein M. (2005). The influence of attitude on behavior. In D. Albarracin, B. T. Johnson & M. P. Zanna (Eds.), *Handbook of attitudes and attitude change: Basic principles* (pp. 173–221). Mahwah, NJ: Erlbaum. doi:10.1093/ijpor/edh109

Amireault, S., Godin, G., Vohl, M.-C., & Pérusse, L. (2008). Moderators of the intention-behaviour and perceived behavioural control-behaviour relationships for leisure-time physical activity. *International Journal of Behavioural Nutrition and Physical Activity, 5,* 7.

Ayres, K., Conner, M. T., Prestwich, A., & Smith, P. (2012). Do implicit measures of attitudes incrementally predict snacking behaviour over explicit affect-related measures? *Appetite, 58,* 835–841.doi:10.1016/j.appet.2012.01.019

Brewer, N. T., DeFrank, J. T., & Gilkey, M. B. (2016). Anticipated regret and health behavior: A meta-analysis. *Health Psychology, 35,* 1264–1275.

Carfora, V., Caso, D., & Conner, M. (2016). Randomized controlled trial of "messaging intervention" to increase fruit and vegetable intake in adolescents: Affective versus instrumental messages. *British Journal of Health Psychology, 21,* 937–955.

Cho, H., & Salmon, C. T. (2006). Fear appeals for individuals in different stages of change: Intended and unintended effects and implications on public health campaigns. *Health Communication, 20*(1), 91–99. doi:10.1207/s15327027hc2001_9

Conner, M. (2013). *Health cognitions, affect and health behaviours.* Keynote presentation at European Health Psychology Society Annual Conference, Bordeaux, France, 17–20 July 2013.

Conner, M., Godin, G., Sheeran, P., & Germain, M. (2013). Some feelings are more important: Cognitive attitudes, affective attitudes, anticipated affect and blood donation. *Health Psychology, 32,* 264–272. doi:10.1037/a0028500

Conner, M., McEachan, R., Taylor, N., O'Hara, J., & Lawton, J. (2015). Role of affective attitudes and anticipated affective reactions in predicting health behaviors. *Health Psychology, 34,* 642–652. doi:10.1037/hea0000143

Conner, M., & Norman, P. (Eds.). (1995). *Predicting health behaviour: Research and practice with social cognition models*. Milton Keynes, UK: Open University Press.

Conner, M., & Norman, P. (Eds.). (2005). *Predicting health behaviour: Research and practice with social cognition models* (2nd ed.). Maidenhead, UK: Open University Press.

Conner, M., & Norman, P. (2015) (Eds.). *Predicting and changing health behaviour: Research and practice with social cognition models* (3rd ed.). Maidenhead, UK: Open University Press.

Conner, M., Godin, G., Sheeran, P., & Germain, M. (2013). Some feelings are more important: Cognitive attitudes, affective attitudes, anticipated affect, and blood donation. *Health Psychology, 32*, 264–272. doi:10.1037/a0028500

Conner, M., McEachan, R., Lawton, J., & Gardner, P. (2016). Basis of intentions as a moderator of the intention-health behavior relationship. *Health Psychology, 35*, 219–227.

Conner, M., McEachan, R., Lawton, J., & Gardner, P. (2017). Applying the reasoned action approach to understanding health protection and health risk behaviors. *Social Science and Medicine, 195*, 140–148.

Conner, M., McEachan, R., Taylor, N., O'Hara, J., & Lawton, R. (2015). Role of affective attitudes and anticipated affective reactions in predicting health behaviors. *Health Psychology, 34*, 642–652. doi:10.1037/hea0000143. Epub 2014 Sep 15.

Conner, M., Prestwich, A., & Ayres, K. (2011). Using explicit affective attitudes to tap impulsive influences on health behavior: A commentary on Hofmann et al. (2008). *Health Psychology Review, 5*, 145–149. doi:10.1080/17437199.2010.539969

Conner, M., Rhodes, R., Morris, B. McEachan, R., & Lawton, R. (2011). Changing exercise through targeting affective or cognitive attitudes. *Psychology and Health, 26*, 133–14958. doi:10.1080/08870446.2011.531570

Conner, M., Sandberg, T., McMillan, B., & Higgins, A. (2006). Role of anticipated regret in adolescent smoking initiation. *British Journal of Health Psychology, 11*, 85–101.

Conner, M., Sandberg, T., Nekitsing, C., Hutter, R., Wood, C., Jackson, C., Godin, G., & Sheeran, P. (2017). Varying cognitive targets and response rates to enhance the question-behaviour effect: An 8-arm randomized controlled trial on influenza vaccination uptake. *Social Science and Medicine, 180*, 135–142.

Conner, M., Sutherland, E., Thorn, K., Kennedy, F., Grearly, C., & Berry, C. (2008). Impact of alcohol on sexual decision making: Differential effects for men and women. *Psychology and Health, 23*, 909–934.

Cox, D., Sturm, L., & Cox, A. D. (2014). Effectiveness of asking anticipated regret in increasing HPV vaccination intention in mothers. *Health Psychology, 33*, 1074–1083.

Dunton, G. F., & Vaughan, E. (2008). Anticipated affective consequences of physical activity adoption and maintenance. *Health Psychology, 27*, 703–710.

Elliott, M. A., Thomson, J. A., Robertson, K., Stephenson, C., & Wicks, J. (2013). Evidence that changes in social cognitions predict changes in self-reported driver behavior: Causal analyses of two-wave panel data. *Accident Analysis and Prevention, 50*, 905–916.

Ferrer, R. A., Taber, J. M., Klein, W. M. P., Harris, P. R., Lewis, K. L., & Biesacker, L. G. (2014). The role of current affect, anticipated affect and spontaneous self-affirmation in decisions to receive self-threatening genetic risk information. *Cognition and Emotion, 29*, 1456–1465.

Fishbein, M., & Ajzen, I. (2010). *Predicting and changing behavior: The reasoned action approach*. New York, NY: Psychology Press.

Gibbons, F. X., & Gerrard, M. (1995). Predicting young adults' health risk behavior. *Journal of Personality and Social Psychology, 69*, 505–517.

Giner-Sorolla, R. (2001). Guilty pleasures and grim necessities: Affective attitudes in dilemmas of self-control. *Journal of Personality and Social Psychology, 80*, 206–221.

Glasman, L. R., & Albarracin, D. (2006). Forming attitudes that predict future behavior: A meta-analysis of the attitude-behavior relation. *Psychological Bulletin, 132*, 778–822.

Godin, G. (1987). Importance of the emotional aspect of attitude to predict intention. *Psychological Reports, 61*, 719–723.

Godin, G., Sheeran, P., Conner, M., & Germain, M. (2008). Asking questions changes behavior: Mere measurement effects on frequency of blood donation. *Health Psychology, 27*, 179–184.

Helfer, S. G., Elhai, J. D., & Geers, A. L. (2015). Affect and exercise: Positive affective expectations can increase post-exercise mood and exercise intentions. *Annals of Behavioral Medicine, 49*, 269–279.

Keer, M., Conner, M., Van den Putte, B., & Neijens, P. (2014). The temporal stability and predictive validity of affect-based and cognition-based intentions. *British Journal of Social Psychology, 53*, 315–327. doi:10.1111/bjso.1203

Kellar, I., & Abraham, C. (2005). Randomized controlled trial of a brief research-based intervention promoting fruit and vegetable consumption. *British Journal of Health Psychology, 10*, 543–558. doi:10.1348/135910705X42940

Kiviniemi, M. T., Jandorf, L., & Erwin, D. O. (2014). Disgusted, embarrassed, annoyed: Affective associations relate to uptake of colonoscopy screening. *Annals of Behavioral Medicine, 48*, 112–119. doi:10.1007/s12160-013-9580-9

Kiviniemi, M. T., Voss-Humke, A. M., & Seifert, A. L. (2007). How do I feel about behavior? The interplay of affective associations with behaviors and cognitive beliefs as influences on physical activity behavior. *Health Psychology, 26*, 152–158.

Lawton, R. J., Ashley, L., Dawson, S., Waiblinger, D., & Conner, M. (2012). Employing an extended theory of planned behaviour to predict breastfeeding intention, initiation and maintenance in White British and South Asian mothers living in Bradford. *British Journal of Health Psychology, 17*, 854–871. doi:10.1111/j.2044-8287.2012.02083.x

Lawton, R., Conner, M., & McEachan, R. (2009). Desire or reason: Predicting health behaviors from affective and cognitive attitudes. *Health Psychology, 28*, 56–65. doi:10.1037/a0013424

Lawton, R., Conner, M., & Parker, D. (2007). Beyond cognition: Predicting health risk behaviors from instrumental and affective beliefs. *Health Psychology, 26*, 259–267. doi:10.1037/0278-6133.26.3.259

Liao, Q., Wong, W. S., & Fielding, R. (2013). How do anticipated worry and regret predict seasonal influenza vaccination uptake among Chinese adults? *Vaccine, 31*, 4084–4090.

Lowe, R., Eves, F., & Carroll, D. (2002). The influence of affective and instrumental beliefs on exercise intentions and behavior: A longitudinal analysis. *Journal of Applied Social Psychology, 32,* 1241–1252.

Manstead, A. S. R., & Parker, D. (1995). Evaluating and extending the theory of planned behaviour. *European Review of Social Psychology, 6,* 69–95.

McEachan, R. R. C, Conner, M., Taylor, N. J., & Lawton, R. J. (2011). Prospective prediction of health-related behaviors with the theory of planned behavior: A meta-analysis. *Health Psychology Review, 5,* 97–144. doi:10.1080/17437199.2010.521684

McEachan, R., Taylor, N., Harrison, R., Lawton, R., Gardner, P., & Conner, M (2016). Meta-analysis of the reasoned action approach (RAA) to understanding health behaviors. *Annals of Behavioral Medicine, 50,* 592–612.

Morris, B., McEachan R., Hurling, R., & Conner, M. (2015). Changing self-reported physical activity using different types of affectively and cognitively framed health messages, in a student population. *Psychology, Health and Medicine, 9,* 1–10. doi:10.1080/13548506.2014.997762

Nasuti, G., & Rhodes, R. E. (2013). Affective judgment and physical activity in youth: Review and meta-analyses. *Annals of Behavioral Medicine, 41,* 18–24. doi:10.1007/s12160-012-9462-6

Parrott, M. W., Tennant, L. K., Olejnik, S., & Poudevigne, M. S. (2008). Theory of planned behaviour: Implications for an email-based physical activity intervention. *Psychology of Sport and Exercise, 9,* 511–526.

Rhodes, R. E., Blanchard, C. M., & Matheson, D. H. (2006). A multi-component model of the theory of planned behaviour. *British Journal of Health Psychology, 11,* 119–137.

Rhodes R. E., & Conner, M. (2010). Comparison of behavioral belief structures in the physical activity domain. *Journal of Applied Social Psychology, 40,* 2105–2120. doi:10.1111/j.1559-1816.2010.00652.x

Rhodes, R., Fiala, B., & Conner, M. (2010). A review and meta-analysis of affective judgments and physical activity in adult populations. *Annals of Behavioral Medicine, 38,* 180–204. doi:10.1007/s12160-009-9147-y

Richard, R., van der Pligt, J., & de Vries, N. K. (1996). Anticipated regret and time perspective: Changing sexual risk-taking behavior. *Journal of Behavioral Decision Making, 9,* 185–199.

Rivis, A., Sheeran, P., & Armitage, C. (2009). Expanding the normative and affective components of the theory of planned behaviour: A meta-analysis of anticipated affect and moral norms. *Journal of Applied Social Psychology, 39,* 2985–3019. doi:10.1111/j.1559-1816.2009.00558.x

Russell, J. T. (2003). Core affect and the psychological construction of emotion. *Psychological Review, 110,* 145–172. doi:10.1037/0033-295X.110.1.145

Sandberg, T., & Conner, M. (2008). Anticipated regret as an additional predictor in the theory of planned behaviour: A meta-analysis. *British Journal of Social Psychology, 47,* 589–606.

Sandberg, T., & Conner, M. (2009). A mere measurement effect for anticipated regret: Impacts on cervical screening attendance. *British Journal of Social Psychology, 48,* 221–236. doi:10.1348/014466608X347001

Sandberg, T., & Conner, M. (2011). Using self-generated validity to promote exercise behaviour. *British Journal of Social Psychology, 50*, 769–783. doi:10.1111/j.2044-8309.2010.02004.x

Sandberg, T., Hutter, R., Richetin, J., & Conner, M. T. (2016). Testing the role of action and inaction anticipated regret on intentions and behaviour. *British Journal of Social Psychology, 55*, 407–425. doi:10.1111/bjso.12141

Sheeran, P., Harris, P. R., & Epton, T. (2014). Does heightened risk appraisals change people's intentions and behaviour? A meta-analysis of experimental studies. *Psychological Bulletin, 140*, 511–543. doi:10.1037/a0033065.

Sheeran, P., Maki, A., Montanaro, E., Caldwell, A. E., Bryan, A. D., & Rothman, A. J. (2016). The impact of changing attitudes, norms, or self-efficacy on health-related intentions and behaviour: A meta-analysis. *Health Psychology, 35*, 1178–1188.

Sirriyeh, R. H., Lawton, R. J., & Ward, J. K. (2010). Physical activity and adolescents: An exploratory randomised controlled trial (RCT) investigating the influence of affective and instrumental text messages. *British Journal of Health Psychology, 15*, 825–840. doi:10.1348/135910710x486889

Smith, C. T., & De Houwer, J. (2015). Hooked on a feeling: Affective anti-smoking messages are more effective than cognitive messages at changing implicit evaluations of smoking. *Frontier in Psychology, 6*, 1488.

Strack, F., & Deutsch, R. (2004). Reflective and impulsive determinants of social behavior. *Personality and Social Psychology Review, 8*, 220–247.

Trafimow, D., & Sheeran, P. (1998). Some tests of the distinction between cognitive and affective beliefs. *Journal of Experimental Social Psychology, 34*, 378–397.

Trafimow, D., Sheeran, P., Lombardo, B., Finlay, K. A., Brown, J., & Armitage, C. J. (2004). Affective and cognitive control of persons and behaviors. *British Journal of Social Psychology, 43*, 207–224.

Van den Berg, H., Manstead, A. S. R., van der Pligt, J., & Wigboldus, D. (2005). The role of affect in attitudes toward organ donation and donor-relevant decisions. *Psychology and Health, 20*, 789–802.

Van der Pligt, J., Zeelenberg, M., van Dijk, W. W., de Vries, N. K., & Richard, R. (1998). Affect, attitudes and decisions: Let's be more specific. *European Review of Social Psychology, 8*, 33–66.

Walsh, E. M., & Kiviniemi, M. T. (2014). Changing how I feel about the food: experimentally manipulated affective associations with fruit change fruit choice behaviors. *Journal of Behavioral Medicine, 37*, 322–331.

Wardle, J., Williamson, S., McCarffery, K., Edwards, R., Sutton, S., Taylor, T., Edwards, R., & Atkin, W. (2003). Increasing attendance at colorectal cancer screening: Testing the efficacy of a mailed, psychoeducational intervention in a community sample of older adults. *Health Psychology, 22*(1), 99–105. doi:10.1037/0278-6133.22.1.99

Wood, C., Conner, M., Sandberg, T., Taylor, N., Godin, G., Miles, E., & Sheeran, P. (2016). The impact of asking intention or self-prediction questions on subsequent behavior: A meta-analysis. *Personality and Social Psychology Review, 20*, 245–268. doi:10.1177/1088868315592334

4

Perceived Satisfaction with Health Behavior Change

AUSTIN S. BALDWIN AND MARGARITA SALA

Multiple theories of health behavior propose that initiating a behavior change is determined, in part, by the expected outcomes that result from the change and the belief in one's ability to make the change (i.e., self-efficacy) (theory of planned behavior: Ajzen & Madden, 1986; social cognitive theory: Bandura, 1986; health belief model: Becker, 1974; protection motivation theory: Rosenstock et al., 1974; transtheoretical model: Prochaska & Diclemente, 1983; see Noar & Zimmerman, 2005, for a review). However, more recent theorizing proposes that the maintenance of behavior change is determined by perceived satisfaction with the change (Rothman, 2000; Rothman, Baldwin, Hertel, & Fuglestad, 2011). Perceived satisfaction is defined as the overall assessment of the various positive and negative experiences and outcomes that result from engaging in the target behavior. A central part of this assessment is how the behavior change makes one feel, including both momentary experiences with and outcomes from the behavior (Rothman,

2000; Rothman et al., 2011). Therefore, perceived satisfaction can be conceptualized as an affective determinant of health behavior. In this chapter, we first review theoretical work about perceived satisfaction and its relevance to behavior change maintenance. We follow this by reviewing how perceived satisfaction has been measured and briefly discussing measurement implications for understanding perceived satisfaction and its influence on health behavior. We then provide a review of the empirical literature on (1) perceived satisfaction as a predictor of health behavior and (2) the determinants of perceived satisfaction. Finally, we conclude with recommendations for future directions in research on perceived satisfaction.

PERCEIVED SATISFACTION AND BEHAVIOR CHANGE MAINTENANCE

Perceived satisfaction is a particularly promising intervention target to improve the maintenance of health behavior changes (e.g., regular exercise, smoking cessation) given that the various health benefits that result from changing unhealthy behavioral practices to healthy ones are contingent on the changes being maintained over time. As a result, interventions targeting perceived satisfaction are a promising path to improve individual and public health.

Multiple health behavior theories (e.g., Ajzen & Madden, 1986; Bandura, 1986; Prochaska & Diclemente, 1983) propose that initiating a behavior change is determined, in part, by the expected outcomes that result from the change and belief in one's ability to make the change. For example, initiating a routine of regular exercise can be motivated by the belief that regular exercise will lead one to feel better and be more physically fit. Likewise, the decision to attempt to quit smoking can be motivated by the expectation that doing so will reduce the risk of future disease and will improve the smell of one's clothing. Both decisions are also determined by the belief that one is capable of doing what is required to make the change (i.e., self-efficacy). After initiating such changes, however, beliefs about whether the changes lead to improvements in health or feeling better are no longer expectations. Instead, behavior changes that have recently been initiated provide individuals with evidence about the relevant experiences and outcomes of the behavior change. For example, someone who has recently begun a routine of regular exercise can assess the extent to which she feels better or her fitness has improved as a result of the exercise; or someone who has recently quit smoking might assess the extent to which his clothing does in fact smell better after quitting. Current theoretical work (Rothman, 2000; Rothman et al., 2011) suggests that the decision to maintain behavior change is determined by this type of assessment of relevant experiences and outcomes that occurs post behavior change. The assessment is indexed by individuals' perceived satisfaction with the new behavior. Put another way, the maintenance of a behavior change is no longer a question of what one expects or whether one can do what it takes to change behavior; instead, it is a question of whether one is satisfied with the changes and wants to continue. Feelings of satisfaction are proposed to be critical to maintenance because they are thought to indicate that the initial decision to change behavior was correct and they help sustain and motivate the efforts needed to continue to monitor behavior and minimize vulnerability to relapse (Rothman, 2000).

How is satisfaction with behavior change determined? First, people monitor how the change influences how they feel while engaging in the behavior, or as a result of changing their behavior, and the various outcomes that result from the change, such as improvements in health and appearance or feedback from other people. Baldwin and colleagues (Baldwin, Baldwin, Loehr, Kangas, & Frierson, 2013; Baldwin, Rothman, Hertel, Keenan, & Jeffery, 2009; Baldwin, Rothman, & Jeffery, 2009) have conducted a series of studies in smoking cessation, weight loss, and regular exercise demonstrating across these domains that people's satisfaction with the change they have made is systematically associated with their experiences and outcomes with the behavior. The experiences and outcomes that matter for perceived satisfaction are domain specific (e.g., improvement in fit of clothes in weight loss, frequency of cravings in smoking cessation), but the general process of monitoring experiences and outcomes is similar across domains. Second, it is thought that people compare their experiences and outcomes to their initial expectations when determining their satisfaction with the new behavior. Experiences and outcomes that meet or exceed expectations will lead to greater satisfaction and motivation to maintain the new behavior. Experiences and outcomes that fail to meet expectations will lead people to feel less satisfied (Foster, Wadden, Vogt, & Brewer, 1997; Neff & King, 1995; Sears & Stanton, 2001; Wilcox, Castro, & King, 2006).

One challenge in considering how expectations might influence perceived satisfaction is that expectations are dynamic and are influenced by recent experiences with the behavior (Loehr, Baldwin, Rosenfield, & Smits, 2014). Therefore, the initial expectations people have at the outset of a behavior change may not be the same expectations they have after a few weeks of engaging in the new behavior. Relatedly, there are individual differences that may affect the extent to which people adapt their expectations during the behavior change process. For example, there is evidence that people who are high in dispositional optimism are more likely to maintain their positive expectations even when faced with difficult challenges (Carver, Scheier, & Segerstrom, 2010; Geers & Lassiter, 2002; Gibson & Sanbonmatsu, 2004). The implications for understanding perceived satisfaction is that it is not clear which expectations people are likely to use as a comparison standard for their experiences and outcomes: their initial expectations or more recent expectations that may have changed since initiating the new behavior. Weight loss goals may be the best example of initial expectations that can have a strong effect on perceived satisfaction. Foster and colleagues (1997) observed a very strong association between people's perceived satisfaction with weight loss and the discrepancy between their initial weight loss goals and the actual weight loss achieved at the end of a year-long weight loss program. The larger the discrepancy between the amount of weight people lost and their initial expectations, the less satisfied they were.

It is important to note that although perceived satisfaction is theorized to be central to behavior change maintenance, its assessment begins upon initiating the behavior change. Experiences and outcomes that occur within the first weeks after undergoing a behavior change are associated with perceived satisfaction (Baldwin et al., 2013), and satisfaction assessed as soon as 2 (Fleig, Lippke, Pomp, & Schwarzer, 2011) to 4 weeks (Baldwin et al., 2006) after initiating a change has been shown to predict maintenance. It is also important to recognize that individuals may reach a point in the behavior change process where their perceived satisfaction with the behavior no longer matters. When individuals reach the point that they engage in the behavior automatically and habitually, they may no longer deliberately monitor and evaluate the positive and negative aspects of the behavior to determine its value and whether they want to continue (i.e., their perceived satisfaction). At this point, the new behavior is responsive to automatic cues and processes rather than deliberate ones (Rothman, Sheeran, & Wood, 2009), and thus perceived satisfaction with the new behavior should no longer matter to its continuation or maintenance. There is evidence in the domain of smoking cessation that is consistent with this premise (Baldwin et al., 2006).

Finally, perceived satisfaction is conceptually distinct from other related constructs (e.g., affective associations, affective attitudes, enjoyment, decisional balance). Drawing on its conceptual definition, perceived satisfaction is a comprehensive assessment of the positive *and* negative experiences and outcomes associated with the relevant behavior change. Therefore, it is not just an assessment of the positive aspects of the behavior change, such as enjoyment. However, in some domains, such as regular exercise, where the affective experiences with the behavior may be particularly important to its maintenance, there may be a strong overlap between the constructs of enjoyment and perceived satisfaction (Rhodes & Quinlan, 2015). This is an issue that needs to be clarified empirically in future work. In addition, perceived satisfaction is not just a reflection of the affective experiences or associations with the behavior but it is also theorized to reflect an assessment of the outcomes of the behavior change. For example, smoking cessation may be somewhat affectively unpleasant, especially initially, but positive outcomes from the behavior change (breathing better, clothes not smelling like smoke) may lead to being satisfied with the change, on balance. Finally, perceived satisfaction is an assessment of experiences and outcomes that *result* from engaging in the target behavior. Therefore, it is not just a decisional balance, which reflects an assessment of the pros and cons *before* changing. Ultimately, clear empirical distinctions between perceived satisfaction and other related constructs are needed in order to fully understand the constructs, what they share in common, and how they are distinct.

MEASUREMENT OF PERCEIVED SATISFACTION

Perceived satisfaction has been assessed in a variety of ways. The most common assessment method, and the one closest to its conceptual definition, is to directly ask about satisfaction with the behavior change. This has been done with a single item that asks for a global assessment of perceived satisfaction (Baldwin et al., 2013; Baldwin, Rothman, Hertel, et al., 2009; Fleig et al., 2011; Hertel et al., 2008; Kassavou, Turner, Hamborg, & French, 2014; West et al., 2011). For example, in the domain of smoking cessation, perceived satisfaction has been measured with an item that reads, "As of today, how satisfied are you with what you have experienced as a result of quitting smoking?" A global assessment of perceived satisfaction has also been done with multi-item measures that ask about satisfaction with specific outcomes (Sears & Stanton, 2001; Williams et al., 2008). For example, Sears and Stanton (2001) asked women who had recently initiated regular exercise to report on how satisfied they were with exercise outcomes such as improved appearance, improved strength, and their ability to cope with stress and anxiety.

Satisfaction can also be assessed by examining the extent to which the outcomes of behavior change meet or fail to meet expectations (i.e., expectancy violation) (Foster et al., 1997; Neff & King, 1995; Wilcox et al., 2006). Although expectancy violations may not represent the entirety of one's assessment of perceived satisfaction, it is theorized to be a central component (Rothman, 2000). As an example of an expectancy violation measure, Wilcox, Castro, and King (2006) asked participants who had initiated a routine of regular exercise to report 6 months later how much improvement they perceived in outcomes such as physical fitness, physical appearance, and confidence. They then compared these reports to the expectations for improvement that participants reported at baseline.

There are two additional measures that have been used that may reflect perceived satisfaction in specific domains. As previously noted, in the domain of exercise, perceived enjoyment may have strong overlap with perceived satisfaction. Enjoyment has frequently been assessed with a multi-item measure of the extent to which exercise is perceived to be enjoyable or fun (Kendzierski & DeCarlo, 1991). It has also been assessed as a part of affective attitudes (Conner, Rhodes, Morris, McEachan, & Lawton, 2011) and intrinsic regulation (Mullan, Markland, & Ingledew, 1997). In domains such as smoking cessation, medication adherence, and dietary changes, enjoyment with the new behavior may be less relevant than in exercise. And in the domain of smoking cessation, the extent to which one values aspects of the old behavior (i.e., smoking) may be the converse of perceived satisfaction with the new behavior (i.e., quitting smoking). Dijkstra and Borland (2003) used a multi-item measure of the extent to which ex-smokers missed aspects of smoking. For example, they asked participants to report whether their ability to relax was better or worse compared to when they were still smoking. Dietary changes may be another behavioral domain in which valuing the previous behavior may be central to perceived satisfaction. In contrast, in domains such as exercise or sunscreen use, missing the old, unhealthy behavior may be less relevant.

Optimal measurement of perceived satisfaction is an issue that has not been adequately addressed to date (see Chmielewski, Sala, Tang, & Baldwin, 2016). Perceived satisfaction is likely a multidimensional construct (e.g., affective experiences, instrumental outcomes), and measures of it should reflect that. Future work on the measurement and construct validity of perceived satisfaction with behavior change in various domains is needed.

EVIDENCE FOR SATISFACTION AS A PREDICTOR OF BEHAVIOR CHANGE AND FOR ITS DETERMINANTS

Given that perceived satisfaction is a particularly promising intervention target to improve the maintenance of health behavior changes, it is important both to understand the effect of perceived satisfaction as a predictor of behavior change maintenance and to understand the determinants of perceived satisfaction. In the framework depicted in Figure 4.1, perceived satisfaction can be conceptualized as a putative mediator of the effect of interventions on behavior change maintenance, and thus an important intervention target.

In the review that follows, we have organized the findings with this framework in mind. Specifically, we have organized the findings in two sections: evidence for perceived satisfaction as a predictor of behavioral maintenance (path b) and evidence for the determinants of satisfaction (path a). Neither section contains an exhaustive review of the literature. Instead, we have identified exemplar studies that address evidence for both pathways.

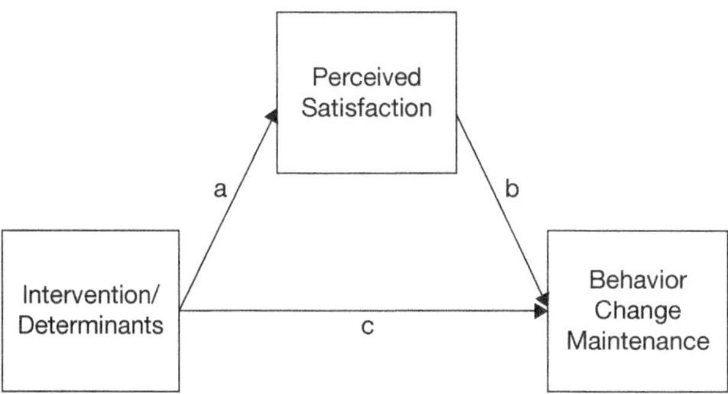

Figure 4.1. Perceived satisfaction as an intervention target for behavior change maintenance.

Perceived Satisfaction as a Predictor of Behavioral Maintenance

In reviewing the literature for evidence of perceived satisfaction as a predictor of behavior, we used three criteria to identify studies that would provide the clearest evidence for its predictive effect. First, examination of the prospective association between perceived satisfaction and behavior, as this type of evidence allows for conclusions about direction of the effect. Second, examination of the continuation or maintenance of the behavior change, as theory suggests that satisfaction is most relevant to behavior change maintenance. Third, the analytic models include at least one other variable in addition to perceived satisfaction in the prediction of behavior (e.g., enjoyment, outcome expectations), as multivariate models allow for an examination of the extent to which perceived satisfaction explains unique variance in the outcome that is not overlapping with other predictors. We have also included studies in this review that met only the first two criteria. Although the evidence for the predictive effect of perceived satisfaction on behavior is not as compelling when it is the lone predictor in a model, we have included these studies as they make up a considerable portion of the evidence. We did not include any cross-sectional studies in the review due to the limited conclusions about prediction that can be drawn from those data.

We identified five studies that met all three criteria. Three of the studies examined regular exercise maintenance as the outcome. First, Sears and Stanton (2001) examined the extent to which satisfaction with outcomes from regular exercise met initial expectations (i.e., expectancy violation) during the first 6 weeks of regular exercise. Expectancy violations were measured by subtracting expected satisfaction for the first 6 weeks of exercise assessed at baseline from current satisfaction assessed after 6 weeks of regular exercise. The investigators used the expectancy violations to predict continuation of exercise during the next 6 weeks. They found that the extent to which people's satisfaction with outcomes failed to meet their expectations did *not* predict average weekly exercise minutes over the next 6 weeks for those who remained in the study. However, it did predict the likelihood of dropping out of the study after controlling for exercise minutes during the first 6 weeks. The larger the discrepancy between people's current satisfaction and what they expected to experience, the more likely they were to dropout. Study dropout likely measured discontinuation of exercise as all dropout participants who responded to a follow-up questionnaire indicated that they had stopped exercising.

In a second study, Williams and colleagues (2008) examined various theoretical predictors of physical activity initiation and maintenance in a physical activity promotion trial. Perceived satisfaction and other psychosocial variables, including enjoyment, were measured at 6 months, and were used to predict physical activity maintenance at 12 months among individuals who were active at 6 months. Satisfaction was measured with a scale adapted from Sears and Stanton (2001), whereas physical activity enjoyment was measured with the Physical Activity Enjoyment Scale (PACES; Kendzierski & DeCarlo, 1991). Physical activity maintenance at 12-month follow-up was operationalized as participants who were active (i.e., participating in at least 150 minutes of at least moderate intensity physical activity per week or at least 60 minutes of vigorous intensity physical activity per week) or not active at follow-up. Consistent with hypotheses, they found that perceived satisfaction trended toward predicting physical activity maintenance at 12 months among those who were active at 6 months, but did not predict physical activity adoption at 12 months among those who were inactive at 6 months. Of interest, enjoyment but not satisfaction at 6 months predicted physical activity status at 12 months in a model when all active and inactive participants were included, although satisfaction trended toward significance.

In a third study, Fleig and colleagues (2011) examined the psychological mechanisms that contribute to exercise behavior maintenance after a cardiac and orthopedic rehabilitation that included exercise therapy. At the end of rehabilitation, which ranged from 14 to 38 days, participants reported their satisfaction with their experiences as a result of exercising, assessed with a single-item measure of global satisfaction. They also reported their plans for exercise over the next month. Both perceived satisfaction and planning were examined as predictors of exercise maintenance. They found that perceived satisfaction with exercise prospectively predicted the amount of exercise participants engaged in during the next month, over and above the effects of planning.

We identified two studies in smoking cessation that have examined perceived satisfaction as a predictor of smoking cessation maintenance. Baldwin and colleagues (2006) examined the relative influence of satisfaction and self-efficacy in predicting smoking cessation initiation and maintenance using data from smokers who enrolled in an 8-week smoking cessation program and were then followed for 15 months. In this study, satisfaction was assessed with a one-item global satisfaction question asking participants to evaluate their experiences with quitting smoking at the end of the program, and at 2- and 9-month follow-ups. Self-efficacy was also assessed at the same time points. The predictive effect of perceived satisfaction on cessation at 2, 9, and 15 months after the end of the program was examined in models that included self-efficacy, and also controlled for the number of cigarettes smoked at baseline and current smoking behavior. The models were run separately for maintainers (i.e., participants who had quit smoking for at least 3 consecutive months) and initiators (i.e., participants who did not meet maintainer criteria). As predicted, the results indicated that satisfaction predicted future cessation for maintainers at 2- and 9-month follow-ups, but self-efficacy did not. The reverse was true in the models run on initiators.

In another smoking cessation study, Dijkstra and Borland (2003) assessed the extent to which ex-smokers still value aspects of smoking (the converse of satisfaction with quitting smoking) and examined its effect on smoking cessation relapse. The measure assessed the extent to which participants feel better or worse than when they were smokers on several dimensions (e.g., negative affect, social situations, physical dependence, relaxation). Higher scores on this measure prospectively predicted smoking cessation relapse 7 months later, over and above self-efficacy to remain smoke-free. Taking these five studies together, there is some promising evidence that perceived satisfaction can predict unique variance in behavioral maintenance, above and beyond other relevant predictors.

We also identified five studies that met the first two criteria we established (prospective predictor, behavior maintenance as outcome), but not the third (additional predictor in the model). In a study of walking for exercise, Kassavou and colleagues (2014) examined the extent to which satisfaction with health outcomes, satisfaction with social outcomes, and overall satisfaction predicted continued attendance at walking groups among participants who had attended the walking groups for at least 3 months. Each version of perceived satisfaction was assessed with two or three questions and examined as a predictor of walking maintenance over the subsequent 3 months. They found that satisfaction with social outcomes, satisfaction with health outcomes, and overall satisfaction each uniquely predicted continued attendance, but only satisfaction with health outcomes significantly predicted continued attendance after accounting for clustering within the walking groups.

Neff and King (1995) examined whether expectancy violations, a type of satisfaction, prospectively predicted exercise adherence in a group of middle-aged adults. Expectancy violations were measured by asking participants to complete a questionnaire assessing expected physical and psychological benefits from exercise. Six months later, participants completed another questionnaire measuring perceptions of change in these dimensions. Participants were then grouped into four categories: (1) individuals who scored below the median on expected benefits at baseline and above the median on perceived change at 6-month follow up (i.e., surprised pessimists); (2) individuals who scored above the median on expected benefits and below the median on perceived change (i.e., disappointed optimists); (3) individuals who scored above the median on both expected benefits and perceived change (i.e., optimistic realists); and (4) individuals who scored below the median on expected benefits and perceived change (i.e., pessimistic realists). They found that surprised pessimists adhered to exercise at a higher rate in the last 6 months of the program compared to the other three groups. Disappointed optimists had the lowest exercise adherence. In a similar study, Wilcox and colleagues (2006) examined whether expectancy violations at 6 months were associated with physical activity participation in the subsequent 6 months in a sample of older women. They found a similar pattern of results. Disappointed optimists had the lowest subsequent physical activity participation, whereas surprised pessimists and optimistic realists had the highest rate of subsequent participation. In other words, exercise maintenance was highest when experiences met or exceeded expectations, and lowest when they failed to meet expectations.

Two studies from the weight loss and smoking cessation literature are consistent with the findings from the exercise behavior literature. Finch and colleagues (2005) examined how satisfaction with weight loss outcomes and satisfaction with changes experienced from weight loss influence weight loss maintenance in a randomized trial. Satisfaction with weight loss was measured on a monthly basis after the end of the weight-loss program with a single item asking participants to report satisfaction with the weight they gained or lost over the past month. Satisfaction with the changes afforded by weight loss was measured by asking participants about how multiple areas of their life (e.g., self-control, positive feedback from others) had changed. They found that increased satisfaction with weight loss and increased satisfaction with changes afforded by weight loss were associated with continued maintenance of weight loss over the follow-up period. Hertel and colleagues (2008) examined whether satisfaction with the outcomes afforded by smoking cessation influence smoking cessation maintenance in an 8-week smoking cessation trial. Satisfaction with smoking cessation was measured with a single item asking about satisfaction with experiences of quitting smoking at the end of program, 3-, and 6-month follow-ups. They found that satisfaction with smoking cessation at the end of the program predicted smoking cessation maintenance at 6 months.

In summary, the findings from these 10 studies provide compelling evidence that perceived satisfaction is a predictor of health behavior maintenance across several different behavioral domains. These findings suggest that increasing people's satisfaction with health behavior change would be an effective way to promote health behavior maintenance.

Determinants of Perceived Satisfaction

In reviewing the literature for evidence of determinants of satisfaction, we identified interventions that have attempted to influence perceived satisfaction as a primary mediating process of the behavioral intervention (Figure 4.1 path a). Identifying interventions that increase perceived satisfaction is critical to developing interventions that can effectively improve behavior change maintenance. Because perceived satisfaction is theorized to be a multidimensional construct, we also identified longitudinal and cross-sectional studies that have examined correlates of perceived satisfaction during the behavior change process.

We identified three intervention studies that have attempted to change perceived satisfaction as a primary mediating process of the intervention by modifying people's expectations for the behavior change. The common hypothesis across all these studies is that modifying people's expectations for the behavior change to be more realistic will lead to greater satisfaction as it will be easier for people to meet or exceed their expectations. Finch and colleagues (2005) conducted a randomized trial that assigned overweight individuals to an 8-week weight loss program focused on either the positive aspects of weight loss only or a program giving equal importance to positive and negative aspects of weight loss. However, they found there were no differences in perceived satisfaction with weight loss between the two intervention groups. Hertel and colleagues (2008) conducted an 8-week smoking satisfaction intervention that assigned participants to groups that focused on either optimistic or modest expectations about smoking cessation. Similarly, there were no differences in perceived satisfaction between the two intervention groups. In a weight loss intervention, Jeffery, Linde, Finch, Rothman, and King (2006) tested the effects on perceived satisfaction with weight loss between two intervention groups who either compared their experienced outcomes to the expectation of future ideal outcomes or their experienced outcomes to their pretreatment status. They also found that the intervention did not produce any differences in perceived satisfaction between the two groups. Overall, the evidence from these interventions suggests that it is difficult to intervene on perceived satisfaction. We return to this issue in the concluding section of the chapter.

Four longitudinal studies have examined how people determine their satisfaction with health behavior change in regular exercise, weight loss, and smoking cessation. Baldwin, Baldwin, et al. (2013) examined associations between ongoing experiences with recently initiated physical activity and satisfaction over the course of 28 days in a sample of previously sedentary adults. Perceived satisfaction was measured with a single item asking about satisfaction with what participants had experienced as a result of exercising. They found that individuals reporting higher levels of positive experiences, higher levels of progress toward goals, and lower levels of thinking about negative aspects of exercise reported higher levels of satisfaction. Moreover, daily fluctuations in positive experiences and perceived progress toward goals that vary within individuals were most strongly associated with satisfaction. Baldwin, Rothman, Hertel, et al. (2009) examined longitudinal correlates of satisfaction with smoking cessation. They found that relationships with nonsmokers, the extent to which belongings smell like smoke, ability to cope with stress, feedback from others, frequency of cravings, ability to detect different tastes and smells, and irritability over the past week were all systematically associated with satisfaction with smoking cessation. Baldwin, Rothman, and Jeffery (2009) examined the extent to which people's satisfaction with weight loss covaries with ongoing changes in outcomes (i.e., improvements in clothes fitting, positive feedback from others, negative feedback from others, perceived attractiveness, and perceived self-control) and experiences (i.e., amount of frustration experienced, amount of effort following the plan, approach to thinking about efforts, missing food high in calories and/or fat, self-weighing) that occur during weight loss. They measured satisfaction at eight different time points by asking participants how satisfied they were with the weight they had gained or lost during the past month. In multivariate analyses controlling for the amount of weight lost, they found that improvement people experienced in the way clothes fit, the amount of frustration they experienced, the amount of self-control and the amount of effort required to control their weight were the strongest correlates of satisfaction. And in a weight loss intervention study mentioned earlier, Foster and colleagues (1997) observed evidence for the relation between satisfaction with outcomes of behavior change and expectancy violation. Specifically, they observed a very strong association between people's perceived satisfaction with weight loss and the discrepancy between their initial weight loss goals and the actual weight loss achieved at the end of a year-long weight loss program. The larger the discrepancy, the less satisfaction participants reported.

Three cross-sectional studies have examined correlates of satisfaction with health behavior change. In the context of cardiac and orthopedic rehabilitation that included exercise therapy, Fleig and colleagues (2011) measured exercise experiences and satisfaction at the end of rehabilitation. They found that participants who had positive experiences as a result of exercise were also more likely to be satisfied with exercise. McArthur and Raedeke (2009) found that individuals who placed more importance on health/fitness, mental health, and intrinsic motives reported enjoying exercise more than those who placed less importance on these motives. Tsafou, De Ridder, van Ee, and Lacroix (2015) found that mindfulness during physical activity is associated with increased satisfaction with physical activity. It may be that mindfully monitoring the positive experiences and outcomes of exercise is what drives this relation. Of note, the relation between mindfulness and satisfaction was stronger for participants with weak habit compared to strong habit, consistent with the theoretical premise that satisfaction may be less relevant for those who engage in the behavior habitually (Rothman et al., 2011).

In summary, these longitudinal and cross-sectional studies suggest that there are a variety of experiences and outcomes associated with a behavior change that are correlated with perceived satisfaction with that change. Although these studies do not provide evidence about how to change perceived satisfaction, they do identify potential dimensions that may underlie the construct and suggest what experiences and outcomes might be targeted to change satisfaction.

CONCLUSIONS AND FUTURE DIRECTIONS

The studies we reviewed suggest that there is good evidence that perceived satisfaction predicts behavioral maintenance (Figure 4.1 path b). In some cases, satisfaction predicts unique variance in maintenance above and beyond other relevant predictors. This evidence points to the promise perceived satisfaction holds as a target for interventions designed to improve behavior change maintenance. However, the evidence to date for the determinants of perceived satisfaction is more mixed (Figure 4.1 path a). There are interesting and consistent findings across both longitudinal and cross-sectional studies that various domain-specific experiences and outcomes associated with behavior change are systematically associated with perceived satisfaction. However, the evidence we reviewed from interventions suggests that knowing how to intervene to increase satisfaction with behavior change remains elusive. In sum, the findings we reviewed suggest that perceived satisfaction is an important predictor of behavior change maintenance, but we do not yet clearly understand why people are satisfied with the changes they make or how to intervene to increase satisfaction. If perceived satisfaction is to be an effective intervention target for behavior change maintenance, a primary focus of future research on the construct needs to be on understanding its determinants and how to intervene to change it.

Addressing the measurement of perceived satisfaction with behavior change may be key to understanding how to change it. The construct is theorized to be multidimensional (i.e., positive and negative affective experiences and outcomes; Baldwin et al., 2013; Rothman et al., 2011), and there is evidence that various experiences and outcomes are longitudinally associated with satisfaction (Baldwin et al., 2013; Baldwin, Rothman, Hertel et al., 2009; Baldwin, Rothman, & Jeffery, 2009). These findings may tell us something about the potential dimensions that underlie satisfaction. However, the different dimensions that underlie perceived satisfaction and how to optimally measure the construct and its dimensions has not been thoroughly addressed empirically to date. Doing so would clarify the reasons why people are satisfied with the behavioral changes they make and on what dimensions to intervene to increase satisfaction. This can lead to more effective interventions aimed at improving behavior change maintenance. Addressing the measurement of perceived satisfaction would also help to clarify its distinctions from other constructs (see Chmielewski et al., 2016).

Other future directions for research on perceived satisfaction with behavior change include a better understanding of how it influences behavioral maintenance. For example, it is possible that the effect of satisfaction is nonlinear. One possibility is that people may need to reach a certain threshold of satisfaction before it has an effect on their decision to maintain a behavior change. Moving from very dissatisfied to somewhat dissatisfied may have little to no effect on behavior, but it may begin to influence behavior once people become somewhat satisfied with the change. Alternatively, it is possible that once people reach a threshold of satisfaction, additional increases in satisfaction may have little effect. Another issue to consider is what aspect of behavioral maintenance perceived satisfaction influences. It is possible that satisfaction has a stronger effect on the decision people make to maintain the behavior at all compared to its effect on how much of the behavior people engage in. For example, if people are satisfied with regular exercise, it may have a strong effect on their decision to engage in exercise at all, but may have little effect on how much exercise they do in a given week (see Baldwin, Fellingham, & Baldwin, 2016). These two issues should be addressed in future research.

Perceived satisfaction, an overall assessment of the various positive and negative experiences and outcomes that result from engaging in the target behavior, is an important determinant of maintaining behavior changes. Given the importance of maintaining healthy behavioral changes over time, perceived satisfaction is a particularly promising intervention target for a variety of health behaviors. Additional research is needed to better understand the determinants of perceived satisfaction and how to intervene to change it.

REFERENCES

Ajzen, I., & Madden, T. J. (1986). Prediction of goal-directed behavior: Attitudes, intentions, and perceived behavioral control. *Journal of Experimental Social Psychology, 22*, 453–474.

Baldwin, A. S., Baldwin, S. A., Loehr, V. G., Kangas, J. L., & Frierson, G. M. (2013). Elucidating satisfaction with physical activity: An examination of the day-to-day associations between experiences with physical activity and satisfaction during physical activity initiation. *Psychology and Health, 28*, 1424–1441. http://doi.org/10.1080/08870446.2013.822078

Baldwin, S. A., Fellingham, G. W., & Baldwin, A. S. (2016). Statistical models for multilevel skewed physical activity data in health research and behavioral medicine. *Health Psychology, 35*, 552.

Baldwin, A. S., Rothman, A. J., Hertel, A. W., Keenan, N. K., & Jeffery, R. W. (2009). Longitudinal associations between people's cessation-related experiences and their satisfaction with cessation. *Psychology and Health, 24*, 187–201. http://doi.org/10.1080/08870440701639377

Baldwin, A. S., Rothman, A. J., Hertel, A. W., Linde, J. A., Jeffery, R. W., Finch, E. A., & Lando, H. A. (2006). Specifying the determinants of the initiation and maintenance of behavior change: An examination of self-efficacy, satisfaction, and smoking cessation. *Health Psychology, 25*, 626–634. http://doi.org/10.1037/0278-6133.25.5.626

Baldwin, A. S., Rothman, A. J., & Jeffery, R. W. (2009). Satisfaction with weight loss: Examining the longitudinal covariation between people's weight-loss-related outcomes and experiences and their satisfaction. *Annals of Behavioral Medicine, 38*, 213–224. http://doi.org/10.1007/s12160-009-9148-x

Bandura, A. (1986). *Social foundations of thought and action: A social cognitive theory.* Englewood Cliffs, NJ: Prentice-Hall.

Becker, M. H. (1974). The health belief model and sick role behavior. *Health Education Monographs, 2*, 409–419.

Carver, C. S., Scheier, M. F., & Segerstrom, S. C. (2010). Optimism. *Clinical Psychology Review, 30*, 879–889. http://doi.org/10.1016/j.cpr.2010.01.006

Chmielewski, M., Sala, M., Tang, R., & Baldwin, A. S. (2016). Examining the construct validity of affective judgments of physical activity measures. *Psychological Assessment, 28*, 1128–1141.

Conner, M., Rhodes, R. E., Morris, B., McEachan, R., & Lawton, R. (2011). Changing exercise through targeting affective or cognitive attitudes. *Psychology and Health, 26*, 133–149. http://dx.doi.org/10.1080/08870446.2011.531570

Dijkstra, A., & Borland, R. (2003). Residual outcome expectations and relapse in ex-smokers. *Health Psychology, 22*, 340–346. http://doi.org/10.1037/0278-6133.22.4.340

Finch, E. A., Linde, J. A., Jeffery, R. W., Rothman, A. J., King, C. M., & Levy, R. L. (2005). The effects of outcome expectations and satisfaction on weight loss and maintenance: Correlational and experimental analyses—a randomized trial. *Health Psychology, 24*, 608–616. http://doi.org/10.1037/0278-6133.24.6.608

Fleig, L., Lippke, S., Pomp, S., & Schwarzer, R. (2011). Exercise maintenance after rehabilitation: How experience can make a difference. *Psychology of Sport and Exercise, 12*, 293–299. http://doi.org/10.1016/j.psychsport.2011.01.003

Foster, G. D., Wadden, T. A., Vogt, R. A., & Brewer, G. (1997). What is a reasonable weight loss? Patients' expectations and evaluations of obesity treatment outcomes. *Journal of Consulting and Clinical Psychology, 65*, 79–85. http://doi.org/10.1037//0022-006X.65.1.79

Geers, A. L., & Lassiter, G. D. (2002). Effects of affective expectations on affective experience: The moderating role of optimism-pessimism. *Personality and Social Psychology Bulletin*, *28*, 1026–1039. http://doi.org/10.1177/01461672022811002

Gibson, B., & Sanbonmatsu, D. M. (2004). Optimism, pessimism, and gambling: The downside of optimism. *Personality and Social Psychology Bulletin*, *30*, 149–160. http://doi.org/10.1177/0146167203259929

Hertel, A. W., Finch, E. A., Kelly, K. M., King, C., Lando, H., Linde, J. A., . . . Rothman, A. J. (2008). The impact of expectations and satisfaction on the initiation and maintenance of smoking cessation: An experimental test. *Health Psychology*, *27*, S197–206. http://doi.org/10.1037/0278-6133.27.3(Suppl.).S197

Jeffery, R. W., Linde, J. A., Finch, E. A., Rothman, A. J., & King, C. M. (2006). A satisfaction enhancement intervention for long-term weight loss. *Obesity*, *14*, 863–869.

Kassavou, A., Turner, A., Hamborg, T., & French, D. P. (2014). Predicting maintenance of attendance at walking groups: Testing constructs from three leading maintenance theories. *Health Psychology*, *33*, 752–756. http://doi.org/10.1037/hea0000015

Kendzierski, D., & DeCarlo, K. J. (1991). Physical activity enjoyment scale: Two validation studies. *Journal of Sport and Exercise Psychology*, *13*(1), 50–64.

Loehr, V. G., Baldwin, A. S., Rosenfield, D., & Smits, J. A. (2014). Weekly variability in outcome expectations: Examining associations with related physical activity experiences during physical activity initiation. *Journal of Health Psychology*, *19*, 1309–1319. http://doi.org/10.1177/1359105313488981

Mullan, E., Markland, D., & Ingledew, D. K. (1997). A graded conceptualization of self-determination in the regulation of exercise behaviour: Development of a measure using confirmatory factor analytic procedures. *Personality and Individual Differences*, *23*, 745–752. http://dx.doi.org/10.1016/S0191-8869(97)00107-4

McArthur, L. H., & Raedeke, T. D. (2009). Race and sex differences in college student physical activity correlates. *American Journal of Health Behavior*, *33*, 80–90. http://doi.org/10.5993/AJHB.33.1.8

Neff, K. L., & King, A. C. (1995). Exercise program adherence in older adults: The importance of achieving one's expected benefits. *Medicine, Exercise, Nutrition, and Health*, *4*, 355–362.

Noar, S. M., & Zimmerman, R. S. (2005). Health behavior theory and cumulative knowledge regarding health behaviors: Are we moving in the right direction? *Health Education Research*, *20*, 275–290. http://doi.org/10.1093/her/cyg113

Prochaska, J., & Diclemente, C. (1983). Stages and processes of self-change of smoking: Toward an integrative model of change. *Journal of Consulting and Clinical Psychology*, *51*, 390–5.

Rhodes, R. E., & Quinlan, A. (2015). Predictors of physical activity change in observational designs. *Sports Medicine*, *45*, 423-441

Rosenstock, I. M. (1974). The health belief model and preventive health behavior. *Health Education Monographs*, *2*, 354–386.

Rothman, A. J. (2000). Toward a theory-based analysis of behavioral maintenance. *Health Psychology*, *19*, 64–69. http://doi.org/10.1037//0278-6133.19.Suppl1.64

Rothman, A. J., Sheeran, P., & Wood, W. (2009). Reflective and automatic processes in the initiation and maintenance of dietary change. *Annals of Behavioral Medicine*, *38*, 4–17.

Rothman, A. J., Baldwin, A. S., Hertel, A. W., & Fuglestad, P. (2011). Self-regulation and behavior change: Disentangling behavioral initiation and behavioral maintenance. In K. D. Vohs & R. F. Baumeister (Eds.), *Handbook of self-regulation: Research, theory, and applications*. New York, NY: Guilford.

Sears, S. R., & Stanton, A. L. (2001). Expectancy-value constructs and expectancy violation as predictors of exercise adherence in previously sedentary women. *Health Psychology, 20*, 326–333. http://doi.org/10.1037//0278-6133.20.5.326

Tsafou, K.-E., De Ridder, D. T., van Ee, R., & Lacroix, J. P. (2015). Mindfulness and satisfaction in physical activity: A cross-sectional study in the Dutch population. *Journal of Health Psychology*. http://doi.org/10.1177/1359105314567207

West, D. S., Gorin, A. A., Subak, L. L., Foster, G., Bragg, C., Hecht, J., . . . Wing, R. R. (2011). A motivation-focused weight loss maintenance program is an effective alternative to a skill-based approach. *International Journal of Obesity, 35*, 259–269.

Wilcox, S., Castro, C. M., & King, A. C. (2006). Outcome expectations and physical activity participation in two samples of older women. *Journal of Health Psychology, 11*, 65–77. http://doi.org/10.1177/1359105306058850

Williams, D. M., Lewis, B. A., Dunsiger, S., Whiteley, J. A., Papandonatos, G. D., Napolitano, M. A., . . . Marcus, B. H. (2008). Comparing psychosocial predictors of physical activity adoption and maintenance. *Annals of Behavioral Medicine, 36*, 186–194. http://doi.org/10.1007/s12160-008-9054-7

5

Self-Regulation of Affect–Health Behavior Relations

PASCHAL SHEERAN, THOMAS L. WEBB, PETER M. GOLLWITZER, AND GABRIELE OETTINGEN

A good deal of research indicates that affect influences health behaviors (see, e.g., as indicated throughout this volume). However, the impact of affect on health behavior is not inevitable, as people can use a variety of strategies to regulate unwanted affect (e.g., Gross, 2015a, 2015b; Gross & Thompson, 2007; Koole, Webb, & Sheeran, 2015; Webb, Miles, & Sheeran, 2012). The present chapter begins by considering three key kinds of affect that warrant regulation in order to promote health behavior—*experienced affect, anticipated affect*, and *implicit affect*. We describe previous research geared at regulating these kinds of affect before outlining a self-regulation perspective on the relationship between affect and health behaviors. Specifically, we propose that the self-regulation of affect–health behavior relations can be improved by using if-then plans or *implementation intentions* (Gollwitzer, 1999, 2014; Gollwitzer & Sheeran, 2006).

If-then plans can be used to modify the impact of affect on health behaviors in two ways (see Figure 5.1). First, if-then plans can be used to

Path A: If-then plan to regulate affect

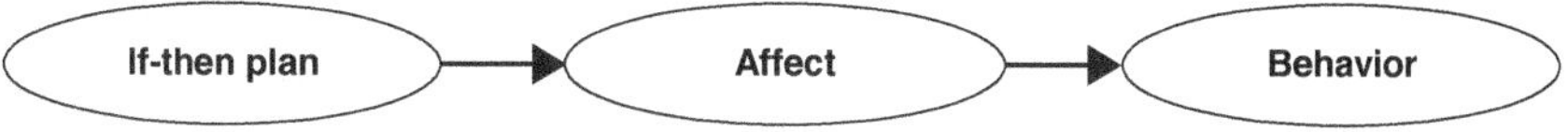

Path B: If-then plan to regulate the impact of affect

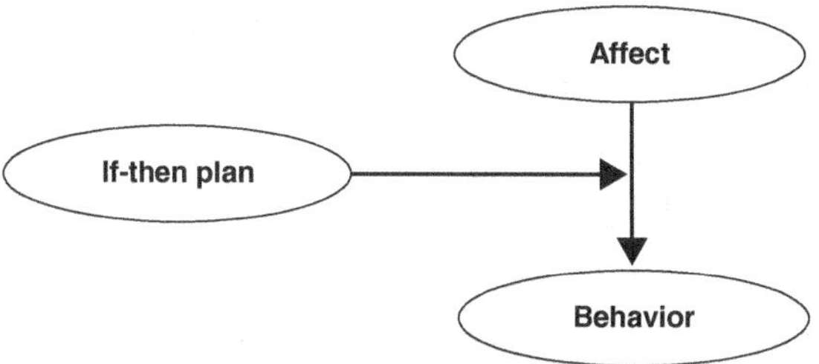

Figure 5.1. Two ways that if-then plans can be used to regulate affect-health behavior relations.

regulate affect, that is, directly alter the strength of the affective response such that it is weaker. Here, the if-then plan targets the affect itself in order to reduce its impact on behavior (Path A). Second, if-then plans can be used to *regulate affective influence*, that is, alter the impact of affect on behavior so that action is no longer disrupted by unwanted affect. Here, the if-then plan is geared, not at modifying the strength of the affective response but at attenuating its motivational force or ensuring that the action unfolds in the manner specified in the plan. In so doing, performance of the behavior should proceed in a manner that circumvents the impact of affect (Path B).

KINDS OF AFFECT

Larsen and Prizmic (2004) defined affect as "the feeling tone a person is experiencing at any particular point in time" (p. 40). The key dimensions of this feeling tone are valence (positive-negative) and arousal (aroused-sleepy) and can be captured, for instance, by Russell, Weiss, and Mendelsohn's (1989) affect grid. Affect encompasses both discrete emotions (e.g., fear, anger, sadness, disgust, happiness, and surprise) and moods. Emotions and moods differ in terms of the strength of the feeling tone (emotions are experienced more strongly than moods), whether the cause is identifiable (emotions have a recognizable cause whereas moods may not), and degree of awareness (emotions are a focus of awareness whereas moods are in the background of awareness). Affective scientists also distinguish between integral and incidental affect. Integral affect refers to affective responses to a focal stimulus such as a particular object, decision, or behavior (e.g., Loewenstein & Lerner, 2002). Depending on the nature of the focal stimulus, integral affective responses may also include what Williams and Evans (2014) termed "affectively charged motivation" or affective reactions such as fear, desire, or cravings that have clear implications for action. Incidental affect, on the other hand, refers to affective responses that are unrelated to the focal stimulus (e.g., the mood that one was in prior to encountering the stimulus) that may nonetheless influence judgments and decisions (e.g., Schwarz & Clore, 2004). Incidental affect and integral affect may combine additively or via principles of mood congruence/incongruence to influence decisions and action (Västfjäll et al., 2016) though interactive relationships have also been observed (e.g., as when negative affect enhances the enjoyment of tobacco; McKee et al., 2011). Regardless of the specific combinatorial rule, for present purposes, both kinds of affect can be seen to represent *experienced affect* or how the person feels at a particular juncture due to both integral and incidental influences.

Experienced affect is not the only kind of affect that can influence health behavior. Indeed, a provocative review by Baumeister, Vohs, DeWall, and Zhang (2007) argued that it is an "increasingly untenable view that the direct causation of behavior is the primary function of emotion" (p. 167). According to Baumeister et al., experienced affect predominantly influences behavior indirectly via *anticipated affect* and *implicit affect.* Experienced affect, in this analysis, is a feedback mechanism that enables the person to learn from past performance of a behavior. Such learning can be explicit or implicit. At the explicit level, affect may stimulate retrospective appraisal of actions and so lead the person to conscious evaluations that promote pursuit or avoidance behaviors based on their likely affective outcomes (i.e., anticipated affect). At the implicit level, the accumulation of experiences forges associations between mental representations of behavior and affect such that encountering the relevant stimulus activates the associated affective concepts (i.e., implicit affect) via the process of spreading activation.

Baumeister et al.'s (2007) analysis of anticipated affect and implicit affect is consistent with findings from research on attitudes. Principal components analyses of responses to attitude questions and memory paradigms have supported a distinction between affective and cognitive attitudes (e.g., Trafimow & Sheeran, 1998). Whereas cognitive attitudes refer to anticipated utilitarian outcomes (e.g., reduced likelihood of disease or illness), affective attitudes refer to anticipated affective outcomes (e.g., pleasure, satisfaction). Considerable research indicates that anticipated affect (affective attitude) is an important predictor of health-related intentions and behavior (see, e.g., Conner, this volume; Rhodes, Fiala, & Conner, 2009). For instance, in a study of 14 health behaviors, anticipated affect better predicted outcomes than did cognitive attitude, and was associated with behavior even after intentions were taken into account (Lawton, Conner, & McEachan, 2009). Similarly, researchers have distinguished between explicit (i.e., self-reported) attitudes and implicit attitudes or "automatic affective reactions resulting from the particular associations that are activated automatically when one encounters a relevant stimulus" (Gawronski & Bodenhausen, 2006, p. 693). Several meta-analyses indicate that implicit affect is associated with health behaviors even after explicit attitude is taken into account (Greenwald, Poehlman, Ulman, & Banaji, 2009; Reich, Below, Goldman, 2010; Rooke, Hine, & Thorsteinsson, 2008). In sum, a comprehensive analysis of the impact of affect on health behaviors needs to take account of three kinds of affect—experienced affect, anticipated affect, and implicit affect—as each has been observed to influence health decisions and actions.

THE ACTION CONTROL MODEL OF AFFECT REGULATION

There are many examples of the impact of experienced affect on health-related intentions and behavior. For instance, fear can motivate people to engage in protective behavior (e.g., Ferrer, Klein, Persoskie, Avishai-Yitshak, & Sheeran, 2016), disgust can undermine uptake of fecal occult blood tests to detect colorectal cancer (e.g., Reynolds, Consedine, Pizarro, & Bissett, 2013), and experiences of craving or distress can lead to smoking relapse (e.g., Ferguson & Shiffman, 2014; Piasecki, Jorenby, Smith, Fiore, & Baker, 2003). But what determines the levels of fear, disgust, or distress that a particular person experiences in response to a particular stimulus in a particular context? One relatively neglected process in research on health behaviors is *affect regulation*—that is, the person's own efforts to alter their affective response. Affect regulation refers to the set of processes involved in modifying the occurrence, intensity, and duration of feeling states (Gross & Thompson, 2007). The dominant account of affect regulation is Gross's (1998, 2014) process model. The model distinguishes five affect regulation processes on a temporal dimension according to when each one is deployed. Antecedent-focused processes occur before appraisals give rise to a full-blown affective response, and includes four strategies: situation selection, situation modification, attentional deployment, and cognitive change.

For instance, a person wanting to regulate their desire for the delicious but unhealthy pastries for sale in a local coffee shop, could choose a different outlet from which to buy coffee (situation selection), or could bring only enough cash to purchase a coffee but not a pastry too (situation modification). Often, however, it is not possible to avoid or modify the affect-eliciting situation. In such cases, cognitive strategies are needed to regulate desire. The first of these strategies specified by the process model concerns how attention is deployed—whether the person distracts her/himself from, or concentrates on, the emotion-eliciting stimulus. Distraction involves altering the focus of attention so that the relevant stimulus no longer elicits unwanted affect (e.g., avoiding looking at the pastries, or counting backward from 250 in sevens in order to prevent elaboration of the desire). Concentrating or focusing attention on the emotion-eliciting stimulus, on the other hand, magnifies the affective response and undermines resistance to temptations (e.g., Mischel, Shoda, & Rodriguez, 1989).

Strategic deployment of attention is not always feasible, however (e.g., it may be impossible to order coffee without also seeing the pastries). If distraction is not possible, then a cognitive change strategy is needed—"changing how we appraise the situation we are in to alter its emotional significance" (Gross & Thompson, 2007, p. 14). Cognitive change involves reappraisal of the stimulus either by coming up with an alternative interpretation of the stimulus (e.g., "That pastry is just a lump of sugar and fat!") or by adopting a detached or third-person perspective (e.g., "I will observe my purchases in the coffee shop as if I were an obesity researcher!"). Whereas situation selection, situation modification, attentional deployment, and cognitive change are each deployed before the affective response has become fully fledged, response-focused strategies are deployed once affect has unfolded. The key response-focused strategy is suppression, which involves trying to hide feelings or pushing them out of one's mind ("I must not feel any desire for pastries!").

Relatively little research has tested the effects of selecting or modifying situations on emotional outcomes (Webb, Miles, et al., 2012; but see Webb, Lindquist, Jones, Avishai-Yitshak, & Sheeran, 2016) whereas numerous primary studies and several meta-analyses have assessed the impact of distraction, concentration, reappraisal, and suppression on experienced affect (see, e.g., Aldao, Nolen-Hoeksema, & Schweizer, 2010; Augustine & Hemenover, 2009; Webb, Miles, et al., 2012, for reviews). In a synthesis of 306 experimental comparisons, Webb, Miles, et al. (2012) reported that distraction, reappraisal of the stimulus, and reappraisal via perspective taking each were effective emotion regulation strategies ($d_+ = 0.27$, 0.36, and 0.45, respectively). Concentration was a counterproductive strategy that exacerbated the affective response ($d_+ = -0.26$), whereas suppression had no effect on self-reported affect ($d_+ = 0.03$). These findings are consistent with predictions from the process model concerning the likely effectiveness of different affect regulation strategies.

The process model offers a comprehensive analysis of *how* people regulate experienced affect—what strategies can be used and the likely effectiveness of using each strategy. Webb, Schweiger Gallo, Miles, Gollwitzer, and Sheeran (2012) pointed out, however, that knowing how to regulate affect is only one of several difficulties that people face in controlling their emotions and moods. Borrowing from research on striving for behavioral goals (e.g., Gollwitzer & Sheeran, 2006), Webb, Schweiger Gallo, et al. (2012) proposed an action control perspective on affect regulation that specified three tasks that need to be accomplished if people are to effectively control affect: Identifying the need to regulate affect (the *identification* task), choosing an affect regulation strategy (the *selection* task), and enacting the selected strategy (the *implementation* task). Recent research indicates that people encounter difficulties in identifying when to regulate affect less frequently than in choosing how to regulate affect or in implementing the affect regulation strategy. However, people encounter difficulties with implementing a strategy just as often as they do with selecting a strategy (Isselhard et al., 2016). Moreover, competence at the task of strategy implementation is a more powerful predictor of affective outcomes compared to competence at either the identification or selection tasks. In a formal test, strategy implementation mediated the relationship between emotional vulnerability (indexed by competence at emotion regulation and emotional reactivity) and negative affective outcomes (indexed by depression, anxiety, and scores on the negative affect schedule) whereas competence at the identification and selection tasks did not (Isselhard et al., 2016). Thus, it is not enough to know which affect regulation strategy to deploy and when to deploy it; effective self-regulation of affect demands that the strategy is implemented when it is needed.

The action control model of affect regulation exploits the distinction between goal intentions and implementation intentions (Gollwitzer, 1993, 1999, 2014; Gollwitzer & Sheeran, 2006, 2009) in order to understand and promote the implementation of affect regulation strategies. In the present context, goal intentions specify whether or how one will control affect (i.e., the decision to engage in affect regulation and which affect regulation strategy to adopt). The process model construes affect regulation in terms of specifying particular strategies in goal intentions (e.g., "I will adopt a detached perspective in response to the images that are presented!" or "I will distract myself in response to the presented images!"). The action control model, on the other hand, acknowledges that there is often a "gap" between goal intentions for affect regulation and subsequent affect control, in the same way as an intention-behavior gap has been observed for behavioral goals (e.g., Sheeran, 2002; Sheeran & Webb, in press; Webb & Sheeran, 2006; see also Rhodes, this volume). Indeed, the relatively modest effect sizes observed for affect regulation strategies on emotional outcomes ($d_+ < 0.5$ for all strategies in Webb, Miles, et al.'s, 2012, review) is consistent with this analysis. To close the gap between goal intentions and affect control, and to promote the effective implementation of affect regulation strategies, the action control model proposes that the person should form implementation intentions (Gollwitzer, 1999) in the wake of forming goal intentions to regulate affect.

IMPLEMENTATION INTENTIONS

Implementation intentions are if-then plans that specify precisely what one will do and when one will do it in a contingent (e.g., if-then) format in order to realize goal intentions. Thus, whereas a goal intention might specify, "I will adopt a detached perspective in response to disgusting images!", a corresponding implementation intention might be "If I see a disgusting image, then I will view it as if I were a medical doctor!" The if-part of the plan identifies the opportunity to regulate affect (e.g., the stimulus that evokes affect, the onset of the feeling or mood) whereas the then-part of the plan specifies the response that the person anticipates will be effective in regulating affect (e.g., the precise strategy that they will use). It is well established that forming implementation intentions improves rates of behavioral performance and goal attainment compared to forming mere goal intentions. Gollwitzer and Sheeran (2006) observed an effect size of medium-to-large magnitude ($d_+ = 0.65$) in a quantitative synthesis of 94 behavioral studies, and meta-analyses of specific health behaviors also found reliable effects of if-then plans on diet (Adriaanse, Vinkers, de Ridder, Hox, & de Wit, 2011) and physical activity (Bélanger-Gravel, Godin, & Amireault, 2013).

How do if-then plans exert these powerful effects? Implementation intentions do not strengthen goal intentions or enhance self-efficacy (Webb & Sheeran, 2008). Nor can the greater specificity of if-then plans explain their effectiveness as forming implementation intentions still improved performance compared to goal intentions even when the content of the two kinds of intention was formally identical and differed only in the use of an if-then format (e.g., Oettingen, Hönig, & Gollwitzer, 2000; Palayiwa, Sheeran, & Thompson, 2010; Wieber, von Suchodoletz, Heikamp, Trommsdorff, & Gollwitzer, 2011). Rather, the effectiveness of if-then plans accrues from psychological processes to do with the if-part and then-part of the plans. Forming an implementation intention is the mental act of linking an anticipated critical situation with an effective goal-directed response. These mental links facilitate goal attainment in two ways. First, the mental representation of the opportunity specified in the if-part of the plan becomes highly activated, and hence more accessible (Gollwitzer, 1999). This heightened accessibility of the if-part of the plan has been demonstrated in several studies (e.g., Aarts, Dijksterhuis, & Midden, 1999; Parks-Stamm, Gollwitzer, & Oettingen, 2007; Webb & Sheeran, 2007, 2008) and means that people who form if-then plans are in a good position to identify and take notice of the critical cue when they subsequently encounter it (e.g., Parks-Stamm et al., 2007; Webb & Sheeran, 2004). Second, forming implementation intentions forges a strong association between the specified opportunity and the specified response (Aarts & Dijksterhuis, 2000; Webb & Sheeran, 2007, 2008). The upshot of these strong links is that the initiation of the goal-directed response specified in the if-then plan becomes relatively automatic; that is, more immediate (e.g., Gollwitzer & Brandstätter, 1997, Experiment 3), more efficient (e.g., Brandstätter, Lengfelder, & Gollwitzer, 2001), and needless of conscious intent at the moment of acting (e.g., Bayer, Achtziger, Gollwitzer, & Moskowitz, 2009; Sheeran, Webb, & Gollwitzer, 2005, Study 2). These component processes of implementation intentions (enhanced cue detection, increased automatization of responding) mean that if-then planners are in a good position both to see and to seize good opportunities to move toward their goals. Forming an if-then plan should thus *strategically automate* affect regulation (Gollwitzer & Schaal, 1998; Schweiger Gallo, Keil, McCulloch, Rockstroh, & Gollwitzer, 2009) because people delegate control of strategy implementation to preselected situational cues that serve to trigger responses swiftly and effortlessly. Neurophysiological evidence supports the idea that response initiation by if-then plans operates in a cue-driven (bottom-up) rather than goal-driven (top-down) fashion (e.g., Gilbert, Gollwitzer, Cohen, Oettingen, & Burgess, 2009; Hallam et al., 2015).

SELF-REGULATION OF EXPERIENCED AFFECT

Path A: Regulating Experienced Affect

Does the strategic automaticity afforded by if-then planning improve strategy implementation and lead to improved affect? Several studies and a recent meta-analysis (Webb, Schweiger Gallo, et al., 2012) suggest that this is the case. Schweiger Gallo and colleagues (Schweiger Gallo & Gollwitzer, 2007; Schweiger Gallo et al., 2009) offered the first demonstrations that forming an implementation intention engenders better affective outcomes compared to forming goal intentions. Furnishing a goal intention ("I will not get frightened!") with an if-then plan ("And if I see a spider, then I remain calm and relaxed!") attenuated negative affective reactions to spider images compared to both goal-intention-only and no-instruction conditions (Schweiger Gallo & Gollwitzer, 2007). These findings emerged even though participants (1) exhibited dispositional fear of spiders, and (2) were under cognitive load as they rated the images (i.e., engaged in a secondary task that consumed working memory); the findings thus speak to the idea that implementation intentions serve to automate control of affect. Electrocortical data also supported the idea that forming implementation intentions help to regulate affective responses. The P1 index typically shows greater positivity about 120 ms after detecting threatening stimuli (e.g., Carretié, Hinojosa, Mercado, & Tapia, 2005) and before conscious efforts to regulate affect are initiated (at about 300 ms). Forming implementation intentions proved effective in down-regulating this ERP component in response to spider images, and led to significantly reduced P1 positivity compared to forming mere goal intentions (Schweiger Gallo et al., 2009).

Subsequent research observed that forming implementation intentions is also more effective than goal intentions in up-regulating mood (McCormack et al., 2010, cited in Webb, Schweiger Gallo, et al., 2012), down-regulating distress (Palayiwa et al., 2010), and modulating affective responses to disgusting (Hallam et al., 2015; Schweiger Gallo, McCulloch, & Gollwitzer, 2012) and sad images (Hallam et al., 2015). Implementation intentions also proved effective in reducing clinical levels of anxiety in an 8-week trial (Varley, Webb, & Sheeran, 2011). Moreover, implementation intentions engendered superior emotional outcomes whether the strategy specified in the then-part of the plan was antecedent-focused (e.g., "And if I see blood, then I take the perspective of a physician!"; Hallam et al., 2015; Schweiger Gallo et al., 2009), response-focused (e.g., "And if I see blood, then I stay calm and relaxed!"; Hallam et al., 2015; Schweiger Gallo et al., 2009), or was geared at situation selection (e.g., "If I am deciding what to this weekend, then I will select activities that will make me feel good and avoid doing things that will make me feel bad!"; Webb et al., 2016, Study 2).

Meta-analysis also supports the effectiveness of implementation intentions for affect regulation (Webb, Schweiger Gallo, et al., 2012). Across all affective outcomes, if-then plans led to a medium-sized improvement in affect compared to goal intentions ($d_+ = .53$, $k = 29$) and a large improvement compared to no instructions ($d_+ = .91$, $k = 21$). These findings support the idea that forming if-then plans helps people to regulate affect (i.e., Path A in Figure 5.1). Although no studies to date have appear to have measured health behaviors in the wake of an if-then plan intervention for affect control, the strong effects of if-then plans on affect coupled with the strong associations between affect and health behavior suggest that planning to regulate relevant affect should lead to changes in the respective health behavior.

Path B: Regulating the Impact of Experienced Affect

Path A in Figure 5.1 is a mediational model. The idea is that forming an if-then plan improves experienced affect, which in turn enhances health behavior performance. There may be occasions, however, where there is little that can be done to alter experienced affect (e.g., an unanticipated negative event occurs, the person is unaware of the impact of a stimulus on his/her affect, no if-then plan has been formed, and the person's capacity for affect regulation in situ is compromised by stress or fatigue). A key question therefore is whether the unwanted behavioral consequences of affect are inevitable in such instances, or whether there is something that the person can do to prevent affect from influencing behavior. Path B in Figure 5.1 suggests that forming implementation intentions can also be helpful in these circumstances. Path B is a moderation model. Here, the if-then plan is geared at regulating *affective influence*, that is, blocking or attenuating the impact of experienced affect on behavioral outcomes.

If-then plans could regulate the influence of experienced affect on behavior in two ways—by targeting the motivational force of experienced affect so as to defuse its impact, or by targeting the execution of the behavior so that performance is longer gripped by affect. Webb, Sheeran, Totterdell, et al. (2012, Experiment 1) explored how the impact of negative mood on risky decision-making could be defused. After negative mood was induced, participants either formed if-then plans geared at disrupting the impact of mood on performance (e.g., "If I am in a bad mood, then I . . . [think 'it is only a mood' and I will not let it bother me!/ think how I have successfully dealt with other situations!]") or formed a mere goal intention to regulate their affect ("I will try and stay in a positive mood!"). Findings showed the predicted interaction between mood and type of intention. For participants in the goal intention condition, the negative mood induction led to riskier decisions compared to the neutral mood condition. When participants had formed implementation intentions on the other hand, the mood induction no longer had any effect on decisions—if-then plans broke the link between mood and decision-making.

The second way that if-then plans could moderate the affect–health behavior relation is by ensuring that performance of the behavior unfolds in the exact manner specified by the plan, and is thus no longer disrupted by unwanted affect. Webb, Sheeran, Totterdell, et al. (2012, Experiment 2) tested this idea using a different mood induction (arousal vs. no arousal) and a different task to index risky decision-making. Participants were randomized to a goal intention condition that merely specified that they would try to make good decisions, or to an implementation intention condition that spelled out how to make good decisions (e.g., If I am asked to make a decision, then I will pay close attention to the relevant risks!). Findings showed that arousal reduced sensitivity to risk information and risky decisions—but only when participants had formed goal intentions. Participants who formed if-then plans remained sensitive to risk information even when they were aroused, and made decisions of equivalent, low risk in both the arousal and no-arousal conditions (see also Bayer, Gollwitzer, & Achtziger, 2010). O'Connor, Armitage, and Ferguson (2015) also observed that forming if-then plans to substitute a healthy snack for an unhealthy snack when feeling stressed attenuated the relationship between stress and unhealthy snacking. Although O'Conner et al. did not measure affect, their results are consistent with the idea that if-then plans are effective at regulating affective influence. In sum, accumulated evidence indicates that implementation intentions are effective at regulating experienced affect (and should thus change health behaviors that are influenced by experienced affect), and at regulating the impact of experienced affect on health decisions and behavior.

SELF-REGULATION OF ANTICIPATED AFFECT

Path A: Regulating Anticipated Affect

Evidence supports the distinction between affective attitude or *anticipated affect* (e.g., "Doing X would be enjoyable/pleasant/fun") and cognitive attitude (e.g., "Doing X would be wise/worthwhile /valuable") (e.g., Trafimow

& Sheeran, 1998), and it is well established that anticipated affect better predicts health-related intentions and behavior compared to cognitive attitude (e.g., Conner, this volume; Lawton et al., 2009; Rhodes et al., 2009). Surprisingly little research has been specifically concerned with modifying levels of anticipated affect in order to promote health-related behaviors (i.e., Path A in Figure 5.1), and most work is concerned with persuading people that performing particular health behaviors is more likely to have positive affective outcomes than they currently anticipate (see, e.g., Conner, Rhodes, Morris, McEachan, & Lawton, 2011). Recently, however, evidence has emerged that affect regulation exerts an important influence on anticipated affect. Sheeran, Webb, Jones, and Avishai-Yitshak (2016) used the Difficulties in Emotion Regulation Scale (Gratz & Roemer, 2004) to index competence at affect regulation and measured anticipated affect ("How [enjoyable/pleasant] would engaging in behavior X be for you?") and participants' behavioral intentions ("I intend to engage in behavior X") in relation to physical activity and dietary behaviors (eating a low-fat diet, eating 5 portions of fruit and vegetables per day). Competence at affect regulation predicted greater anticipated affect and stronger intentions in relation to all three behaviors. Moreover, anticipated affect mediated the relationship between competence at affective regulation and intention in each case. Thus, people who are good at regulating their affect expect that performing weight-control behaviors will feel good which, in turn, leads to the formation of stronger intentions to perform those behaviors.

In an experimental test, participants were primed either to experience affect (using scrambled sentences containing words such as "feelings," "emotion," and "passion"), to regulate affect via reappraisal (using scrambled sentences containing words such as "analyze," "scrutinize," and "evaluate"), or were not primed. Next, in a supposedly unrelated study, participants completed measures of anticipated affect ("How positive or negative are your feelings about performing behavior X?"), cognitive attitude ("How positive or negative are the consequences of performing behavior X?"), and behavioral intentions in relation to 22 (predominantly health-related) behaviors. Comparisons across the three conditions indicated that participants in the affect-regulation prime condition attached less weight to anticipated affect and attached greater weight to cognitive attitude during intention formation relative to participants in the other conditions. These findings are consistent with Path A in Figure 5.1 and indicate that affect regulation processes modify not only experienced affect but also anticipated affect concerning health behaviors. Ongoing studies test whether forming if-then plans facilitates the regulation of anticipated affect compared to mere goal intentions to regulate that affect.

Path B: Regulating the Impact of Anticipated Affect

Several studies have tested whether forming if-then plans can overcome the impact of anticipated affect on health behaviors (Sheeran, Aubrey, & Kellett, 2007; Sheeran, Webb, & Gollwitzer, 2016). As was the case for experienced affect, implementation intention interventions have attempted to regulate anticipated affective influence in two ways—by targeting the motivational impact of anticipated affect, or by targeting the execution of the behavior so that performance is no longer gripped by anticipated affect. The first study that used if-then plans to target anticipated affect concerned attendance for psychotherapy (Sheeran et al., 2007). On average, 40% of clients who are offered therapy fail to attend their first appointment (Hampton-Robb, Qualls, & Compton, 2003) and anticipated affect (e.g., believing that attending therapy would be embarrassing, shameful, or stigmatizing) is a key factor that militates against attendance. With this in mind, participants who were offered a first appointment for psychotherapy (N = 479) were randomized to instructions prompting them to form an if-then plan geared at undermining the impact of negative anticipated affect about attendance, or to a treatment-as-usual (TAU) control condition. The if-part of the plan specified the anticipation of negative affect ("As soon as I feel concerned about attending my appointment . . .") and the then-part of the plan specified two responses. The first response was designed to prevent the elaboration of the anticipated negative affect (". . . then I ignore that feeling . . .") and the second response was designed to encourage participants to construe their affect as entirely normal, and so prevent participants from using their affect as information that they should not attend the appointment (". . . and tell myself this is perfectly understandable!").

Forming if-then plans reliably improved rates of attendance at psychotherapy according to both intention-to-treat (64% vs. 50%) and explanatory analyses (83% vs. 57%). Moderated regression analysis revealed a three-way interaction between if-then planning, anticipated affect, and anticipated benefits. Decomposition of the interaction showed that anticipated affect was a powerful, negative predictor of attendance among participants in the TAU condition. However, for participants who had formed an if-then plan *and* also anticipated that attendance would be beneficial, anticipated negative affect was not significantly related to behavior—anticipated feelings of shame or embarrassment no longer prevented these participants attending their scheduled psychotherapy appointment. Sheeran, Webb, and Gollwitzer (2016, Study 2) observed equivalent findings in an intervention to reduce frequency of drunkenness among young people.

Two further studies attempted to overcome the impact of anticipated affect on health behavior by using if-then plans to spell out exactly how the behavior would be performed. The expectation was that controlling action via the cues specified in the plan would circumvent the impact of anticipated affect. Findings confirmed this expectation (Sheeran, Webb, & Gollwitzer, 2016). In the first study, participants nominated a snack food that they wanted to consume less of, and formed an implementation intention that specified exactly where and when they would consume a limited number of snacks (our prediction was that precommitting to indulgence in specific contexts would prevent overindulgence). Control participants did not form a plan. Participants who formed an if-then plan consumed fewer snacks compared to controls during the subsequent week. For control participants, anticipated affect but not cognitive attitudes predicted consumption. For treatment participants, on the other hand, forming if-then plans seemed to resolve the conflict between anticipated affect and cognitive attitude in favor of participants' cognitive attitude. When participants who formed implementation intentions anticipated feeling bad about reducing their snack consumption, then cognitive attitudes predicted less snack consumption—that is, if participants thought it was a good idea to reduce consumption and had formed if-then plans to avoid overindulgence, then consumption was reduced.

The second study was a reanalysis of a randomized controlled trial concerning cervical cancer screening. The original report indicated that forming an if-then plan that specified when, where, and how one would make an appointment for screening led to improved screening rates (92% vs. 69%; Sheeran & Orbell, 2000). Reanalysis of the data showed that if-then planning moderated the impact of anticipated affect on attendance for screening. Whereas anticipating that screening would be worrying, embarrassing, or unpleasant was strongly associated with nonattendance among control participants, anticipated affect no longer predicted attendance among participants who had formed if-then plans. In sum, affect regulation is important in reducing anticipated affect in relation to health behaviors, and if-then plans have proved effective in emancipating health actions from deleterious effects of anticipated affect.

SELF-REGULATION OF IMPLICIT AFFECT

Path A: Regulating Implicit Affect

Implicit affect is typically measured by speeded classification tasks such as the implicit association test (IAT; Greenwald, McGhee, & Schwartz, 1998) that require participants to classify target stimuli (e.g., words or images representing, for instance, high-fat foods or physical activity) with concepts related to affect (e.g., pleasant-unpleasant, approach-avoid). The extent to which participants are faster to classify target stimuli in the same category as concepts with positive valence (relative to how fast they classify target stimuli with negative concepts) is assumed to index participants' implicit affect towards targets. Findings indicate that implicit affect is only modestly related to explicit attitudes (e.g., $r_+ = .21$ in Greenwald et al.'s, 2009, meta-analysis), and implicit affect predicts unique variance in behavioral outcomes even after explicit attitudes have been taken into account (e.g., Greenwald et al., 2009; Reich et al., 2010; Rooke et al., 2008).

Can if-then plans help to regulate implicit affect? Several studies suggest that this is the case (e.g., Hofmann, Deutsch, Lancaster, & Banaji, 2010; Webb, Sheeran, & Pepper, 2012). In four experiments on social stereotyping, Webb, Sheeran, and Pepper (2012) observed that forming if-then plans (for instance, to associate the social group "Muslims" with the concept of "peace") led to weaker outgroup bias on the IAT and another implicit measure. Hofmann et al. (2010) compared whether goal intentions to reappraise chocolate (i.e., ". . . imagine the chocolate in a strange or novel way unrelated to the purpose of consumption") or if-then plans to resist chocolate consumption specified by the participant (e.g., "If my friend offers me chocolate during the film, then I will say 'no thanks' and concentrate on the film!") could reduce implicit affect toward chocolate compared to a no-instruction control condition. Hofmann et al. found that goal intentions to reappraise led to weaker associations between chocolate and positive affect compared to the control condition. However, forming if-then plans reduced the positivity of implicit affect to a significantly greater extent than did goal intentions. Thus, implementation intention formation can alter the valence of implicit affect, and should thus change behaviors for which implicit affect is a key determinant.

Path B: Regulating the Impact of Implicit Affect

Two studies have tested whether if-then plans can overcome the impact of implicit attitudes on behavior (Sheeran, Miles et al., 2016). The first study aimed to defuse the motivational impact of implicit attitudes by causing participants to deliberate about their consumption of chocolate at the critical juncture ("And if I am tempted to have chocolate, then I ask myself, 'Do I really want to do this?'"). Participants completed an IAT designed to measure implicit affect toward chocolate and also completed a measure of explicit attitudes prior to randomization to if-then plan versus no-plan control conditions. One week later, participants reported their chocolate consumption. Forming if-then plans led to a 30% reduction in the amount of chocolate that participants consumed. Whereas implicit affect was a strong predictor of consumption for control participants, among participants who formed if-then plans, the influence of implicit affect depended on their explicit attitudes. If participants' explicit attitude favored a reduction in consumption, then implicit affect was *negatively* related to consumption. Participants ate the least chocolate (less than one-half of a unit) when they had formed an if-then plan, thought that it was a good idea to reduce their consumption, *and* had positive implicit affect toward chocolate.

The second study aimed to regulate the impact of implicit affect by spelling out exactly how the focal behavior would be performed. Participants were informed that the study concerned attitudes toward mental illness and that they would later have a conversation with John, who had a diagnosis of schizophrenia. Participants completed a battery of explicit measures and an IAT that measured their implicit affect in relation to schizophrenia. Participants were then randomized to a no-instruction control condition, a goal intention condition, or an if-then plan condition. The no-instruction condition comprised an information sheet that simply explained that participants would meet John. Participants in the goal intention condition received the same information sheet but were also informed that, "Your goal is to be friendly and warm to this person!" Finally, the if-then plan condition was the same as the goal intention condition save for inclusion of an implementation intention ("As soon as I get a chance to be friendly and warm to this person, then I'll take it!"). Next, participants were directed to a meeting room in which two chairs were set side-by-side against the back wall. Participants were instructed to set out the chairs for the meeting with John while the experimenter (ostensibly) went downstairs to get him. Upon returning, the experimenter probed participants for suspicion (none of the participants guessed the true purpose of the study), and then measured the distance between the two chairs that the participants had set out. Seating distance was used as the measure of behavioral avoidance.

Findings showed that participants who formed if-then plans chose to sit closer to John than participants in both the goal intention and control condition. The latter conditions were combined to analyze the impact of implicit affect among participants in the if-then plan versus no plan conditions. Implicit affect was a reliable predictor of seating distance for participants in the no-plan condition, such that more positive implicit affect was associated with greater interpersonal closeness. For participants who formed if-then plans, however, implicit affect no longer predicted behavioral avoidance. Participants elected to sit close to John, and implicit affect toward people with schizophrenia did not affect their behavior. In sum, the findings from studies on implementation intentions and implicit affect parallel the findings observed for experienced affect and implicit affect. If-then plans can serve both to regulate implicit affect itself, and to regulate the impact of implicit affect on behavior.

CONCLUSION

The impact of affect on health decisions and actions is not inevitable. The present chapter offers evidence concerning the important role of self-regulation processes in mitigating the influence of three kinds of affect—experienced, anticipated, and implicit–on health behaviors. For each of these three kinds of affect, we observed that forming if-then plans or implementation intentions could emancipate health actions from unwanted influence by affect. This emancipation could be achieved in two ways—by directly targeting the affect itself so as to undermine the strength of the affective response, or by targeting the relationship between affect and health behavior so that the translation of affect into action is reduced or blocked. We acknowledge that there are gaps in the evidence base, and that if-then planning interventions that measure health behaviors in the wake of changes in experienced affect and interventions that target levels of anticipated affect, in particular, are needed. Larger scale trials with more representative and clinical samples over longer follow-up periods would also help to make the case for using if-then plans to regulating affect-health behavior relations even more compelling. Notwithstanding these limitations, however, the self-regulation approach advocated here holds considerable promise for both theory and practice. Further research using this approach therefore seems warranted.

REFERENCES

Aarts, H., & Dijksterhuis, A. (2000). Habits as knowledge structures: automaticity in goal-directed behavior. *Journal of Personality and Social Psychology, 78*(1), 53–63.

Aarts, H., Dijksterhuis, A. P., & Midden, C. (1999). To plan or not to plan? Goal achievement or interrupting the performance of mundane behaviors. *European Journal of Social Psychology, 29*, 971–979.

Adriaanse, M. A., Vinkers, C. D. W., de Ridder, D. T. D., Hox, J. J., de Wit, J. B. F. (2011). Do implementation intentions help to eat a healthy diet? A systematic review and meta-analysis of the empirical evidence. *Appetite, 56*, 183–193.

Aldao, A., Nolen-Hoeksema, S., & Schweizer, S. (2010). Emotion regulation strategies across psychopathology: A meta-analytic review. *Clinical Psychology Review, 30*, 217–237.

Augustine, A. A., & Hemenover, S. H. (2009). On the relative effectiveness of affect regulation strategies: A meta-analysis. *Cognition and Emotion, 23*, 1181–1220.

Baumeister, R. F., Vohs, K. D., DeWall, C. N., & Zhang, L. (2007). How emotion shapes behavior: Feedback, anticipation, and reflection, rather than direct causation. *Personality and Social Psychology Review, 11*, 167–203.

Bayer, U. C., Achtziger, A., Gollwitzer, P. M., & Moskowitz, G. B. (2009). Responding to subliminal cues: Do if-then plans facilitate action preparation and initiation without conscious intent? *Social Cognition, 27*, 183.

Bayer, U. C., Gollwitzer, P. M., & Achtziger, A. (2010). Staying on track: Planned goal striving is protected from disruptive internal states. *Journal of Experimental Social Psychology, 46*, 505–514.

Bélanger-Gravel, A., Godin, G., & Amireault, S. (2013). A meta-analytic review of the effect of implementation intentions on physical activity. *Health Psychology Review, 7*, 23–54.

Brandstätter, V., Lengfelder, A., & Gollwitzer, P. M. (2001). Implementation intentions and efficient action initiation. *Journal of Personality and Social Psychology, 81*, 946.

Carretié, L., Hinojosa, J. A., Mercado, F., & Tapia, M. (2005). Cortical response to subjectively unconscious danger. *NeuroImage, 24*, 615–623.

Conner, M., Rhodes, R. E., Morris, B., McEachan, R., & Lawton, R. (2011). Changing exercise through targeting affective or cognitive attitudes. *Psychology and Health, 26*, 133–149.

Ferguson, S. G., & Shiffman, S. (2014). Effect of high-dose nicotine patch on craving and negative affect leading up to lapse episodes. *Psychopharmacology, 231*, 2595–2602.

Ferrer, R. A., Klein, W. M. P., Persoskie, A., Avishai-Yitshak, A., & Sheeran, P. (2016). The tripartite model of risk perception (TRIRISK): Evidence that perceived risk has deliberative, affective, and experiential components. *Annals of Behavioral Medicine, 50*(5), 653–663.

Gawronski, B., & Bodenhausen, G. V. (2006). Associative and propositional processes in evaluation: An integrative review of implicit and explicit attitude change. *Psychological Bulletin, 132*, 692–731.

Gilbert, S. J., Gollwitzer, P., Cohen, A.-L., Oettingen, G., & Burgess, P. W. (2009). Separable brain systems supporting cued versus self-initiated realization of delayed intentions. *Journal of Experimental Psychology: Learning, Memory and Cognition, 35*, 905–915.

Gollwitzer, P. M. (1993). Goal achievement: The role of intentions. *European Review of Social Psychology, 4*, 141–185.

Gollwitzer, P. M. (1999). Implementation intentions: Strong effects of simple plans. *American Psychologist, 54*, 493–503.

Gollwitzer, P. M. (2014). Weakness of the will: Is a quick fix possible? *Motivation and Emotion, 38*, 305–322.

Gollwitzer, P. M., & Brandstätter, V. (1997). Implementation intentions and effective goal pursuit. *Journal of Personality and Social Psychology, 73*, 186.

Gollwitzer, P. M., & Schaal, B. (1998). Metacognition in action: The importance of implementation intentions. *Personality and Social Psychology Review, 2*, 124–136.

Gollwitzer, P. M., & Sheeran, P. (2006). Implementation intentions and goal achievement: A meta-analysis of effects and processes. *Advances in Experimental Social Psychology, 38*, 69–120.

Gollwitzer, P. M., & Sheeran, P. (2009). Self-regulation of consumer decision making and behavior: The role of implementation intentions. *Journal of Consumer Psychology, 19*, 593–607.

Gratz, K. L., & Roemer, L. (2004). Multidimensional assessment of emotion regulation and dysregulation: Development, factor structure, and initial validation of the Difficulties in Emotion Regulation Scale. *Journal of Psychopathology and Behavioral Assessment, 26*, 41–54.

Greenwald, A. G., McGhee, D. E., & Schwartz, J. L. (1998). Measuring individual differences in implicit cognition: The implicit association test. *Journal of Personality and Social Psychology, 74*, 1464–1480.

Greenwald, A. G., Poehlman, T. A., Uhlmann, E. L., & Banaji, M. R. (2009). Understanding and using the Implicit Association Test: III. Meta-analysis of predictive validity. *Journal of Personality and Social Psychology, 97*, 17–41.

Gross, J. J. (1998). The emerging field of emotion regulation: An integrative review. *Review of General Psychology, 2*, 271.

Gross, J. J. (2014). Emotion regulation: Conceptual and empirical foundations. *Handbook of Emotion Regulation, 2*, 3–20.

Gross, J. J. (2015a). Emotion regulation: Current status and future prospects. *Psychological Inquiry, 26*, 1–26.

Gross, J. J. (2015b). The extended process model of emotion regulation: Elaborations, applications, and future directions. *Psychological Inquiry, 26*, 130–137.

Gross, J. J., & Thompson, R. A. (2007). Emotion regulation: Conceptual foundations. In J. J. Gross (Ed.), *Handbook of emotion regulation* (pp. 3–24). New York, NY: Guilford.

Hallam, G. P., Webb, T. L., Sheeran, P., Miles, E., Wilkinson, I. D., Hunter, M. D., . . . Farrow, T. D. (2015). The neural correlates of emotion regulation by implementation intentions. *PLoS One, 10*.

Hampton-Robb, S., Qualls, R. C., & Compton, W. C. (2003). Predicting first-session attendance: The influence of referral source and client income. *Psychotherapy Research, 13*, 223–233.

Hofmann, W., Deutsch, R., Lancaster, K., & Banaji, M. R. (2010). Cooling the heat of temptation: Mental self-control and the automatic evaluation of tempting stimuli. *European Journal of Social Psychology, 40*, 17–25.

Isselhard, A., Sheeran, P., Webb, T. L., Jones, K., Avishai-Yitshak, A., & Alberts, A. (2016). *Problems in regulating emotions: Their nature, consequences, and resolution.* Unpublished manuscript, University of North Carolina at Chapel Hill.

Koole, S. L., Webb, T. L., & Sheeran, P. (2015). Implicit emotion regulation: Feeling better without knowing why. *Current Opinion in Psychology, 3*, 6–10.

Larsen, R. J., & Prizmic, Z. (2004). Affect regulation. In R. Baumeister & K. Vohs (Eds.), *Handbook of self-regulation research* (pp. 40–60). New York, NY: Guilford.

Lawton, R., Conner, M., & McEachan, R. (2009). Desire or reason: Predicting health behaviors from affective and cognitive attitudes. *Health Psychology, 28*, 56.

Loewenstein, G., & Lerner, J. S. (2002). The role of affect in decision making. In R. J. Davidson, H. H. Goldsmith, & K. R. Scherer (Eds.), *The handbook of affective science.* Oxford: Oxford University Press.

McKee, S. A., Sinha, R., Weinberger, A. H., Sofuoglu, M., Harrison, E. L., Lavery, M., & Wanzer, J. (2011). Stress decreases the ability to resist smoking and potentiates smoking intensity and reward. *Journal of Psychopharmacology, 25*, 490–502.

Mischel, W., Shoda, Y., & Rodriguez, M. L. (1989). Delay of gratification in children. *Science, 244*, 933–938.

O'Connor, D. B., Armitage, C. J., & Ferguson, E. (2015). Randomized test of an implementation intention-based tool to reduce stress-induced eating. *Annals of Behavioral Medicine, 49*, 331–343.

Oettingen, G., Hönig, G., & Gollwitzer, P. M. (2000). Effective self-regulation of goal attainment. *International Journal of Educational Research, 33*, 705–732.

Palayiwa, A., Sheeran, P., & Thompson, A. (2010). "Words will never hurt me!": Implementation intentions regulate attention to stigmatizing comments about appearance. *Journal of Social and Clinical Psychology, 29*, 575.

Parks-Stamm, E., Gollwitzer, P. M., & Oettingen, G. (2007). Action control by implementation intentions: Effective cue detection and efficient response initiation. *Social Cognition, 25*, 248–266. doi:10.1521/soco.2007.25.2.248

Piasecki, T. M., Jorenby, D. E., Smith, S. S., Fiore, M. C., & Baker, T. B. (2003). Smoking withdrawal dynamics: I. Abstinence distress in lapsers and abstainers. *Journal of Abnormal Psychology, 112*, 3–13.

Reich, R. R., Below, M. C., & Goldman, M. S. (2010). Explicit and implicit measures of expectancy and related alcohol cognitions: A meta-analytic comparison. *Psychology of Addictive Behaviors, 24*, 13.

Reynolds, L. M., Consedine, N. S., Pizarro, D. A., & Bissett, I. P. (2013). Disgust and behavioral avoidance in colorectal cancer screening and treatment: A systematic review and research agenda. *Cancer Nursing, 36*, 122–130.

Rhodes, R. E., Fiala, B., & Conner, M. (2009). A review and meta-analysis of affective judgments and physical activity in adult populations. *Annals of Behavioral Medicine, 38*, 180–204.

Rooke, S. E., Hine, D. W., & Thorsteinsson, E. B. (2008). Implicit cognition and substance use: A meta-analysis. *Addictive Behaviors, 33*, 1314–1328.

Russell, J. A., Weiss, A., & Mendelsohn, G. A. (1989). Affect grid: A single-item scale of pleasure and arousal. *Journal of Personality and Social Psychology, 57*, 493–502.

Schwarz, N., & Clore, G. L. (2004). Mood as information: 20 years later. *Psychological Inquiry, 14*, 296–303.

Schweiger Gallo, I., & Gollwitzer, P. M. (2007). Implementation intentions: Control of fear despite cognitive load. *Psicothema, 19*, 280–285.

Schweiger Gallo, I., Keil, A., McCulloch, K. C., Rockstroh, B., & Gollwitzer, P. M. (2009). Strategic automation of emotion regulation. *Journal of Personality and Social Psychology, 96*, 11.

Schweiger Gallo, I., McCulloch, K. C., & Gollwitzer, P. M. (2012). Differential effects of various types of implementation intentions on the regulation of disgust. *Social Cognition, 30*, 1.

Sheeran, P. (2002). Intention-behaviour relations: A conceptual and empirical review. *European Review of Social Psychology, 12*, 1–36.

Sheeran, P., Aubrey, R., & Kellett, S. (2007). Increasing attendance for psychotherapy: Implementation intentions and the self-regulation of attendance-related negative affect. *Journal of Consulting and Clinical Psychology, 75*, 853–863.

Sheeran, P., Miles, E., Baird, H., Tidwell, K., Webb, T. L., Harris, P. R., & Gollwitzer, P. M. (2016). *Self-control over the influence of implicit associations on behavior*. Unpublished raw data, University of North Carolina at Chapel Hill.

Sheeran, P., & Orbell, S. (2000). Using implementation intentions to increase attendance for cervical cancer screening. *Health Psychology, 19*, 283.

Sheeran, P., & Webb, T. L. (in press). The intention-behavior gap. *Social and Personality Psychology Compass*.

Sheeran, P., Webb, T. L., & Gollwitzer, P. M. (2005). The interplay between goal intentions and implementation intentions. *Personality and Social Psychology Bulletin, 31*, 87–98.

Sheeran, P., Webb, T. L., & Gollwitzer, P. M. (2016). *Self-regulation of the impact of thoughts versus feelings on behavior*. Manuscript under review.

Sheeran, P., Webb, T. L., Jones, K., & Avishai-Yitshak, A. (2016). *Control of behavior by thoughts versus feelings: The role of emotion regulation*. Unpublished raw data, University of North Carolina at Chapel Hill.

Trafimow, D., & Sheeran, P. (1998). Some tests of the distinction between cognitive and affective beliefs. *Journal of Experimental Social Psychology, 34*, 378–397.

Varley, R., Webb, T. L., & Sheeran, P. (2011). Making self-help more helpful: A randomized controlled trial of the impact of augmenting self-help materials with implementation intentions on promoting the effective self-management of anxiety symptoms. *Journal of Consulting and Clinical Psychology, 79*, 123–128.

Västfjäll, D., Slovic, P., Burns, W. J., Erlandsson, A., Koppel, L., Asutay, E., & Tinghög, G. (2016). The arithmetic of emotion: Integration of incidental and integral affect in judgments and decisions. *Frontiers in Psychology, 7*(e46240), 448–10.

Webb, T. L., Lindquist, K. A., Jones, K., Avishai-Yitshak, A., & Sheeran, P. (2016). Situation selection is an effective emotion regulation strategy, especially for people who need help regulating their emotions. Manuscript under review.

Webb, T. L., Miles, E., & Sheeran, P. (2012). Dealing with feeling: A meta-analysis of the effectiveness of strategies derived from the process model of emotion regulation. *Psychological Bulletin, 138*, 775–808.

Webb, T. L., Schweiger Gallo, I., Miles, E., Gollwitzer, P. M., & Sheeran, P. (2012). Effective regulation of affect: An action control perspective on emotion regulation. *European Review of Social Psychology, 23*, 143–186. doi:10.1080/10463283.2012.718134

Webb, T. L., & Sheeran, P. (2004). Identifying good opportunities to act: Implementation intentions and cue discrimination. *European Journal of Social Psychology, 34*, 407–419.

Webb, T. L., & Sheeran, P. (2006). Does changing behavioral intentions engender behavior change? A meta-analysis of the experimental evidence. *Psychological Bulletin, 132*, 249–268.

Webb, T. L., & Sheeran, P. (2007). How do implementation intentions promote goal attainment? A test of component processes. *Journal of Experimental Social Psychology, 43*, 295–302.

Webb, T. L., & Sheeran, P. (2008). Mechanisms of implementation intention effects: The role of goal intentions, self-efficacy, and accessibility of plan components. *British Journal of Social Psychology, 47*, 373–395.

Webb, T. L., Sheeran, P., & Pepper, J. (2012). Gaining control over responses to implicit attitude tests: Implementation intentions engender fast responses on attitude-incongruent trials. *British Journal of Social Psychology, 51*, 13–32.

Webb, T. L., Sheeran, P., Totterdell, P., Miles, E., Mansell, W., & Baker, S. (2012). Using implementation intentions to overcome the effect of mood on risky behaviour. *British Journal of Social Psychology, 51*, 330–345.

Wieber, F., von Suchodoletz, A., Heikamp, T., Trommsdorff, G., & Gollwitzer, P. M. (2011). If-then planning helps school-aged children to ignore attractive distractions. *Social Psychology, 42*, 39–47.

Williams, D. M., & Evans, D. R. (2014). Current emotion research in health behavior science. *Emotion Review, 6*, 277–287.

6

Affective Dynamics in Temporal Self-Regulation Theory

Social Forces Meet Neurobiological Processes

PETER A. HALL, GEOFFREY T. FONG, AND CASSANDRA J. LOWE

The idea that human behavior is tricky to predict and explain is supported by the fact that we still struggle to do so after more than 100 years of applying the scientific method. The proliferation of theoretical perspectives on human behavior over this past century is reflective of both the universally appreciated importance of understanding human behavior and our continued dissatisfaction with our ability to do so. Health behaviors have attracted a disproportionate amount of attention within psychology over the past half-century, and much of the new theory development about human behavior has taken place in this arena. Many of the current wave of health behavior models incorporate social, cognitive and neurobiological processes (e.g., Bickel, Moody, Quisenberry, Ramey, & Sheffer, 2014; Hall & Fong, 2007; Hofmann et al., 20012; McClure & Bickel, 2014), with neurobiological processes being the most unique contribution in relation to more traditional models of health behavior offered in the late part of the 20th century.

In many such models, explicit mention of emotion—and affect more broadly—are conspicuously absent. However, upon closer examination it is apparent that many (if not all) models indeed assume affect to be of central importance, but that its effects are translated through (or accounted for by) the other constructs. A specific description of how and why affect is relevant is useful, as it cannot always be gleaned by a glance at a graphical representation of any of these models. This chapter presents temporal self-regulation theory (TST; Hall & Fong, 2007, 2015) as one of several recent theories of health behavior and describes mechanisms by which affective processes play out within the confines of the model.

The TST model (Figure 6.1) was first introduced in 2007 (Hall & Fong, 2007), with revisions occurring in two subsequent iterations. The current version of the model is described in Hall and Fong (2015) with a specific application to physical activity behavior, and is also outlined in general form in Hall and Marteau (2014). This version of the TST model has retained all of its original constructs, with several clarifications added regarding the nature of recursive feedback loops, in order to better account for the repeated nature of many behaviors over time.

The TST model begins with the premise that behavior is a joint function of neurobiological, social ecological, and motivational processes. Behavioral intention, executive control processes, and behavioral prepotency are central determinants of behavior, with the latter two constructs moderating the influence of intention on behavior. Ambient contingencies (i.e., costs and benefits, etc.) supplied by the ecological context are predicted to moderate the influence of all other constructs on behavior, with explicit consideration of temporal frame. Specifically, environments that afford subtle (but immediate) costs for a given target behavior, despite more substantial long-term benefits, impel inconsistency in behavior (a common problem for health protective behaviors); environments that supply subtle but immediate benefits for a given target behavior, despite long-term costs, are thought to impel unwanted consistency in behavior (a common problem for health risk behaviors).

Despite intentions being a central construct in the model, there are several factors that are hypothesized to be ultimately more distal yet

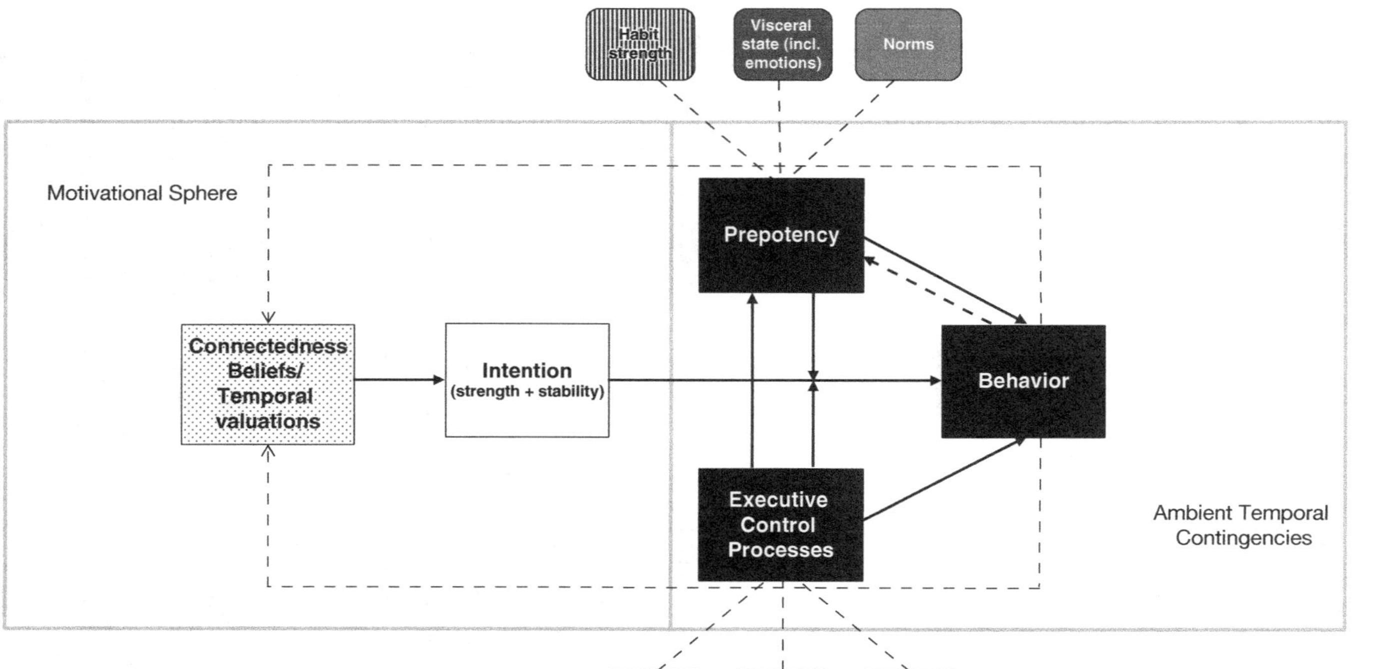

Figure 6.1. Graphical depiction of temporal self-regulation theory (TST).

highly important. Connectedness beliefs are beliefs that refer to the extent to which a target behavior will result in an array of outcomes (positive, negative, and neutral). These are each weighted with reference to temporal proximity of the anticipated outcome, with temporally immediate outcomes weighted disproportionately more heavily than those that are more distal. Essentially, this is a temporally weighted expectancy-value calculation that is not intended to determine behavior directly, but rather the prebehavior construct of intention. The latter may be considered in terms of absolute magnitude as well as with reference to stability. The intention–behavior relationship is not expected to be uniform, but instead modified by prepotency and executive control system activation.

EXECUTIVE CONTROL

The inclusion of executive control as a focal construct in the TST model represents a significant departure from any major model of health behavior that existed prior to its introduction in 2006, as the lead article in the inaugural issue of *Health Psychology Review*. Based on theorizing and empirical findings from cognitive psychology and cognitive neuroscience, the executive control system is thought to be rooted in the neurobiology of the prefrontal cortex (e.g., dorsolateral, ventromedial, and ventrolateral subregions most centrally), the parietal lobe, and connections between these cortical nodes and lower reward and emotion generation centers (e.g., ventral striatum; limbic system; Miller, 2000; Miller & Cohen, 2001; Miyake & Friedman, 2012; Yarkoni, Poldrack, Nichols, Van Essen, & Wager, 2011). The executive control system is thought to have significance for implementation of behaviors that are counter to highly routinized processes such as habit, competing cues from the environment, and other factors that lower the prior probability of a target behavior being performed. The role of executive control within TST may be to both moderate the intention–behavior link, and to influence behavior more directly via non-intentional channels (Hall & Fong, 2015).

The TST model was informed at the construction phase by a very large and diverse evidence base from a number of fields, including economics, social psychology, personality, cognitive neuroscience, and cognitive psychology. For a review of this evidence base, the interested reader is directed toward the original article (Hall & Fong, 2007), as an exhaustive review is beyond the scope of the current chapter. However, it is informative to highlight some encouraging recent findings regarding the causal association between executive control and health behavior, particularly in relation to diet (see Hall, 2016, for a summary). Using a variant of repetitive transcranial magnetic stimulation called continuous theta burst stimulation (cTBS; a cortical excitation-reducing protocol), Lowe, Hall, and Staines (2014) showed that temporary down-regulation of the dorsolateral prefrontal cortex (dlPFC)—an important node in the executive control network—resulted in amplified cue-induced food cravings, and increased actual consumption of foods during a subsequent taste test. One notable aspect of the findings was that the food consumption effects were highly selective to high-calorie (appetitive) snack foods, and did not generalize to food in general (i.e., a general tendency to consume all foods, regardless of caloric content), consistent with the postulates of the TST model. Importantly, a mediational analysis confirmed that the cTBS effects on the food outcomes were mediated by cTBS-induced decreases in Stroop performance. Although consumption effects have been less consistent in other studies using less reliable neuromodulation methods involving dlPFC up-regulation, a subsequent meta-analysis confirmed a reliable effect of dlPFC modulation on food cravings across studies and stimulation modalities (Lowe Vincent, & Hall, 2017; Hall, Lowe, & Vincent, 2017).

With respect to exercise behavior, two forthcoming studies have documented prospective associations between volumetric parameters of brain structures implicated in executive control and adherence to structured exercise programming (Best, Chiu, Hall, & Liu-Ambrose, 2017; Gujral, McAuley, Oberlin, Kramer, & Erickson, 2017). A second set of observational studies has documented reliable prospective effects of executive function (defined with reference to performance on an executive control task) on exercise adherence (Daly, McMinn, & Allan, 2015; Best,

Nagamatsu, & Liu-Ambrose, 2014). One of these studies documented recursive feedback loops between exercise and executive function in a multiwave analysis of the English Longitudinal Study of Aging; interestingly, the effects of function on adherence were 50% larger than those of exercise on executive function (Daly et al., 2015). In the second study, structured exercise training resulted in improved executive task performance, and such task performance gains subsequently predicted exercise adherence in the unstructured follow-up interval (Best et al., 2014).

Importantly, several of these findings have been produced with use of neuroimaging and neuromodulation methods, such as structural magnetic resonance imaging (MRI) and repetitive transcranial magnetic stimulation (rTMS). These methods that have not typically been deployed for validation of health behavior theories, but may prove tremendously valuable, as they are increasingly integrated with social and behavioral research methods already within the domain of health behavior research. They have indeed been used fruitfully in the domain of emotion regulation research described later.

Nonetheless, the central question at hand is the following: how and when do affective processes fit into the TST model? This question is examined mostly with reference to health-related behaviors, given that they have been the primary application of the TST model to date. However, essentially the same mechanisms would be proposed to underlie behaviors outside of the health domain. In all cases, the interaction of affective processes is hypothetical, but could be tested directly in subsequent research.

AFFECT, EMOTIONS, AND THE HUMAN BRAIN

For the purposes of this review, affect is considered to comprise a broad spectrum of phenomena ranging from mood states to fundamental emotional experiences, as well as more complex social cognitive reactions to events (e.g., relief, disgust). The focus here is on emotional states as specific instances of affect, often more palpable and biologically mediated than other examples of affect, with correspondingly clearer points of intersection with the TST model.

In contrast with other more elusive mental phenomena, the neurobiological bases of emotional processes in the brain is somewhat well understood, at least in relation to negatively valenced emotional states such as anxiety (Denny et al., 2015; Ochsner, Silvers, & Buhle, 2012; Wilcox, Pommy, & Adinoff, 2016; Yarkoni et al., 2011). The limbic system plays a key role both in negative emotional reactivity (i.e., emotional responses elicited by external stimuli) and in emotional modulation. However the latter, including the ability to intervene or circumvent the emotional reactivity, is enabled by interconnectivity of the limbic system with higher cognitive control networks in the prefrontal and parietal regions. An example of the latter potential is illustrated by the influence of cognitive reevaluation of stimuli in order to preempt reactive negative emotionality. Other functions of the PFC include modulation of emotion after appearance, in a slightly more downstream form of raw inhibition. In short, the executive control system can play a role in both the emergence of emotional response and the modulation of the magnitude of such a response once it surfaces.

Despite the potential for executive control to influence all phases of response, there is good reason to believe that the effects of the PFC on the *emergence* of strong visceral states (cravings, emotional states, etc.) is more effective. For example, studies involving the use of noninvasive brain stimulation to experimentally manipulate PFC function show that such modulation has more potent effects on drive states than on the behavioral expression of such drive states (Jansen et al., 2013; Lowe, Vincent & Hall, 2016). This has been largely supported by work in the specific area of emotional regulation as well (Martin & Ochsner, 2016; Ochsner et al., 2012; Silvers, Buhle, & Ochsner, 2014; Silvers, Wager, Weber, & Ochsner, 2015; Wilcox et al., 2016).

It is difficult to envision being interested in human behavior—particularly behaviors that are prone to problems of self-control—and not being also interested in the function of the PFC. There are other interesting interactions between the PFC and emotional states beyond those described earlier. Although stress is not in itself an emotion, it is concomitant with anxiety, and it has been demonstrated that stress tends to impair dlPFC function. For instance in a recent fMRI study, cognitively stressful challenges induced decreased function of the dlPFC and also resulted in amplification of delay discounting of reward (Aranovich et al., 2016). Such findings show the potential for some affective dynamics to impair function of brain centers that are critical for behavioral self-control.

Behavioral Intentions, Prepotency, and Affect

In addition to executive control, the TST model posits that behavior is a joint function of intentional processes and behavioral prepotency, the latter being defined as the psychological "inertia" of the behavior, as a function of three nonexclusive factors: (1) past performance history in similar contexts, (2) the presence of strong cues to action in the environment, or (3) the emergence of behavior-impelling visceral states (including emotional states). Emotional responses are thought to contribute to behavior to the extent that they constitute visceral states and to the extent that they might influence the intentional sphere (i.e., motivation to perform a given behavior).

With respect to intention, it is possible that the experience of a strong negative emotional state might hijack the motivational system such that myopia for the present may occur, supplanting any nonimmediate goals or objectives that might otherwise be active. The influence of emotional states might be disproportionately observed when there are nonimmediate (or long-term) objectives that cannot be deliberated over effectively due to the crowding of working memory with thoughts and images pertaining to the current emotional state.

With respect to prepotency, the experience of strong emotional states could also result in stronger prepotency for some behaviors over others. For instance, when feeling acutely anxious, the prepotency associated with avoidance behaviors—which function to reduce the unpleasant state of being acutely anxious—might become much more probable than competing behaviors that involve engagement of the situation or others involved in the interpersonal interaction.

EMOTIONAL STATES AND INTENTION STABILITY

One of the primary criticisms of models that include intention as a central construct—for example, the theory of planned behavior (Ajzen & Madden, 1986)—is the lack of stability of intentions over time (Sheeran, 2002). This phenomenon is particularly well illustrated in the health behavior domain, wherein most of the population is familiar with the tendency to make resolutions to exercise more and snack less, only to be subject to the temptation of sedentary screen time and high-calorie snacks when they become immediately available. The empirical literature largely confirms the imperfect nature of the intention–behavior link, with a particular emphasis on intention instability as a key culprit (Conner & Godin, 2007; Conner, Norman, & Bell, 2002; Cooke & Sheeran, 2004, 20013; Rhodes & Dickau, 2012; Sheeran, 2002; Sheeran & Abraham, 2003; Sheeran & Webb, 2016; Webb & Sheeran, 2006). Such changes from healthy preferences to unhealthy ones in the heat of the moment are potentially a problem for intention-based models, to the extent that they assume that intentions are stable.

Intertemporal choice paradigms provide a mechanistic account of how the earlier preference intention instability can occur, with reference to value changes as a function of temporal proximity. According to Ainslie (1975, 2013), in the case of two competing behaviors, preferences for the initially more valuable alternative become inverted as a more temporally proximal but initially less valued alternative presents itself. For instance, when both options are removed in time, there may very well be strong preference for exercise over sedentary behavior, but when one is more accessible in a temporal sense (i.e., an opportunity for sedentary screen time), the rank ordering of the preferences for exercise and sedentary screen time reverses. This dynamic flipping of preference is thought to be one factor that underlies what seems to be intention instability (i.e., strong intentions to exercise followed by weaker intentions later on, when a choice point is reached). This phenomenon is thought to be a function of the human tendency to very steeply discount rewards that are removed in time; the shape of the value curve is hyperbolic, reflecting a steeper tendency to discount than an exponential curve that might reflect more classically rational temporal discounting (Figure 6.2). Delay discounting does tend to predict both intention stability and many behavioral tendencies that have health implications (Bickel & Marsch, 2001; Epstein, Salvy, Carr, Dearing, & Bickel, 2010).

Ultimately, the intention instability introduced by delay discounting may lead to imperfect prediction of behavior by intention, or lack of a causal effect of intention on behavior. A meta-analysis of experimental studies on intention-behavior causal effects revealed that while experimental manipulations that increase intentions do indeed work, the translation of such intention changes into changes in actual behavior is modest, particularly when such behavior is measured objectively (Webb &

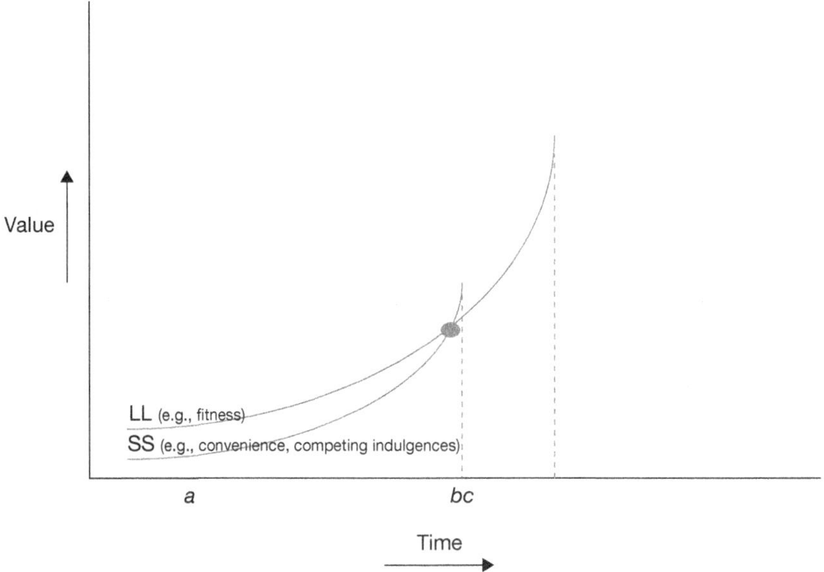

Figure 6.2. Hyperbolic discount curves depicting preference reversal in favor of sedentary activity over fitness.

Sheeran, 2006). Within the TST model, there are several moderators of the intention-behavior link, as it is indeed assumed to be imperfect.

One such moderator includes emotional states that might make preference reversals more likely to occur. For instance, when resolving to only eat healthy foods (an intention to avoid high-calorie snacks), one might still succumb to the temptation of potato chips following a stressful conversation with a significant other, or when otherwise in need of an indulgence of distraction. Although such dynamics involving eating may not be the norm, they are only one example of an emotional state that may temporarily highjack initial preferences. Many examples involving exercise, relationships, and financial behaviors exist as well. All of these suggest that emotions may make the intention-behavior link subject to momentary disruption.

Within the TST model, such disruptive influences could be conceptualized within the behavioral prepotency construct as mentioned earlier, but it could also be argued that momentary preferences may surge due to imperfect or ineffectively deployed executive control, motivated reasoning (i.e., a change in the intentional process itself, leading to new intention formation), or environmental circumstances that effect both the emergence of the emotional state and the ease of implementation of the intended behavior.

CONNECTEDNESS BELIEFS

Downstream from intention and behavior in the TST model are the constructs of connectedness beliefs and temporal valuations, the latter assumed to operate on the hyperbolic discounting rules described earlier. Connectedness beliefs are belief-based expectancies (derived from past experience, and other sources) that certain consequences will result from engaging in the target behavior. These can include expectancies of physical, relational, financial, or affective outcomes. Each outcome is rendered disproportionately more influential based on how proximal it will be, with those experienced during behavior being assumed to be most potent (i.e., highest immediacy = highest value, as per Ainslie's temporal discounting theory). Most health-related behaviors are thought to be performed with inconsistency because the bulk of the most immediate aspects of experience are negative (e.g., inconvenience, discomfort leading up to and in the early stages of the exercise bout), despite the nonimmediate benefits (e.g., improved appearance, mood, and health outcomes over time). However, the stark classifying of benefits into nonimmediate and costs into immediate in this example is not what is proposed by TST, but rather a consideration of the relative balance of expected outcomes, each weighted by temporal proximity. The positive emotional experience of exercise might indeed be influential on behavior precisely because of its immediacy, and such effects might explain why people exercise at all. To the extent that emotional experiences fuel both what people expect to occur upon future performance and when they expect those outcomes to occur, positive emotional responses to exercise (the "what" part of the equation) might be experienced during exercise (the "when" part of the equation) and might lend emotion some special significance in relation to the intention sphere of influence.

Indeed there is evidence that anticipated emotional reactions may influence behavior by determining the stability of the intention-behavior link. Conner, McEachan, Lawton, and Gardner (2016) demonstrated, in a prospective analysis of 20 behaviors, that intentions based on anticipated emotional consequences of engaging in a given behavior were a particularly potent determinant of intention stability. As applied to the TST model, it may be that expected positive affect might engender intentions that are more robust in relation to the prepotency of competing behavior. Rhodes and Kates (2015) recently found that exercise-related mood enhancements predicted future exercise behavior, consistent with the notion that experience-generated expectancies may improve the chances at behavior being repeated.

EMOTIONAL DISPOSITIONS

While the effects of some personality traits per se are reliable predictors of behaviors (including health behaviors; Murray & Booth, 2015), the magnitude of such relationships is sometimes overstated, a problem that has been long appreciated in the field (Mischel, 1968, 2009). This does not negate the possibility that individual differences more broadly may still interact at some meaningful level with the components of theoretical models of behavior that are predominantly social-cognitive in nature, and that such individual differences might have a link with underlying neurobiology (Berman et al., 2013; Hall, Fong, & Epp, 2014; Shoda, Mischel, & Wright, 1994). Indeed, individual differences in cognitive processes may account for some of the apparent link between personality traits and health-related behaviors (Hall, Fong, & Epp, 2014).

Individual differences in emotional temperament may have effects on moment-to-moment cognitive and behavioral processes included in the TST model. Overall level of emotional reactivity and cognitive ability (specifically executive control) might be important individual differences to consider as background forces, particularly when acting in concert with each other. A combination of high emotional reactivity and low executive control might render the environment a powerful force driving preference reversals, may reduce both intentional control over behavior in "strong" situations, and may imbue some reactive behaviors with more prepotency, regardless of intentions.

CONCLUSIONS

In conclusion, there are several indirect ways in which the TST model accounts for the influence of emotional states and dispositions on behavior. The first is in relation to the influence of emotions on intentional processes: strong negative emotions might preempt some goals and plans that are not consistent with a present-oriented focus. Second, emotions—as one type of visceral state—can abruptly alter the prepotency of a target behavior, thereby rendering behavior less likely in a direct sense, or via changes in intentional stability. Finally, emotional states—particularly negative mood states and stress—can reduce the effectiveness of executive control systems, rendering behavior more responsive to the environment.

To the extent that emotional processes affect several or all of these simultaneously, they may be especially relevant to behavioral performance. Although emotional processes are not represented directly, they are accounted for at several levels of the TST model, ranging from conscious cognition, to visceral experience, to neurobiological control substrates.

What makes emotions worthy of special consideration, among the host of other factors is the possibility that emotions may in some cases be particularly prominent actors, as demonstrated by Conner et al. (2016). With the advent of advanced neuroimaging techniques (fMRI; fNIR) that allow for identification of emotional state onset without conscious reporting, and neural correlates of emotional dispositions, there is much to be gained by integrating the science of human behavior with the science of the brain as a biological entity. It is likely that the most productive lines of inquiry will be those that consider both behavior and brain within social context.

REFERENCES

Aranovich, G., McClure, S. M., Fryer, S., Shanbhag, H., Roach, B. J., & Mathalon, D. H. (2016). The effect of cognitive stress on delay discounting. *NeuroImage, 124*, 733–739.

Ainslie, G. (1975). Specious reward: A behavioral theory of impulsiveness and impulse control. *Psychological Bulletin, 82*, 463–496.

Ainslie, G. (2013). *Picoeconomics in neural and evolutionary contexts*. In P. A. Hall (Ed.), *Social neuroscience and public health* (pp. 3–18). New York, NY: Springer.

Ajzen, I., & Madden, T. J. (1986). Prediction of goal-directed behavior: Attitudes, intentions and perceived behavioral control. *Journal of Experimental Social Psychology, 22*, 453–474.

Berman, M. G., Yourganov, G., Askren, M. K., Ayduk, O., Casey, B. J., Gotlib, I. H., . . . Jonides, J. (2013). Dimensionality of brain networks linked to life-long individual differences in self-control. *Nature Communications, 4*, 1373.

Best, J. R., Nagamatsu, L. S., & Liu-Ambrose, T. (2014). Improvements to executive function during exercise training predict maintenance of physical activity over the following year. *Frontiers in Human Neuroscience, 8*, 353. doi: 10.3389/fnhum.2014.00353

Best, J. R., Chiu, B. K., Hall, P. A., & Liu-Ambrose, T. (2017). Larger lateral prefrontal cortex volume predicts better exercise adherence among older women: Evidence from two exercise training studies. *Journals of Gerontology Series A: Biological Sciences and Medical Sciences, 72*, 804–810.

Bickel, W. K., & Marsch, L. A. (2001). Toward a behavioral economic understanding of drug dependence: Delay discounting processes. *Addiction, 96*, 73–78.

Bickel, W. K., Moody, L., Quisenberry, A. J., Ramey, C. T., & Sheffer, C. E. (2014). A competing neurobehavioral decision systems model of SES-related health and behavioral disparities. *Preventative Medicine, 68*, 37–43.

Cooke, R., & Sheeran, P. (2004) Moderation of cognition-intention and cognition-behaviour relations: A meta-analysis of properties of variables from the theory of planned behaviour. *British Journal of Social Psychology, 43*, 159–186.

Cooke, R., & Sheeran, P. (2013). Properties of intention: Component structure and consequences for behavior, information processing, and resistance. *Journal of Applied Social Psychology, 43*, 749–760.

Conner, M., & Godin, G. (2007). Temporal stability of behavioural intention as a moderator of intention–health behaviour relationships. *Psychology and Health, 22*, 875–897.

Conner, M., McEachan, R., Lawton, R., & Gardner, P. (2016). Basis of intentions as a moderator of the intention-health behavior relationship. *Health Psychology, 35*, 219–227.

Conner, M., McEachan, R., Taylor, N., O'Hara, J., & Lawton, R. (2016). Role of affective attitudes and anticipated affective reactions in predicting health behaviors. *Health Psychology, 34*, 642–652.

Conner, M., Norman, P., & Bell, R. (2002). The theory of planned behavior and healthy eating. *Health Psychology, 21*, 194–201.

Daly, M., McMinn, D., & Allan, J. (2015). A bidirectional relationship between physical activity and executive function in older adults. *Frontiers in Human Neuroscience, 8*, 1044.

Denny, B. T., Inhoff, N. C., Zerubavel, N., Davachi, L., & Ochsner, K. N. (2015). Getting over it: Long-lasting effects of emotion regulation on amygdala response. *Psychological Science, 26*, 1377–1388.

Epstein, L. H., Salvy, S. J., Carr, K. A., Dearing, K. K., & Bickel, W. K. (2010). Food reinforcement, delay discounting and obesity. *Physiology and Behavior, 100*, 438–445.

Gujral, S., McAuley, E., Oberlin, L., Kramer, A., Erickson, K. (2017, in press). The role of brain structure in predicting adherence to a physical activity regimen. *Psychosomatic Medicine*.

Hall, P. A. (2016). Executive-control processes in high-calorie food consumption. *Current Directions in Psychological Science, 25*, 91–97.

Hall, P. A., & Fong, G. T. (2007). Temporal self-regulation theory: A model for individual health behavior. *Health Psychology Review, 1*, 6–52.

Hall, P. A., & Fong, G. T. (2015). Temporal self-regulation theory: A neurobiologically informed model for physical activity behavior. *Frontiers in Human Neuroscience, 9*, 117.

Hall, P. A., Fong, G. T., & Epp, L. J. (2014). Cognitive and personality factors in the prediction of health behaviors: An examination of total, direct and indirect effects. *Journal of Behavioral Medicine, 37*, 1057–1068.

Hall, P. A., Lowe, C. J., & Vincent, C. M. (2017). Brain stimulation effects on food cravings and consumption: An update on Lowe et al. (2017) and a response to Generoso et al. (2017). *Psychosomatic Medicine, 79*, 839–842.

Hall, P. A., & Marteau, T. M. (2014). Executive function in the context of chronic disease prevention: Theory, research and practice. *Preventive Medicine, 68*, 44–50.

Hofmann, W., & Lotte Van Dillen. (2012). Desire: The new hot spot in self-control research. *Current Directions in Psychological Science, 21*(5), 317–322.

Jansen, J. M., Daams, J. G., Koeter, M. W., Veltman, D. J., van den Brink, W., & Goudriaan, A. E. (2013). Effects of non-invasive neurostimulation on craving: A meta-analysis. *Neuroscience and Biobehavioral Reviews, 37*, 1480–2472.

Lowe, C. J., Hall, P. A., & Staines, W. R. (2014). The effects of continuous theta burst stimulation to the left dorsolateral prefrontal cortex on executive function, food cravings, and snack food consumption. *Psychosomatic Medicine, 76*, 503–511.

Lowe, C. J., Vincent, C. M., & Hall, P. A. (2017). Effects of noninvasive brain stimulation on food cravings and consumption: A meta-analytic review. *Psychosomatic Medicine, 79*, 2–13.

Martin, R. E., & Ochsner, K. N. (2016). The neuroscience of emotion regulation development: Implications for education. *Current Opinion in Behavioral Sciences, 10*, 142–148.

McClure, S. M., & Bickel, W. K. (2014). A dual systems perspective on addiction: Contributions from neuroimaging and cognitive training. *Annals of the New York Academy of Sciences, 1327*, 62–78.

Miller, E. K. (2000). The prefrontal cortex and cognitive control. *Nature Reviews Neuroscience, 1*, 59–66.

Miller, E. K., & Cohen, J. D. (2001). An integrative theory of prefrontal cortex function. *Annual Review of Neuroscience, 24*, 167–202.

Miyake, A., & Friedman, N. P. (2012). The nature and organization of individual differences in executive functions four general conclusions. *Current Directions in Psychological Science, 21*, 8–14.

Mischel, W. (1968). *Personality and assessment*. New York: Wiley.

Mischel, W. (2009). From personality and assessment (1968) to personality science, 2009. *Journal of Research in Personality, 43*, 282–290.

Murray, A., & Booth, T. (2015). Personality and physical health. *Current Opinion in Psychology, 5*, 50–55.

Ochsner, K. N., Silvers, J. A., & Buhle, J. T. (2012). Functional imaging studies of emotion regulation: A synthetic review and evolving model of the cognitive control of emotion. *Annals of the New York Academy of Sciences, 1251*, E1–E24.

Rhodes, R. E., & Dickau, L. (2012). Experimental evidence for the intention–behavior relationship in the physical activity domain: A meta-analysis. *Health Psychology, 31*, 724–727.

Rhodes, R. E., & Kates, A. (2015). Can the affective response to exercise predict future motives and physical activity behavior? A systematic review of published evidence. *Annals of Behavioral Medicine, 49*, 715–731.

Sheeran, P. (2002). Intention–behavior relations: A conceptual and empirical review. *European Review of Social Psychology, 12*, 1–36.

Sheeran, P., & Abraham, C. (2003). Mediator of moderators: Temporal stability of intention and the intention-behavior relation. *British Journal of Health Psychology, 29*, 205–215.

Sheeran, P., & Webb, T. L. (2016). The intention–behavior gap. *Social and Personality Psychology Compass, 10*, 503–518.

Shoda, Y., Mischel, W., & Wright, J. C. (1994). Intraindividual stability in the organization and patterning of behavior: Incorporating psychological situations into the ideographic analysis of personality. *Journal of Personality and Social Psychology, 67*, 674–687.

Silvers, J. A., Buhle, J. T., & Ochsner, K. N. (2014). The neuroscience of emotion regulation: Basic mechanisms and their role in development, aging and psychopathology. In K. N. Ochsner & S. M. Kosslyn (Eds.), *The Oxford handbook of cognitive neuroscience*, Vol. 2: *The cutting edges* (pp. 53–78). New York, NY: Oxford University Press.

Silvers, J. A., Wager, T. D., Weber, J., & Ochsner, K. N. (2015). The neural bases of uninstructed negative emotion modulation. *Social Cognitive and Affective Neuroscience, 10*, 10–18.

Webb, T. L., & Sheeran, P. (2006). Does changing behavioral intentions engender behavior change? A meta-analysis of the experimental evidence. *Psychological Bulletin, 132*, 249–268.

Wilcox, C. E., Pommy, J. M., & Adinoff, B. (2016). Neural circuitry of impaired emotion regulation in substance use disorders. *American Journal of Psychiatry, 173*, 344–361. doi: 10.1176/appi.ajp.2015.15060710.

Yarkoni, T., Poldrack, R. A., Nichols, T. E., Van Essen, D. C., & Wager, T. D. (2011). Large-scale automated synthesis of human functional neuroimaging data. *Nature methods, 8*, 665–670.

7

Affect in the Context of Self-Determination Theory

MARTIN S. HAGGER AND CLEO PROTOGEROU

INTRODUCTION

Self-determination theory (Deci & Ryan, 1985, 2000) is an established theory of motivation that has been applied extensively to the prediction and understanding of health-related behavior. Although the theory is positioned in the organismic, humanistic tradition, researchers have demonstrated that it is closely related with the antecedents of health-related behavior from multiple theories based on the social cognitive tradition (Biddle, Hagger, Chatzisarantis, & Lippke, 2007; Hagger & Chatzisarantis, 2009; Wilson, Rodgers, Blanchard, & Gessell, 2003). However, unlike the belief-based, information-processing perspective that pervades social cognitive approaches, self-determination theory focuses on psychological needs and motivational quality as central factors that determine motivation toward, engagement in, and persistence with health-related behavior (Ryan & Deci, 2000). The theory has been shown to be efficacious in explaining variance in numerous health-related behaviors and also for guiding interventions to promote greater participation in health behaviors (e.g., Chatzisarantis, Hagger, Biddle, Smith, & Wang, 2003; Ng et al., 2012; Teixeira et al., 2016). In addition, self-determination theory has also focused on predicting a number of adaptive outcomes related to motivation and behavioral engagement, including positive emotional and affective outcomes. A growing body of research has demonstrated the effect of motivational constructs from self-determination theory on affective responses in health-related contexts, as well as adaptive emotion-related outcomes that are important for overall health, such as psychological well-being and life satisfaction (Deci & Ryan, 2008; Ng et al., 2012; Williams, Frankel, Campbell, & Deci, 2000). There is also evidence to suggest that emotional responses, particularly positive affect and psychological well-being, are integral to motivation itself within self-determination theory (Deci & Ryan, 2000; Ryan, Huta, & Deci, 2006). In the current chapter, we outline the general tenets of self-determination theory, identify the role that emotion and affect plays in self-determination theory as an outcome and a process, review the research applying self-determination theory in health behavior contexts, outline possible future research on affect and self-determination theory applied to health contexts, and summarize the importance of affect in the development of behavioral interventions based on self-determination theory to promote better health.

THE THEORY

Self-determination theory (Deci & Ryan, 1985, 2000) is a broad, empirically based theory of motivation that focuses on fundamental processes that relate to salient outcomes in everyday life, including psychological needs and aspirations, goal setting and attainment, self-regulation, interpersonal relations, emotions and affect, cultural and societal influences, and nonconscious processes. The theory has been applied to explain motivation in numerous contexts including education (Black & Deci,

2000; Hagger, Sultan, Hardcastle, & Chatzisarantis, 2015), the workplace (Chan & Hagger, 2012; Gagné & Deci, 2005), sport (Chan et al., 2015; Jõesaar, Hein, & Hagger, 2012; Wallhead, Hagger, & Smith, 2010), health (Teixeira, Carraca, Markland, Silva, & Ryan, 2012; Williams, Minicucci, et al., 2002), economics (Webb, Soutar, Mazzarol, & Saldaris, 2013), and interpersonal relations (Deci & Ryan, 2008).

Basic Needs and the Organismic Dialectic

Central to self-determination theory is the concept of basic psychological needs. The theory specifies three psychological needs—*competence, relatedness*, and *autonomy*—that are seen as innate, fundamental prerequisites or "nutriments" for optimal growth and happiness in humans (Deci & Ryan, 2000). The need for competence, also referred to as effectance, is the individual's need to have an impact on their environment and to experience a sense of mastery over actions. The need for competence is satisfied through the learning and mastering of new skills, setting goals, and successful goal attainment. The need for relatedness is the desire to connect with others, to love and care for others, and to be loved and cared for by others. The need for relatedness is satisfied through functional group membership and close relationships. The need for autonomy is the propensity to be agentic and to experience a sense of ownership and volition when acting. The need for autonomy is satisfied through the experience of voluntary initiation, execution, and control of behavior. While the theory views competence, relatedness, and autonomy as basic and universal, it also assumes individual differences in the ways people interact in their social environments to satisfy their needs. Basic psychological needs are viewed as the driving force behind motivated action and are viewed as a unifying concept within self-determination theory (Ryan & Deci, 2000). From the perspective of the theory, the important question is not the existence of needs per se—Deci and Ryan point to research demonstrating their existence and universality (Sheldon, Elliot, Kim, & Kasser, 2001)—but rather the extent to which needs are satisfied. The type and quality of motivation toward actions in a given context will determine whether psychological needs are satisfied and the extent to which needs are satisfied will motivate individuals to seek out those actions and experiences in future.

Self-determination theory puts forth the *organismic dialectic* as a fundamental lifelong human process, which exemplifies an *active* dialogue between the individual and others, and functions to produce a coherent and consistent sense of self through the satisfaction of the basic psychological needs (Deci & Ryan, 2000). The organismic dialectic that underpins the theory is firmly in line with philosophical precursors immersed in the humanistic and philosophical traditions that focus on the optimally functioning organism. The term "organismic" is derived from the Greek word "organismós" and refers to an entity comprising mutually interdependent parts and, more loosely, to a living creature. The word "dialectic" is a direct translation of the Greek word "dialektikḗ," which means engaging in logical discourse or conversation, with the aim to find truth and meaning. The organismic dialectic assumes that people are born with innate, natural tendencies to "engage interesting activities, to exercise capacities, to pursue connectedness in social groups, and to integrate intrapsychic and interpersonal experiences into a relative unity" (Deci & Ryan, 2000, p. 229). These inherent developmental tendencies are not satisfied automatically or easily, rather, they require the individual to actively seek "nutriments" and supports in the social environment that scaffold their development. In the context of self-determination theory, these nutriments are represented through the needs of autonomy, relatedness, and competence. However, it is important to stress that the theory does not attribute the organismic dialectic to a need deficit, as previous motivation theorists have postulated (e.g., Hull, 1943; Maslow, 1943). Rather, self-determination theory assumes that seeking need satisfaction in the environment is a natural and organic process. The theory, therefore, suggests that individuals seek to develop overall coherence and consistency in motives and action such that goals and behaviors are consistent with the optimally functioning, genuine sense of self.

Motivational Regulations and a Graded Continuum of Motivation

Beyond individual differences, Deci and Ryan (2000) suggest that individuals engage in activities in given contexts for reasons that are broadly autonomous or self-determined, or broadly controlled or non-self-determined. They propose a set of motivational styles or *regulations* that reflect the extent to which actions or behaviors satisfy psychological needs and have been partly or wholly internalized into an individual's repertoire of need-satisfying behaviors. Three autonomous regulations have been identified: intrinsic motivation (engaging in activities because they are inherently interesting and satisfying, even in the apparent absence of any external controlling contingency), integration (engaging in activities that are consistent with goals and values that are characteristic of the individual's genuine sense of self), and identification (engaging in activities that are self-endorsed and lead to self-relevant outcomes with which they strongly identify). Controlled regulations reflect non-self-determined reasons for acting, such that behavior is determined by contingencies that are perceived to be, or are actually, external to the individual. Two forms of controlled regulation have been proposed: introjection (engaging in activities driven by a desire to be approved by external agents in the environment) and external regulation or extrinsic motivation (engagement in activities in order to gain external rewards and avoid potential punishment). Finally, amotivation reflects the absence of any autonomous or controlled form of motivation. In an amotivated state, the person is not inclined to act due to a sense of diminished efficacy in relation to desired outcomes, or because the person does not find value in the outcome. Autonomous regulations have been consistently associated with better physical and emotional health and, critically, positive affect (Deci & Ryan, 2000; Ng et al., 2012).

The regulatory motives are conceptualized as delineating a self-determination *continuum* (Howard, Gagné, & Bureau, 2017). Intrinsic motivation and external regulation are represented at the extremes or "poles" of the continuum and the intermediate motivational regulations are situated along the continuum according to their relative degree of autonomy. Amotivation lies outside the continuum because it reflects a lack of endorsement of any reason for acting. The self-determination continuum reflects individuals' motives for action in line with the organismic dialectic. The type of motivational regulation an individual experiences with respect to goal-oriented actions or behaviors will be positioned on the continuum according to the extent to which the behaviors have been internalized as those that satisfies needs. Actions that are autonomously motivated are considered adaptive, as they are likely to contribute to psychological need satisfaction, increased psychological growth, optimal functioning, and better well-being (Deci & Ryan, 2000; Ng et al., 2012).

Intrinsic motivation is conceptualized as the prototypic form of autonomous motivation, and reflects engaging in behaviors out of the inherent interest, satisfaction, and positive emotion derived from the behavior itself. Importantly, individuals engage in intrinsically motivated actions, even in the apparent absence of any external contingency, and are behaviors that satisfy basic psychological needs. In line with this premise, intrinsically motivated actions play a unique role in self-determination theory as they are viewed as fundamental to lifelong psychological growth and the development of an optimally functioning genuine sense of self (Deci & Ryan, 1985). Importantly, intrinsically motivated actions are associated with optimal self-regulation of actions and persistence on tasks. In contrast, externally motivated behaviors reflect engaging in action for external contingencies such as rewards or praise or to avoid punishment or criticism. External regulation is the prototypical form of extrinsic or controlled motivation. The controlling contingencies in externally regulated action undermine intrinsic motivation and are associated with maladaptive outcomes including diminished creativity, problem-solving, psychological well-being and analytic thought, as well as negative affect and frustration (Deci & Ryan, 2000, 2008).

Of course, not all behaviors are characterized by the prototypical motivational styles of intrinsic motivation and external regulation (Ryan & Deci, 2009). Individuals' actions are frequently regulated by interpersonal styles situated on intermediate positions on the self-determination continuum. The styles reflect actions that are, to some extent, autonomous or controlled. For example, acting out of identified regulation reflects engaging in behaviors for some self-endorsed, personally valued goal or outcome rather than the action itself. In this case, an individual might not particularly enjoy or derive intrinsic satisfaction from engaging in a health behavior like physical activity. However, outcomes derived from the activity, such as the feeling of satisfaction afterward and its role in maintaining fitness that are autonomously valued, lead the behavior to be one that satisfies psychological needs. In this respect, the continuum represents an important property of the organismic dialectic, in that individuals will tend to *internalize* and *integrate* external reasons for engaging in behavior if the behavior is experienced as servicing autonomous goals and satisfying psychological needs (Deci, Eghrari, Patrick, & Leone, 1994; Deci & Ryan, 2000). The internalization process is adaptive as it enables individuals to incorporate more actions into their repertoire of need-satisfying behaviors. This process does not happen immediately but occurs through repeatedly experiencing actions as autonomous and supporting psychological needs in contexts and environmental conditions that are likely to be autonomy supportive. Taking the previous example of physical activity, the behavior is characterized as one that is partially internalized with potential to be fully integrated over the passage of time resulting in a shift in regulatory style toward the autonomous pole. Such a shift may occur over time with experience of the activity as servicing autonomous goals and under conditions that are conducive to supporting autonomy (Deci & Ryan, 2000).

Theoretical Underpinnings and Corollaries

The concept of psychological needs in self-determination theory is consistent with humanistic perspectives of needs as innate and psychological as opposed to exclusively biological (DeCharms, 1968; Maslow, 1943). Needs for autonomy and competence are closely related to control-related constructs (Hagger, 2014) that feature prominently in social-cognitive theories (e.g., Ajzen, 2015; Bandura, 1977). The need for relatedness reflects early attachment perspectives that argue for an innate tendency for humans to form close relationships with others (e.g., Bowlby, 1958). The lifelong human endeavor to satisfy needs in the social environment proposed in the organismic dialectic echoes drive growth processes for competence, effectance, and, ultimately, maturity (e.g., White, 1959). Evidence for autonomy, competence, and relatedness as candidate needs has been identified in research across nations and cultural groups, providing important evidence that the needs are innate and universal (Sheldon et al., 2001). However, there have also been suggestions that self-esteem (Sheldon et al., 2001), benevolence (Martela & Ryan, 2016), and novelty (González-Cutre, Sicilia, Sierra, Ferriz, & Hagger, 2016) are also separate candidate needs, although evidence in support of these needs is in its infancy. Suffice to say that needs as a unifying concept within self-determination theory has some support, but it is important to note that direct evidence is relatively sparse.

AFFECT AND SELF-DETERMINATION THEORY

Affect and emotional responses have an important place within the predictions and corollaries of self-determination theory. Generally, affect has been conceptualized in two ways within the theory: as an outcome and as part of the processes by which psychological need satisfaction and autonomous motivation, as core concepts within the theory, relate to engagement and persistence in action. Next we outline these two functions of affect within self-determination theory and highlight how research on these functions provides insight into the role of affect in the motivation of health behavior.

Affect as an Outcome in Self-Determination Theory

From its inception, affect has been identified as a key outcome of self-determined motivation (Deci & Ryan, 1985; Ryan & Deci, 2001). In cognitive evaluation theory (Deci & Ryan, 1985), a fundamental subtheory of self-determination theory, external contingencies (e.g., rewards, deadlines, threats), are proposed to undermine intrinsic motivation, and result in a concomitant increase in generalized negative affect and related negative emotional responses, such as frustration, reduced positive affect, and reduced interest and enjoyment. In contrast, contingencies in the environment that bolster intrinsic motivation, such as informative feedback, are associated with increased interest, enjoyment, and positive affect and a mitigation of negative affect. These affective responses were evidenced in formative experimental work on cognitive evaluation theory using the free choice paradigm, as a behavioral means to measure intrinsic motivation, and the subsequent development of the intrinsic motivation inventory (Deci, 1972). In free choice experiments, participants provided with rewards exhibited reduced motivation on an inherently interesting task during a free choice period, and also subsequently reported less interest, enjoyment, and engagement in the task. In contrast, participants provided with an informational justification for the task or with contingent feedback were less vulnerable to the undermining effect of external rewards, and were less likely to experience negative affect (Deci, Koestner, & Ryan, 1999).

This general tendency for affective responses to be related to motivational styles and motivational responses to external contingencies has also been observed in the field in health contexts. Consistent with the general tenets of the theory, motivational regulations that reflect greater internalization, including integrated and identified forms of motivation, and, therefore, more autonomous or self-determined forms of motivation with respect to a particular health behavior, are associated with greater intentions to participate in a target health-related behavior and actual future engagement in the behavior. This has been found in research adopting self-determination theory in physical activity (Chatzisarantis et al., 2003; Teixeira et al., 2012), smoking cessation (Williams, Gagne, Ryan, & Deci, 2002), alcohol reduction (Caudwell & Hagger, 2015; Hagger et al., 2012), and occupational risk reduction (Chan, Fung, Xing, & Hagger, 2014; Chan & Hagger, 2012). The research also demonstrates that individuals experiencing their action as self-determined are more likely to persist with the health behavior and less likely to drop out (Sarrazin, Vallerand, Guillet, Pelletier, & Cury, 2002).

Importantly, just as autonomous motivation has been shown to predict intentions and action in health contexts (Hagger & Chatzisarantis, 2016; Pihu, Hein, Koka, & Hagger, 2008), autonomous motivation been shown to predict adaptive emotional responses, including increased positive affect and psychological well-being, in health (Deci et al., 2001; Sheldon et al., 2004). For example, in the context of healthy eating, individuals who adopt autonomous motives like intrinsic motivation (e.g., they enjoy and value healthy eating itself) or identified regulation (e.g., they view healthy eating as important to personal goals such as losing weight, gaining more energy, and feeling less lethargic) are more likely to experience enjoyment, satisfaction, and positive emotions as a consequence of the behavior. In contrast, individuals adopting more controlled reasons such as introjected regulation (e.g., eating healthily out of obligation to others) are likely to feel increased negative affect such as guilt and frustration (Koestner & Losier, 2002). Further, if the perceived introject or obligation is removed, the individual will likely lapse from their healthy eating. Overall, therefore, motivational styles that reflect greater autonomy will be related to behavioral persistence and adaptive affective responses.

Research has shown that need satisfaction is related to a number of adaptive outcomes, including affect-related outcomes and behavioral persistence (Ryan & Deci, 2000). This is consistent with the overall premise that psychological need satisfaction is a unifying construct within self-determination theory. Just as satisfaction of psychological needs has been shown to be related to increased autonomous motivation and behavioral outcomes, need satisfaction has also been shown to relate to positive affective outcomes and reduced negative affect. For example, research in the domain of physical activity has consistently demonstrated that individuals who feel that engaging in a target health behavior satisfies their psychological needs are more likely to report participating for autonomous reasons, and are also more likely to experience the activity as enjoyable, satisfying, and interesting (Sebire, Jago, Fox, Edwards, & Thompson,

2013). In contrast, when the individual experiences his or her needs as being thwarted or frustrated by the context or environment, they are more likely to avoid or desist from physical activity and report heightened levels of frustration and negative affect (Gunnell, Crocker, Wilson, Mack, & Zumbo, 2013).

As an outcome, therefore, research has indicated that engaging in health behaviors for self-determined reasons and experiencing the action as supporting the satisfaction of the three basic psychological needs, is related to not only adaptive behavioral outcomes but also increased positive affect. In some respects, affective responses, as a consequence of autonomous behavioral engagement and need satisfaction, have essentially been treated as emotional byproducts of the motivational regulation. In other words, the emotional responses are considered indicators of autonomous motivation and psychological need satisfaction. However, there is increased recognition that emotional responses are an important health-related outcome in their own right. Emotional responses may have a persistence function that provides essential feedback to the individual indicating the optimal nature of their autonomous actions. The emotional response may, therefore, serve an important function in the continuity of action and reinforcing further persistence with the task in future so as to further satisfy psychological needs.

AFFECT AS A PROCESS IN SELF-DETERMINATION THEORY

Most research investigating the role of self-determination theory in predicting health behavior has focused on affect as an outcome. This is based on the premise that affect indicates the type of motivational regulation experienced by the actor. Positive affect reflects autonomous motivation and the optimal satisfaction of psychological needs, and negative affect reflects controlled motivation and the lack of, or thwarting of, psychological needs. In contrast, research that has focused on the role of affect as a process in the genesis of self-determined action has received relatively less attention. However, Ryan and Deci (2001) have illustrated how well-being and self-determined motivation are inextricably linked, and Vallerand (2008) has illustrated how extreme forms of self-determined motivation lead to participation in behavior that is highly emotive, in research on passion. Furthermore, management and acceptance of affective responses are inextricably linked to the process by which autonomously motivated individuals effectively regulate their behavior (Legault & Inzlicht, 2013). We deal with each of these issues in turn.

Well-Being and Autonomous Motivation

As outlined previously, psychological well-being is considered an important component of health. Psychological well-being is defined as a state of psychological wellness and reflects overall satisfaction with all aspects of mental health and quality of life. It is, therefore, strongly related to indices of emotional health, such as positive affect, and quality of life. Psychological well-being is consistently related to autonomous motivation. However, well-being is also implicated in the process by which autonomous motivation leads to better overall health and future motivation to engage in health behaviors. Ryan and Deci (2001) make the distinction between hedonic and eudaimonic well-being when discussing the importance of affect and emotion as a process in self-determination theory. Consistent with Ryff and Singer's (2000) conceptualization, the concept of hedonic well-being reflects the pursuit of a state of happiness and felt positive emotion as an end goal. In contrast, eudaimonic well-being focuses on obtaining a state of optimal functioning reflecting personal growth of the true self and a sense of consistency between motives and action, self-actualization or realization, and congruence between action and personally held values. Accordingly, hedonic well-being focuses on felt emotions and happiness alone with little meaning or internal value (Ryff & Singer, 2000). The eudaimonic approach eschews the emphasis on felt happiness and positive emotion for its own sake, and focuses on the attainment of outcomes that reflect self-actualization including mastery of actions, perceived ownership and agency in one's actions, personal growth, cohesive and meaningful relations with others, and self-actualization (see Ryff & Keyes, 1995). Well-being itself is inextricably linked to positive emotion, with definitions of well-being focusing on the greater frequency of overall feelings of positive affect, but also, consistent with the eudaimonic perspective, greater quality and meaning of the felt emotions.

According to Ryan and Deci (2001), experiences of competence and autonomy are related to psychological well-being, but well-being and adaptive emotions are also implicated in motivational outcomes. Links between experiences of competence and effectance toward health behaviors and psychological well-being are indicative of the properties of self-determined motivation in promoting self-actualization and optimal functioning. Well-being also operates in the process by which autonomous motivation leads to future action. Research has suggested that congruence between the goals that individuals pursue and their motivation relates to subjective well-being. Goal-motive consistency is indicated in levels of well-being, such that as consistency increases so does well-being and the likelihood of future behavioral persistence (Sheldon & Kasser, 1998). For example, if an individual's reasons for acting are autonomous they are more likely to be consistent with the goals that they endorse and choose, and reflect their genuine self. This is likely to lead to greater feelings of positive affect and an overall sense of well-being. In contrast, acting for controlled reasons are likely to conflict with autonomous goals and the sense of inconsistency will not foster well-being. Similarly, while goal progress may lead to happiness in the short term, it is the fulfilling nature of the goal content that leads to well-being. Pursuit of autonomous goals that are consistent with personal values and a genuine, authentic sense of self are more likely to be related to greater experience of well-being. While these findings implicate indices of positive emotion and overall well-being in the process of motivation toward health behavior, evidence of the effects of these factors on subsequent motivation is relatively limited and more research is needed to explore these reciprocal effects.

Passion and Emotion

A related perspective on emotion and well-being derived from the self-determination theory approach is Vallerand's (2008) dualistic perspective on passion. In his model, Vallerand defines passion as "a strong inclination toward a self-defining activity that one likes (or even loves), finds important, and in which one invests time and energy" (Vallerand, 2008, p. 2). In most respects this definition of passion has parallels with intrinsic motivation as the pursuit of tasks in the absence of external contingencies and to gain a sense of effectance, mastery and competence, self-actualization, and need satisfaction. Vallerand highlights that engaging in activities toward which individuals are passionate is essential to the process of constructing a repertoire of behaviors that satisfy psychological needs and define one's genuine sense of self. Hobbies and leisure-time pursuits are often identified as exemplifying activities that are highly intrinsically motivating and are seen as central to an individual's identity and related to eudaimonic well-being. In many ways, therefore, passion is an extreme form of intrinsic motivation and part of the process by which individuals develop, grow, and attain optimal functioning and promote good psychological health.

However, Vallerand identifies the lighter and darker sides of passion in the distinction between harmonious and obsessive passion. *Harmonious* passion reflects an autonomous, self-endorsed pursuit of an activity that is fully integrated into the individual's true sense of self and identity. Individuals engaging in these activities are met with a sense of effortless control and positive affect. In some respects, this is the prototypical form of passion, and one that is linked to better psychological well-being. In contrast, Vallerand suggests that not all passionately pursued activities are fully integrated into the individuals' repertoire of need-satisfying behaviors. These *obsessive* passions may be pursued due to externally felt contingencies such as the desire to please others or for a sense of contingent self-worth. Or the individual may derive a sense of meaning and satisfaction from the activity, but their engagement in the activity is uncontrollable and not need satisfying or integrated into their true sense of self. An individual engaging in activities for which they are obsessively passionate experiences an inability to control his or her engagement or desistence from the activity. As the pursuit of the activity is ego-involving, the individual engages through rigid persistence, and, as a result, may engage in the activity at the expense of other more important aspects of their life, making their obsession unhealthy and undermining their well-being.

A harmoniously passionate exerciser will engage in physical activity as part of their fully integrated self and, as such, will choose to spend as much free time as possible exercising, but it will not be at the expense of other important activities. In contrast, a person who is obsessively passionate about their exercise routine may feel a sense of frustration and negative affect when exercising when they know they should be focusing their attention on other important life activities, but cannot stop themselves because of their perceived obligation to the activity. Conversely, the person might feel that they should be focusing on other activities but become frustrated when they are not able focus on the activity they are passionate about. In this way, obsessive passion resembles addiction—the person may not view that balancing other elements in their life as a priority as long as they "exercise." As a consequence they experience no sense of balance of "harmony" with respect to their exercise and other aspects of their life.

Vallerand and coworkers (2003) demonstrated the effects of the dual theory of passion in numerous studies using their "passion" scale, which has obsessive and harmonious subscales. Overall, harmonious passion was related to optimal pursuit of tasks and indices of psychological health including psychological well-being, vitality, and life satisfaction in multiple contexts, including health behavior. In contrast, obsessive passion was unrelated or negatively related to these constructs. In addition, research has demonstrated that the mechanism by which harmonious passion relates to adaptive outcomes is through the persistent experience of positive affect. For example, a longitudinal study in a physical activity context indicated that harmonious passion predicted psychological adjustment mediated by positive affect, while obsessive passion was related to negative affect and unrelated to adjustment (Rousseau & Vallerand, 2008). Overall, the research demonstrates the importance of optimal, autonomous engagement in activities that are consistent with psychological needs and that obsessive pursuit of behaviors that are internalized but not integrated can undermine well-being and is associated with lower functioning and psychological adjustment.

Emotion, Self-Determination and Self-Regulation

A final perspective on the role of emotion in self-determination theory applied to health behaviors comes from research on autonomous motivation in the self-regulation of actions. Self-regulation reflects an individual's capacity to override a well-learned "dominant" response or a response that is strongly linked to impulses, urges, and cravings that are often reinforced by intrinsic reward (e.g., sensations of pleasure through dopaminergic pathways in the brain) (Allom, Mullan, & Hagger, 2016; Inzlicht, Schmeichel, & Macrae, 2014). Many health-related behaviors such as healthy eating, physical activity, quitting smoking, reducing alcohol consumption, and condom use require an individual to forego the short-term rewards related to engaging in the undesired health-compromising behavior, in favor of longer-term desired outcomes such as psychological well-being and quality of life (Hagger, Leung, et al., 2013; Hagger, Panetta, et al., 2013; Mpondo, Ruiter, van den Borne, & Reddy, 2015; Muraven & Shmueli, 2006). There are numerous perspectives on self-regulation; many view self-regulation as an individual difference, an enduring trait that increases individuals' capacity to pursue long-term goals over short-term gain in multiple domains (Allom, Panetta, Mullan, & Hagger, 2016; de Ridder, Lensvelt-Mulders, Finkenauer, Stok, & Baumeister, 2012).

There is also research suggesting that individuals provided with autonomous goal pursuit or provided with autonomy support prior to engaging in tasks that require self-control (e.g., controlling impulses, thoughts, and emotions) demonstrate better persistence on the tasks (Moller, Deci, & Ryan, 2006). The research indicated that autonomous motivation led individuals to experience the tasks as important to their internalized or integrated goals rather than focus on the arduousness of the task or the limitations of their capacity for self-control. A recently proposed perspective indicates that autonomously motivated individuals recognize and expect the inherent negative affect and aversive experiences when pursuing challenging tasks toward long-term goals (Legault & Inzlicht, 2013). However, autonomously oriented individuals are able to persist on effortful tasks, and effectively manage the associated aversive affective responses, because they have internalized or integrated the long-term goal or outcome as important to their genuine sense of self and satisfying of their basic psychological needs. Legault and Inzlicht (2013) showed that autonomously oriented individuals were better at engaging in tasks requiring self-regulation. Using an electroencephalogram (EEG), the researchers found that the effect of autonomous orientation on self-regulatory task performance was mediated by error-related negativity (ERN), a neural signal related to error detection on tasks. Legault and Inzlicht replicated and extended their findings in an experimental paradigm where they manipulated autonomy support, and examined its effects on self- regulatory capacity under conditions of ego-depletion, and found the mediating effect of the ERN signals. The ERN signals were interpreted as indicative of autonomous individuals' capacity to recognize and accept aversive feelings like negative affect as part of the task. As a consequence they did not have reactive or defensive responses to threatening self-relevant information, such as failure on the tasks. These better self-regulatory capacities meant they were better able to cope with the aversive nature of the tasks and were, therefore, better able to self-regulate. This research emphasizes the important role that affect and autonomous individuals' means to cope with it plays in self-regulation.

RECOMMENDATIONS FOR FUTURE RESEARCH AND PRACTICE

Self-determination theory has been used as a means to guide health behavior change intervention development (Ryan, Patrick, Deci, & Williams, 2008). The key focus of these interventions has been to promote the autonomy support of leaders and figures of authority that will foster autonomous forms of motivation among the people under their leadership or influence. The resulting autonomy-supportive social environment (also known as a motivational "climate') increases the internalization and integration of the target behavior by the people acting in the environment. Research has identified the components of autonomy support that are likely to promote autonomous motivation (Hardcastle et al., 2017; Hardcastle, Blake, & Hagger, 2012; Koka & Hagger, 2010; Reeve, Bolt, & Cai, 1999), and programs have been developed that aim to train individuals to promote an autonomy supportive social environment (Cheon, Reeve, & Moon, 2012; McLachlan & Hagger, 2010). These components are behaviors that significant others need to adopt to promote an autonomy-supportive social environment with respect to the behavior of interest: providing choice over behavioral options, providing noncontingent positive feedback regarding behavioral engagement, avoiding controlling language (e.g., "should" or "must") when promoting the target behavior, providing a meaningful rationale for the behavior, being responsive to the actors' questions, providing experiences of competence, and making perspective-acknowledging statements.

There have been recent developments in charting the different individual, irreducible, replicable "components" of behavior change intervention in "taxonomies" of behavior change techniques (Michie et al., 2013). These "components" are the content of interventions that lead to behavior change, and are often referred to as the "active ingredients" of interventions. This is important to identify and isolate the components that do the work when it comes to changing behavior. Consistent with this process, researchers are engaging in a process to do the same for the components of autonomy supportive interventions (Teixeira et al., 2016). There is recognition that such components comprise content (i.e., *what* is said or delivered to individuals to change their behavior) and interpersonal style (i.e., *how* content is delivered to interventions). The interpersonal style components have been identified as parameters that affect the delivery and assimilation of content-based techniques while others have identified them as separate "relational" techniques in their own right (Dombrowski & Luszczynska, 2009;

Hagger & Hardcastle, 2014; Hardcastle, Fortier, Blake, & Hagger, 2016). The interpersonal style components include aspects of emotional support and warmth in the interpersonal relations between significant others and the individuals with whom they work. Positive interpersonal relations are an aspect of interpersonal style that will foster greater relatedness and, as a consequence, greater autonomous motivation. A "taxonomy" of autonomy supportive behavior-change techniques is currently under development (Teixeira et al., 2016). The taxonomy will serve as a useful tool for leaders and authority figures in identifying the appropriate behavior that could be adopted to promote autonomy support. The taxonomy will also permit researchers to identify which components are most effective in promoting autonomous motivation and the extent to which they interact in determining health behavior change through the adoption of factorial designs.

To date, research on autonomy supportive interventions has demonstrated their effectiveness in promoting change in physical activity (Chatzisarantis & Hagger, 2009), medication and self-management (Williams, McGregor, Zeldman, & Freedman, 2004), smoking (Williams, Gagne, et al., 2002), and healthy eating (Resnicow et al., 2008) behaviors. The research has also shown that changes in behavior are also met with changes in affect-related outcomes such as psychological well-being, vitality, and positive affect. However, to our knowledge, no intervention has sought to include components to assist in the management of stress and negative affect in self-determination theory based interventions in health contexts. Such emotion-reducing intervention components may act synergistically with autonomy support in promoting better health. Allaying negative emotions or, at least, acknowledging their role as well as supporting autonomy, have both been shown to promote greater autonomous motivation and better self-regulation. Future research should, therefore, investigate the unique and interactive effects of an intervention that leverages these affective components to change behavior using factorial designs. Such an approach will provide evidence as to whether it is the independent effects of these components, or their interaction, or both, that leads to health behavior change.

CONCLUSION

We have provided an overview of the role of affect in self-determination theory applied to health and health behavior. We outlined the key tenets of self-determination theory and identified the importance of psychological well-being and positive affect as outcomes in self-determination theory research. Psychological well-being, in particular, is an important outcome as it as a reflection of the adaptive, self-actualizing optimal functioning brought about by autonomous motivation. However, we have also indicated that affective responses are inextricably tied to the process by which autonomous motivation affects behavioral outcomes in health contexts. Specifically, we have outlined how positive affect may serve as important feedback of need-satisfying behavior, the importance of eudaimonic well-being as a key goal of autonomous engagement in behavior, the experience of harmonious and obsessive passion when individuals engage in absorbing emotionally salient activities, and the important role autonomous motivation plays in the management of aversive affect responses in self-regulation. Overall, current evidence indicates dual roles for affect in the context of self-determination theory applied to health behavior, as an outcome and as part of the motivational process. Future research could examine these roles simultaneously in multiple health behavioral contexts. Finally, we have offered some thoughts on how autonomy supportive interventions based on self-determination theory can promote better health behavior change and the potential role affect may play in such interventions.

ACKNOWLEDGMENT

Cleo Protogerou's contribution was supported by a grant from the University of Cape Town's Research Committee (URC), and Martin S. Hagger's contribution was supported by a Finland Distinguished Professor (FiDiPro) award from Tekes, the Finnish funding agency for innovation.

REFERENCES

Ajzen, I. (2015). The theory of planned behavior is alive and well, and not ready to retire. *Health Psychology Review, 9*, 131–137.

Allom, V., Mullan, B. A., & Hagger, M. S. (2016). Does inhibitory control training improve health behaviour? A meta-analysis. *Health Psychology Review, 10*, 168–186.

Allom, V., Panetta, G., Mullan, B., & Hagger, M. S. (2016). Self-report and behavioural approaches to the measurement of self-control: Are we assessing the same construct? *Personality and Individual Differences, 90*, 137–142.

Bandura, A. (1977). Self-efficacy: Toward a unifying theory of behavioral change. *Psychological Review, 84*, 191–215.

Biddle, S. J. H., Hagger, M. S., Chatzisarantis, N. L. D., & Lippke, S. (2007). Theoretical frameworks in exercise psychology. In G. Tenenbaum & R. C. Eklund (Eds.), *Handbook of sport psychology* (3rd ed., pp. 537–559). New York, NY: Wiley.

Black, A. E., & Deci, E. L. (2000). The effects of instructors' autonomy support and students' autonomous motivation on learning organic chemistry: A self-determination theory perspective. *Science Education, 84*, 740–756.

Bowlby, J. (1958). The nature of the child's tie to his mother. *International Journal of PsychoAnalysis, 34*, 1–23.

Caudwell, K. M., & Hagger, M. S. (2015). Predicting alcohol pre-drinking in Australian undergraduate students using an integrated theoretical model. *Applied Psychology: Health and Well-Being, 7*, 188–213.

Chan, D. K. C., Dimmock, J. A., Donovan, R. J., Hardcastle, S., Lentillon-Kaestner, V., & Hagger, M. S. (2015). Self-determined motivation in sport predicts motivation and intention of anti-doping behaviors: A perspective from the trans-contextual model. *Journal of Science and Medicine in Sport, 18*, 315–322.

Chan, D. K. C., Fung, Y.-K., Xing, S., & Hagger, M. S. (2014). Myopia prevention, near work, and visual acuity of college students: Integrating the theory of planned behavior and self-determination theory. *Journal of Behavioral Medicine, 37*, 369–380.

Chan, D. K. C., & Hagger, M. S. (2012). Autonomous forms of motivation underpinning injury prevention and rehabilitation among police officers: An application of the trans-contextual model. *Motivation and Emotion, 36*, 349–364.

Chatzisarantis, N. L. D., & Hagger, M. S. (2009). Effects of an intervention based on self-determination theory on self-reported leisure-time physical activity participation. *Psychology and Health, 24*, 29–48.

Chatzisarantis, N. L. D., Hagger, M. S., Biddle, S. J. H., Smith, B., & Wang, C. K. J. (2003). A meta-analysis of perceived locus of causality in exercise, sport, and physical education contexts. *Journal of Sport and Exercise Psychology, 25*, 284–306.

Cheon, S. H., Reeve, J., & Moon, I. (2012). Experimentally based, longitudinally designed, teacher-focused intervention to help physical education teachers be more autonomy supportive toward their students. *Journal of Sport and Exercise Psychology, 34*, 365–396.

de Ridder, D. T. D., Lensvelt-Mulders, G., Finkenauer, C., Stok, F. M., & Baumeister, R. F. (2012). Taking stock of self-control: A meta-analysis of how trait self-control relates to a wide range of behaviors. *Personality and Social Psychology Review, 16*, 76–99.

DeCharms, R. (1968). *Personal causation: The internal affective determinants of behavior*. New York, NY: Academic Press.

Deci, E. L. (1972). Intrinsic motivation, extrinsic motivation, and inequity. *Journal of Personality and Social Psychology, 22*, 113–120.

Deci, E. L., Eghrari, H., Patrick, B. C., & Leone, D. R. (1994). Facilitating internalization: The self-determination theory perspective. *Journal of Personality, 62*, 119–142.

Deci, E. L., Koestner, R., & Ryan, R. M. (1999). The undermining effect is a reality after all—Extrinsic rewards, task interest, and self-determination: Reply to Eisenberger, Pierce, and Cameron (1999) and Lepper, Henderlong, and Gingras (1999). *Psychological Bulletin, 125*, 692–700.

Deci, E. L., & Ryan, R. M. (1985). *Intrinsic motivation and self-determination in human behavior*. New York, NY: Plenum Press.

Deci, E. L., & Ryan, R. M. (2000). The "what" and "why" of goal pursuits: Human needs and the self-determination of behavior. *Psychological Inquiry, 11*, 227–268.

Deci, E. L., & Ryan, R. M. (2008). Facilitating optimal motivation and psychological well-being across life's domains. *Canadian Psychology, 49*, 14–23.

Deci, E. L., Ryan, R. M., Gagne, M., Leone, D. R., Usunov, J., & Kornazheva, B. P. (2001). Need satisfaction, motivation, and well-being in the work organizations of a former Eastern Bloc country. *Personality and Social Psychology Bulletin, 27*, 930–942.

Dombrowski, S., & Luszczynska, A. (2009). The interplay between conscious and automatic self-regulation and adolescents' physical activity: The role of planning, intentions, and lack of awareness. *Applied Psychology, 58*, 257–273.

Gagné, M., & Deci, E. L. (2005). Self-determination theory and work motivation. *Journal of Organizational Behavior, 26*, 331–362.

González-Cutre, D., Sicilia, A., Sierra, A. C., Ferriz, R., & Hagger, M. S. (2016). Understanding the need for novelty from the perspective of self-determination theory. *Personality and Individual Differences, 102*, 159–169.

Gunnell, K. E., Crocker, P. R. E., Wilson, P. M., Mack, D. E., & Zumbo, B. D. (2013). Psychological need satisfaction and thwarting: A test of basic psychological needs theory in physical activity contexts. *Psychology of Sport and Exercise, 14*, 599–607.

Hagger, M. S. (2014). Avoiding the "déjà-variable" phenomenon: Social psychology needs more guides to constructs. *Frontiers in Psychology, 5*, 52.

Hagger, M. S., & Chatzisarantis, N. L. D. (2009). Integrating the theory of planned behaviour and self-determination theory in health behaviour: A meta-analysis. *British Journal of Health Psychology, 14*, 275–302.

Hagger, M. S., & Chatzisarantis, N. L. D. (2016). The trans-contextual model of autonomous motivation in education: Conceptual and empirical issues and meta-analysis. *Review of Educational Research, 86*, 360–407.

Hagger, M. S., & Hardcastle, S. J. (2014). Interpersonal style should be included in taxonomies of behaviour change techniques. *Frontiers in Psychology, 5*, 254.

Hagger, M. S., Leung, C. M., Leaver, E., Esser, K., te Pas, N., Keatley, D. A., . . . Chatzisarantis, N. L. D. (2013). Cue-induced smoking urges deplete cigarette smokers' self-control resources. *Annals of Behavioral Medicine, 46*, 394–400.

Hagger, M. S., Lonsdale, A., Hein, V., Koka, A., Lintunen, T., Pasi, H. J., . . . Chatzisarantis, N. L. D. (2012). Predicting alcohol consumption and binge drinking in company employees: An application of planned behaviour and self-determination theories. *British Journal of Health Psychology, 17*, 379–407.

Hagger, M. S., Panetta, G., Leung, C.-M., Wong, G. G., Wang, J. C. K., Chan, D. K.-C., . . . Chatzisarantis, N. L. D. (2013). Chronic inhibition, self-control and eating behavior: Test of a "resource depletion" model. *PLoS ONE, 8*, e76888.

Hagger, M. S., Sultan, S., Hardcastle, S. J., & Chatzisarantis, N. L. D. (2015). Perceived autonomy support and autonomous motivation toward mathematics activities in educational and out-of-school contexts is related to mathematics homework behavior and attainment. *Contemporary Educational Psychology, 41*, 111–123.

Hardcastle, S. J., Fortier, M. S., Blake, N., & Hagger, M. S. (2016). Identifying content-based and relational techniques to change behavior in motivational interviewing. *Health Psychology Review, 11*, 1–16.

Hardcastle, S. J., Blake, N., & Hagger, M. S. (2012). The effectiveness of a motivational interviewing primary-care based intervention on physical activity and predictors of change in a disadvantaged community. *Journal of Behavioral Medicine, 35*, 318–333.

Howard, J. L., Gagné, M., & Bureau, J. S. (2017). Testing a continuum structure of self-determined motivation: A meta-analysis. *Psychological Bulletin, 143*, 1346–1377. doi:10.1037/bul0000125

Hull, C. L. (1943). *Principles of behavior*. New York, NY: Appleton-Century.

Inzlicht, M., Schmeichel, B. J., & Macrae, C. N. (2014). Why self-control seems (but may not be) limited. *Trends in Cognitive Sciences, 8*, 127–133.

Jõesaar, H., Hein, V., & Hagger, M. S. (2012). Youth athletes' perception of autonomy support from the coach, peer motivational climate and intrinsic motivation in sport setting: One-year effects. *Psychology of Sport and Exercise, 13*, 257–262.

Koestner, R., & Losier, G. F. (2002). Distinguishing three ways of being internally motivated: A closer look at introjection, identification, and intrinsic motivation. In E. L. Deci & R. M. Ryan (Eds.), *Handbook of self-determination research* (pp. 101–121). Rochester, NY: University of Rochester Press.

Koka, A., & Hagger, M. S. (2010). Perceived teaching behaviors and self-determined motivation in physical education: A test of self-determination theory. *Research Quarterly for Exercise and Sport, 81*, 74–86.

Legault, L., & Inzlicht, M. (2013). Self-determination, self-regulation, and the brain: Autonomy improves performance by enhancing neuroaffective responsiveness to self-regulation failure. *Journal of Personality and Social Psychology, 105*, 123–138.

Martela, F., & Ryan, R. M. (2016). The benefits of benevolence: Basic psychological needs, beneficence, and the enhancement of well-being. *Journal of Personality, 84*, 750–764.

Maslow, A. (1943). A theory of human motivation. *Psychological Reports, 50*, 370–396.

McLachlan, S., & Hagger, M. S. (2010). Effects of an autonomy-supportive intervention on tutor behaviors in a higher education context. *Teaching and Teacher Education, 26*, 1205–1211.

Michie, S., Richardson, M., Johnston, M., Abraham, C., Francis, J., Hardeman, W., . . . Wood, C. E. (2013). The Behavior Change Technique Taxonomy (v1) of 93 hierarchically clustered techniques: Building an international consensus for the reporting of behavior change interventions. *Annals of Behavioral Medicine*, *46*, 81–95.

Moller, A. C., Deci, E. L., & Ryan, R. M. (2006). Choice and ego depletion: The moderating role of autonomy. *Personality and Social Psychology Bulletin*, *32*, 1024–1036.

Mpondo, F., Ruiter, R. A. C., van den Borne, B., & Reddy, P. S. (2015). Self-determination and gender–power relations as predictors of condom use self-efficacy among South African women. *Health Psychology Open*, *2*, 1–11.

Muraven, M., & Shmueli, D. (2006). The self-control costs of fighting the temptation to drink. *Psychology of Addictive Behaviors*, *20*, 154–160.

Ng, J. Y. Y., Ntoumanis, N., Thøgersen-Ntoumani, C., Deci, E. L., Ryan, R. M., Duda, J. L., & Williams, G. C. (2012). Self-determination theory applied to health contexts. *Perspectives on Psychological Science*, *7*, 325–340.

Pihu, M., Hein, V., Koka, A., & Hagger, M. S. (2008). How students' perceptions of teacher's autonomy-supportive behaviours affect physical activity behaviour: An application of trans-contextual model. *European Journal of Sport Science*, *8*, 193–204.

Reeve, J., Bolt, E., & Cai, Y. (1999). Autonomy-supportive teachers: How they teach and motivate students. *Journal of Educational Psychology*, *91*, 537–548.

Resnicow, K., Davis, R. E., Zhang, G., Konkel, J., Strecher, V. J., Shaikh, A. R., . . . Wiese, C. (2008). Tailoring a fruit and vegetable intervention on novel motivational constructs: Results of a randomized study. *Annals of Behavioral Medicine*, *35*, 159–169.

Rousseau, F. L., & Vallerand, R. J. (2008). An examination of the relationship between passion and subjective well-being in older adults. *International Journal of Aging and Human Development*, *66*, 195–211.

Ryan, R. M., & Deci, E. L. (2000). The darker and brighter sides of human existence: Basic psychological needs as a unifying concept. *Psychological Inquiry*, *11*, 319–338.

Ryan, R. M., & Deci, E. L. (2001). On happiness and human potentials: A review of research on hedonic and eudaimonic well-being. *Annual Review of Psychology*, *52*, 141–166.

Ryan, R. M., & Deci, E. L. (2009). Promoting self-determined school engagement: Motivation, learning, and well-being. In K. R. Wentzel & A. Wigfield (Eds.), *Handbook on motivation at school* (pp. 171–196). New York, NY: Routledge.

Ryan, R. M., Huta, V., & Deci, E. L. (2006). Living well: A self-determination theory perspective on eudaimonia. *Journal of Happiness Studies*, *9*, 139–170.

Ryan, R. M., Patrick, H., Deci, E. L., & Williams, G. C. (2008). Facilitating health behaviour change and its maintenance: Interventions based on self-determination theory. *European Health Psychologist*, *10*, 2–5.

Ryff, C. D., & Keyes, C. L. M. (1995). The structure of psychological well-being revisited. *Journal of Personality and Social Psychology*, *69*, 719–727.

Ryff, C. D., & Singer, B. (2000). Interpersonal flourishing: A positive health agenda for the new millennium. *Personality and Social Psychology Review*, *4*, 30–44.

Sarrazin, P., Vallerand, R. J., Guillet, E., Pelletier, L. G., & Cury, F. (2002). Motivation and dropout in female handballers: A 21-month prospective study. *European Journal of Social Psychology*, *32*, 395–418.

Sebire, S., Jago, R., Fox, K., Edwards, M., & Thompson, J. (2013). Testing a self-determination theory model of children's physical activity motivation: a cross-sectional study. *International Journal of Behavioral Nutrition and Physical Activity, 10*, 111.

Sheldon, K. M., Elliot, A. J., Kim, Y., & Kasser, T. (2001). What is satisfying about satisfying events? Testing 10 candidate psychological needs. *Journal of Personality and Social Psychology, 80*, 325–339.

Sheldon, K. M., Elliot, A. J., Ryan, R. M., Chirkov, V., Kim, Y., Wu, C., . . . Sun, Z. (2004). Self-concordance and subjective well-being in four cultures. *Journal of Cross-Cultural Psychology, 35*, 209–233.

Sheldon, K. M., & Kasser, T. (1998). Pursuing personal goals: Skills enable progress, but not all progress is beneficial. *Personality and Social Psychology Bulletin, 24*, 1319–1331.

Teixeira, P. J., Carraca, E., Markland, D. A., Silva, M., & Ryan, R. M. (2012). Exercise, physical activity, and self-determination theory: A systematic review. *International Journal of Behavioral Nutrition and Physical Activity, 9*, 78.

Teixeira, P. J., Silva, M. N., Marques, M. M., Carraça, E. V., La Guardia, J. G., Williams, G. C., . . . Hagger, M. S. (2016). *Identifying self-determination theory-based techniques aimed at promoting autonomy, competence, and relatedness in health contexts.* Paper presented at the Self-Determination Theory Conference, Victoria, British Columbia, Canada.

Vallerand, R. J. (2008). On the psychology of passion: In search of what makes people's lives most worth living. *Canadian Psychology, 49*, 1–13.

Vallerand, R. J., Blanchard, C., Mageau, G. A., Koestner, R., Ratelle, C. F., Léonard, M., & Marsolais, J. (2003). Les Passions de l'âme: On obsessive and harmonious passion. *Journal of Personality and Social Psychology, 85*, 756–767.

Wallhead, T. L., Hagger, M. S., & Smith, D. T. (2010). Sport education and extra-curricular sport participation: An examination using the trans-contextual model of motivation. *Research Quarterly for Exercise and Sport, 81*, 442–455.

Webb, D., Soutar, G. N., Mazzarol, T., & Saldaris, P. (2013). Self-determination theory and consumer behavioural change: Evidence from a household energy-saving behaviour study. *Journal of Environmental Psychology, 35*, 59–66.

White, R. W. (1959). Motivation reconsidered: The concept of competence. *Psychological Review, 66*, 297–333.

Williams, G. C., Frankel, R. M., Campbell, T. L., & Deci, E. L. (2000). Research on relationship-centered care and healthcare outcomes from the Rochester biopsychosocial program: A self-determination theory integration. *Families, Systems and Health, 18*, 79–90.

Williams, G. C., Gagne, M., Ryan, R. M., & Deci, E. L. (2002). Facilitating autonomous motivation for smoking cessation. *Health Psychology, 21*, 40–50.

Williams, G. C., McGregor, H. A., Zeldman, A., & Freedman, Z. R. (2004). Testing a self-determination theory process model for promoting glycemic control through diabetes self-management. *Health Psychology, 23*, 58–66.

Williams, G. C., Minicucci, D. S., Kouides, R. W., Levesque, C. S., Chirkov, V. I., Ryan, R. M., & Deci, E. L. (2002). Self-determination, smoking, diet and health. *Health Education Research*, *17*, 512–521.

Wilson, P. M., Rodgers, W. M., Blanchard, C. M., & Gessell, J. (2003). The relationship between psychological needs, self-determined motivation, exercise attitudes, and physical fitness. *Journal of Applied Social Psychology*, *33*, 2373–2392.

8

Affect, Dual-Processing, Developmental Psychopathology, and Health Behaviors

REINOUT W. WIERS, KRISTEN G. ANDERSON, BRAM VAN BOCKSTAELE, ELSKE SALEMINK, AND BERNHARD HOMMEL

INTRODUCTION

In this chapter, we develop a broad theoretical framework to account for healthy and unhealthy behaviors and related psychopathology from a developmental perspective. We start with a discussion of dual process models, and argue that from a neurocognitive perspective, dual (or multiple) processes are an emergent property of unfolding and interacting brain processes. Although dual process models have been criticized, we argue that these models can still be useful at the psychological level of description. We then turn to broad developmental and personality inspired models including differences in temperament and socialization in relation to the development of individual differences in outcomes of health-relevant behaviors. The general heuristic model (Gladwin, Figner, Crone, & Wiers, 2011) is illustrated with a description of experiments, on the interplay between bottom-up and top-down processes in relation to health behaviors. In the second part of the chapter, we discuss interventions from this perspective.

AFFECT AND COGNITION, DUAL-PROCESS MODELS, AND BEYOND

Dual process models have been en vogue the past few decades in psychology (Evans, 2008; Smith & DeCoster, 2000; Strack & Deutsch, 2004). They have ancient roots, emphasizing the struggle between passion and reason, or the heart and the head (Hofmann, Friese, & Strack, 2009). Many different names have been given to the different processing modes (sometimes called systems), we here use the terms "impulsive" and "reflective" processes (Strack & Deutsch, 2004). Note that this does not equate to unconscious and conscious, some problem-solving occurs unconsciously (Kounios & Beeman, 2014), and some seemingly rash impulsive behaviors may be entirely goal-directed (see for intriguing examples, Kopetz & Orehek, 2015). As the historical background suggests, affective influences have primarily been associated with impulsive processes and non-affective influences with reflective processes. However, as emotions get a stronger cognitive component (e.g., shame, guilt), they may also fuel reflective processes to inhibit an impulse to prevent (anticipated) shame, regret, or guilt. Some theorists have emphasized different evolutionary origins, with impulsive processes representing evolutionary old processes and reflective processes evolutionary later additions (Evans, 2008; K. B. MacDonald, 2008); some have emphasized different developmental origins, with impulsive processes emerging earlier in life than reflective (effortful control) processes (Nigg, 2006; Rothbart & Posner, 2011); some have distinguished between associative (impulsive) processes and symbolic (reflective) processes (Gawronski & Bodenhausen, 2006; Strack & Deutsch, 2004); and some have distinguished between model-free (impulsive) versus model-based (reflective) learning mechanisms (Ashby,

Alfonso-Reese, Turken, & Waldron, 1998; Daw, Niv, & Dayan, 2005). In addition to general dual-process models, more specific models have been developed to account for the development of common mental disorders, such as addictive behaviors (Bechara, 2005; Wiers & Stacy, 2006), anxiety (Ouimet, Gawronski, & Dozois, 2009), and depression (Beevers, 2005). Dual-process models have also been adapted to account for health behaviors (Hofmann, Friese, & Wiers, 2008; Sheeran, Gollwitzer, & Bargh, 2013). Before we return to dual process models and health, it is important to consider some of the recent criticisms of dual process models, and to consider what can be maintained regarding a general model on cognitive-motivational processes involved in health psychology and related psychopathology.

Neurocognitive Processes and Dual Process Models

In an influential criticism of dual process/systems models, it was argued that there is no evidence for separable neural systems for impulsive and reflective processes (Keren & Schul, 2009). We agree to some extent with the criticisms of those dual process models in which authors have equated specific brain systems with impulsive (or "reflexive") processing (including "emotional" structures like the amygdala and striatum), and other areas, including parts of the prefrontal and parietal cortex as dealing exclusively with reflective processing (e.g., Heatherton & Wagner, 2011; Satpute & Lieberman, 2006), or in more broad, unspecified terms that different brain areas are correlated with impulsive and reflective processes (Evans & Stanovich, 2013). One problem is that this does not prove anything, many other models would be compatible with that observation (Keren, 2013; Hommel & Wiers, 2017).

But is this a fatal blow for dual process models? We argue it is not at the psychological level (Gladwin et al., 2011; Wiers, Gladwin, Hofmann, Salemink, & Ridderinkhof, 2013; Wiers & Gladwin, 2017). What the criticism rules out are dual process models that propose a one-to-one relationship between mental processes and the underlying neurocognitive machinery, but alternatives are conceivable. For instance, the MIMIC (multiple indicators, multiple causes) model is based on the supervenience thesis (Kievit et al., 2011), according to which psychological constructs can be realized by underlying neural structures or processes in multiple ways. The neural indicators determine/constrain the psychological processes, without necessarily having a one-to-one relationship with them. This is in line with findings in cognitive neuroscience that the same neural structures are implicated in many psychological processes (see Kievit et al., 2011).

According to another perspective on the relationship between brain- and mental processes, the processes described in dual process models are emergent properties of the dynamic unfolding interplay between different neural systems (Cunningham & Zelazo, 2007; Gladwin et al., 2011; Hazy, Frank, & O'Reilly, 2007). This perspective suggests that behavior that can be described according to a dual process model might actually arise from interactions among several neural systems, each with their own computational objectives, and that any one of the "processes" reflects a dynamic interaction among these same systems (Frank, Cohen, & Sanfey, 2009; Hommel & Wiers, 2017). Importantly, recent computational models have demonstrated how symbolic processing, characteristic of reflective processing, can arise via dynamic interactions among multiple "loops" connecting the prefrontal cortex and basal ganglia (Collins & Frank, 2013; Kriete, Noelle, Cohen, & O'Reilly, 2013). According to these models, there can still be a first crude pass of information, which in extreme cases may already activate action-tendencies ("impulsive action"). However, typically more loops of information processing take place, which can be described as increasingly reflective *states* of processing (Gladwin et al., 2011). Clearly, this does not allow for specific neural structures (e.g., the dorsolateral prefrontal cortex) to only be involved in reflective processes and other structures (e.g., the amygdala) in impulsive processes (see, for a similar argument regarding emotion and cognition, Pessoa, 2008).

Where does this leave us at the psychological level? At that level of description (i.e., models describing the interactions between psychological constructs, without equating them to underlying neural processes or systems), we would argue that dual process models could still be useful in generating testable predictions for understanding health-related processes. For example, in the case of health psychology, one paradoxical prediction of dual process models is that health prevention messages can backfire, especially when they are negatively phrased (e.g., "alcohol does not make you sexy"). The reason is that negation is a typical example of symbolic processing, and that the presentation with the two concepts (alcohol–sexy) can actually be strengthened by exposure, when over time the "not" part gets lost (Deutsch, Gawronski, & Strack, 2006; Krank, Ames, Grenard, Schoenfeld, & Stacy, 2010).

DEVELOPMENT, COGNITIVE PROCESSES, PSYCHOPATHOLOGY, AND HEALTH

While numerous terms have been used in the literature to describe self-regulatory capacity, these functions generally represent our ability to exert control, inhibit, or regulate attention, behavior, and cognition (Ahadi & Rothbart, 1994; Eisenberg et al., 2013; Nigg, 2000), and are commonly contrasted with dispositional approach tendencies, impulsivity, or disinhibition (Gray, 1994; Whiteside & Lynam, 2003), with both changing substantively across development (Anderson & Briggs, 2016). Before age 2, attentional control is the predominant means of coping with emotional distress with signs of more classical behavioral regulation developing by age 3 (Anderson & Briggs, 2016; Eisenberg, Smith, & Spinrad, 2010). Self-control capacity increases dramatically in the preschool years and continues to do so throughout childhood, with some regulatory functions achieving adult-like levels by adolescence (Luna, Paulsen, Padmanabhan, & Geier, 2013; Posner, Rothbart, Sheese, & Voelker, 2014; Rothbart & Posner, 2011). While adolescents can inhibit responding as well as adults in some contexts, self-regulation within certain rewarding environments, particularly involving peers, may be more challenging and require greater effort (Anderson & Briggs, 2016; Galvan, 2013; Van Duijvenvoorde & Crone, 2013).

Individual differences in effortful and reactive self-control (impulsivity; inhibition to novelty) are evident as early as 2.5 years of age with evidence for differentiation between reactive under- and overcontrol by age 3.5 (Eisenberg et al., 2013). Temperament traits, particularly surrounding self-control, inhibition, and disinhibition, have been related to the development of psychopathology in childhood and beyond (Kagan, 2013; Nigg, 2000, 2006).

Partly based on these developmental findings, Carver and colleagues (Carver, Johnson, & Joormann, 2008, 2014) developed a model in which the relative dominance of impulsive versus reflective processes is modulated by serotonin, with low levels of serotonin relating to a relative dominance of impulsive processing. An elegant aspect of this model is that it can explain effects of both trait-differences (e.g., genetic factors modulating serotonin, for example genetic variability of the serotonin transporter gene, 5HTT), and state modulations of serotonin (e.g., depletion effect through experimental manipulations or natural factors such as sleep loss). Interestingly, a recent study demonstrated that participants with a genetic variant related to relatively low levels of serotonin performed better on a sorting task under conditions that favored model-free learning, while individuals with high levels of serotonin performed better under conditions that favored model-based learning in the same task (Maddox et al., 2015).

From this perspective (Carver et al., 2008, 2014; Ernst, Pine, & Hardin, 2006), individual differences in tendencies to develop certain mental and health problems are related to the interactions of *three* broad neural systems: an impulsive approach-oriented, an impulsive avoidance-oriented, and a reflective effortful control system. This model can explain why low levels of serotonin are related both to externalizing problems (e.g., aggression) and internalizing problems (e.g., anxiety and depression). For example, strong reactive approach coupled with weak control increases chances of reactive aggression, weak approach with weak control increases chances of depressive symptoms, and strong avoidance with weak control increases chances of developing anxiety problems. Important support for this idea comes from the at first sight counterintuitive finding that individuals who have experienced a depressive episode are also more impulsive in response to positive stimuli (Carver, Johnson, & Joormann, 2013).

As another a point in case, the famous Dunedin study, following approximately 1,000 children since birth into adulthood, has demonstrated that indices of effortful control in childhood predicted later outcomes of mental and physical health (Moffitt et al., 2011), replicating and extending earlier findings by Walter Mischel and colleagues (Mischel, Shoda, & Rodriguez, 1989). Interestingly, a paper based on data of the Dunedin study argued that there could be a general factor in psychopathology (labeled the "p-factor") in addition to the two broad classes of internalizing and externalizing behaviors (Caspi et al., 2014). One of the attractive aspects of this conceptualization is that it better fits with the developmental multiple process models described earlier, and indeed the p-factor was found to correlate with working memory capacity, often used as a general index of the capacity to control (Hofmann, Friese, & Wiers, 2011). In addition, the model may explain the counterintuitive positive correlation between internalizing and externalizing disorders, while in clinical practice children typically first develop either an internalizing or an externalizing problem, with occasional overlap often as a secondary diagnosis (e.g., becoming depressed as a consequence of negative social reactions to aggressive behavior). Hence, from this perspective, relatively weak effortful control and the associated tendency of reacting relatively impulsively are associated with the tendency to develop both internalizing and externalizing problems.

The next important developmental period is adolescence, the period in which most psychopathology originates (Paus, Keshavan, & Giedd, 2008), and the period in which many habits develop which impact later healthy and unhealthy lifestyles (smoking, drinking, physical exercise, etc.). With the onset of puberty, testosterone rises, which has been associated with an increase in dopamine in the midbrain and at a behavioral level with sensation seeking (Steinberg, 2010) and risk taking (Peper, Koolschijn, & Crone, 2013). From the present perspective, it would suggest a shift in balance between operating systems toward more impulsive reactions especially to emotional stimuli (Carver et al., 2014), as indeed has been demonstrated both for reactions to both threat and romantic pictures (Quevedo, Benning, Gunnar, & Dahl, 2009). Adolescent risk-taking has been related to a relative immaturity of brain regions involved in control (frontal cortices), combined with a higher reward sensitivity (Steinberg, 2010). However, changes in social and affective brain processes have also been implicated (Crone & Dahl, 2012), indicating that some of adolescents' risk-taking behaviors may be due not to a lack of ability to moderate an impulse but rather to other goals being more important (e.g., making a good impression on peers or potential romantic partners). Similarly, in addictive behaviors in youth, it has often been assumed that they occur because of the relative immaturity of cognitive control systems (making impulsive reactions dominant), but often also these behaviors are goal-driven (Kopetz, Lejuez, Wiers, & Kruglanski, 2013; Kopetz & Orehek, 2015). This is another example of affective goals influencing behavior through reflective rather than impulsive processes. Hence, control of impulses with an impact on addictive and other health behaviors is not only about ability to control but also about motivation to control (Hofmann, Friese, et al., 2008; van Deursen et al., 2015; Wiers et al., 2007).

In a series of studies on the prediction of substance use in adolescents, it was found that in adolescents with relatively weak control capacity (assessed with measures of working memory or of interference control such as the classical Stroop test), substance use and problems were better predicted by relatively automatic or implicit measures (review: Wiers, Boelema, Nikolaou, & Gladwin, 2015). These findings were observed in adolescents both in regular education (Thush et al., 2008) and in special education, both in the Netherlands (Peeters et al., 2012, 2013) and in the United States (Grenard et al., 2008). However, there were also some negative findings (Janssen, Larsen, Vollebergh, & Wiers, 2015), perhaps related to Internet assessment. In some of the studies, the opposite pattern was found for explicit cognitive motivational measures such as alcohol-related expectancies and motives to drink, which were found to be stronger predictors in individuals with relatively strong executive control (EC) capacity (Thush et al., 2008), suggesting that some adolescents (with relatively weak control capacity) are more sensitive for environmental cues to drink or smoke, while others (with stronger control capacity) make more rational decisions regarding substance use. Note that this interaction pattern was found not only for addictive behaviors but also for other health-related behaviors, including dietary behaviors (Hofmann, Gschwendner, Friese, Wiers, & Schmitt, 2008) and aggression after alcohol (Wiers, Beckers, Houben, & Hofmann, 2009). Interestingly, from the present perspective, a similar pattern was also found in adolescents in the prediction of anxiety (Salemink & Wiers, 2012), and including the opposite pattern of stronger prediction of explicit processes in individuals with a strong control system was observed in anxiety (Salemink, Friese, Drake, Mackintosh, & Hoppitt, 2013).

Finally, it should be noted that dual process models in fact would predict a triple interaction, including not only ability to control impulses but also motivation to do so (Hofmann, Friese, et al., 2008; Wiers et al., 2007). Indeed, in a recent study this triple interaction was partly confirmed in a sample of problem drinkers who signed up for online training: implicit alcohol associations were especially predictive of levels of problematic drinking in those who scored low on control capacity and high on motivation to cut down (van Deursen et al., 2015). A similar pattern was also observed in a study that experimentally manipulated motivation to restrain drinking in students (who were told that greater consumption in a taste test would impair performance on a later task where they could win a reward), and found prediction of drinking by implicit associations, in those students in an ego-depletion condition (Ostafin, Marlatt, & Greenwald, 2008).[1] Hence, the overall pattern is consistent with the notion that the impact of impulsive processes on health behaviors depends on the combination of ability and motivation to control.

IMPLICATIONS FOR INTERVENTIONS IN HEALTH: TRAINING AND MOTIVATION

From the multiple processing account laid out already, health interventions can target different processes, either more impulsive or more reflective processes (Friese, Hofmann, & Wiers, 2011), provided that there is some motivation to change the behavior. A number of training interventions have been developed that target either different relatively automatic cue-induced processes in addictive behaviors, such as an attentional bias and an approach-bias for substance-related cues, or cognitive processes related to control over impulses, such as working memory training (see for a review: Wiers et al., 2013). The first types of training are examples of cognitive bias modification (CBM), which targets domain-specific cognitive-motivational processes, such as an attentional bias, affective memory associations, or action tendencies related to disorder or health-domain-specific cues. Hence, CBM in alcohol use disorders or risky drinking will contain stimuli (words or pictures) referring to alcohol, and CBM for smoking will contain cigarette-cues. In order to assess (and modify) disorder-relevant biases, it is important that the stimuli are first validated (see for a protocol: Pronk, van Deursen, Beraha, Larsen, & Wiers, 2015). The second type of training targets domain-general EC processes, like working memory, which has indeed shown promise in relation to addictive behaviors (Bickel, Yi, Landes, Hill, & Baxter, 2011; Houben, Wiers, & Jansen, 2011) and risk for depression (Hoorelbeke, Koster, Vanderhasselt, Callewaert, & Demeyer, 2015). Another strategy concerning training of general control capacity concerns training of inhibition (Dovis, Van Der Oord, Wiers, & Prins, 2015).

One characteristic of domain-general training is that—compared to CBM—many more sessions are needed for this type of training (typically around 25, Klingberg, 2010; while around six sessions usually suffice in CBM, Eberl et al., 2014). This makes motivation to train very important in EC-training. One way to increase this is to embed the training in a game-like program (Dovis et al., 2015). However, it should be noted in the context of substance use, that while gamification may increase motivation to do training, it does not by itself increase motivation to change the addictive behavior (Boendermaker, Prins, & Wiers, 2015). Moreover, when a boring training is introduced as a game, youth will have high expectations, based on their experience with commercial videogames, and the gamified training may briefly be less boring than the original, but subsequently be liked even less, because of a violation of expectancy effect (Boendermaker, Boffo, & Wiers, 2015).

One type of training that is sometimes misclassified from the present logic, concerns what we called selective inhibition training (Wiers et al., 2013), in which a Go/NoGo task is administered including cues of a health-related behavior (e.g., alcohol), which are systematically paired with an inhibitory (NoGo) response in the active condition, while there is no such relationship in the control condition. Because of the specific categories involved, this type of training should be regarded as a variety of CBM rather than as executive control training. Further, effects on behavior have been found after short training (a single session), and effects generalized to affective associations (Houben, Havermans, Nederkoorn, & Jansen, 2012; Houben, Nederkoorn, Wiers, & Jansen, 2011), but not to general inhibition as assessed with another standard task (Houben et al., 2012). Note that in these studies, participants (typically students) were not aware of the manipulation and did not need to have a motivation to change. Effects were short-lived (in a taste-test directly after the manipulation or in the week to follow) and weaker over time (see for a meta-analysis: Allom, Mullan, & Hagger, 2015). However, one study successfully used this paradigm to support overweight people to reduce weight (Veling, Koningsbruggen, Aarts, & Stroebe, 2014). In this study, volunteers in a study investigating different psychological interventions to facilitate dieting, were randomized to either active Go/NoGo training (combining food and drink pictures with a NoGo signal) or control Go/NoGo training (without food and drink pictures). In addition, participants also received an active or control implementation intention condition. In the active condition, participants were instructed to make detailed if-then plans concerning different meals and how to handle the situation in line with the diet goals. Hence, participants received Go/NoGo training (real/sham) and implementation intention training (real/sham). Both interventions had a positive effect on success in dietary restraint (on weight reduction), and only the effect of implementation intentions were moderated by the strength of the dietary goal, suggesting that this intervention strengthens the impact of reflective or goal-directed processes, while Go/NoGo training appears to be more independent of these processes. Note that in the domain of anxiety, there is also a "mixture" type of training. In order to effectively improve cognitive control over emotional information processing, a working memory training in the context of emotional stimuli was developed and improved cognitive control over affective information and emotion regulation stimuli, while a working memory training with neutral stimuli did not (Schweizer, Grahn, Hampshire, Mobbs, & Dalgleish, 2013; Schweizer, Hampshire, & Dalgleish, 2011). A recent study with adolescents was unable to replicate these findings, but participants were unselected adolescents who thus were not selected on motivation for change (de Voogd, Wiers, Zwitser, & Salemink, 2016).

Clinical samples are typically at least somewhat motivated to change and receive therapy in which alternative goals are activated that are incompatible with continued excessive alcohol or drug use (Wiers et al., 2016; Wiers, Boffo, & Field, in press). In this context, varieties of CBM training have been found to generate positive effects. For example, retraining of an approach bias for alcohol was found to increase abstinence rates 1 year after treatment discharge by approximately 10% (Eberl et al., 2013; Wiers, Eberl, Rinck, Becker, & Lindenmeyer, 2011), with the clinical effect being mediated by the change in approach bias (Eberl et al., 2013). Retraining an attentional bias for alcohol in patients also had clinically relevant effects (Schoenmakers et al., 2010). These findings contrast with more modest or null findings in student populations, typically not motivated to change (Christiansen, Schoenmakers, & Field, 2015; Lindgren et al., 2015; Wiers et al., in press). Hence, an important issue concerning the application of CBM to the domain of health is that participants should first be at least somewhat motivated to change for CBM to exert effects. For example, a study in community smokers unmotivated to quit was successful in changing an attentional bias for cigarettes, but did not result in a change in smoking behavior (Kerst & Waters, 2014).

Increasing Motivation to Change

Motivation to change can be effectively increased through motivational interviewing (MI), a technique originally developed in addiction treatment research and now used more widely to increase motivation to change behaviors related to (mental) health (Miller & Rollnick, 2013). Tailored varieties have been developed (combined with CBT elements), to increase motivation to change and motivation to perform the training for alcohol-dependent outpatients (Boffo, Pronk, Wiers, & Mannarini, 2015), and for smoking youth (Kong et al., 2015). Another strategy can be to select people with at least some level of motivation to change. A recent study on smoking cessation provides a point in case. Potential participants signed up at an antismoking website for free online training to support their quit attempt. Importantly, the quit attempt was verified and only those people who made an actual quit attempt were selected to participate in the training study and randomized to real attentional retraining or a placebo variety including the same pictures. Results in this sample demonstrated significantly more success in abstinence half a year after the quit attempt after real training compared with placebo training (Elfeddali, de Vries, Bolman, Pronk, & Wiers, 2016). These findings contrast with largely negative earlier trials in smoking (Christiansen et al., 2015) and with an online trial in problem drinkers who did not want to quit but wanted to reduce drinking and succeeded irrespective of training condition (Wiers, Houben, et al., 2015).

Before we further discuss the important question for health psychology—how to influence people who are not motivated to change, it is worth pointing out that CBM also has potential in treating internalizing disorders and related health problems. Training-induced changes in attentional bias have relatively consistently been associated with changes in anxiety or emotional responsiveness to stressors (Macleod & Clarke, 2015; Van Bockstaele et al., 2014). In a similar vein, experimentally induced changes in interpretation bias (i.e., the tendency to interpret a neutral or ambiguous stimulus as being threatening) have also been shown to reduce anxiety (Hirsch, Meeten, Krahé, & Reeder, 2016). Also in this domain, there are some indications that motivation plays an important role. For example, findings regarding interpretation bias retraining appear to be more promising in a clinical sample. Note that there are also negative findings that led some to conclude that CBM is ineffective (Cristea, Kok, & Cuijpers, 2015).

However, a re-analysis considering whether manipulation of the mediator (the cognitive bias) was successful or not, demonstrated that those studies that did not affect the cognitive bias had no effect on emotional and clinical symptoms, but those studies that did succeed in changing the bias resulted in a medium to large effect in emotional and clinical symptoms (Macleod & Clarke, 2015; Grafton et al., 2017). Important for the domain of health psychology is that the negative studies were often conducted over the Internet.

Cognitive Bias Modification and Emotion Regulation

Improved emotion regulation is likely to be the mechanism behind these beneficial effects of CBM in anxiety. Indeed, according to the influential emotion regulation model of Gross (Gross & Thompson, 2007), two important strategies to regulate emotions are attention deployment and reappraisal. Attention deployment refers to people's ability to selectively attend to specific positive, neutral, or negative aspects of a situation, whereas reappraisal refers to people's ability to select or change the meaning that is attached to a situation. As such, attentional bias modification procedures have been argued to improve attention deployment (MacLeod & Grafton, 2014; Todd, Cunningham, Anderson, & Thompson, 2012), and interpretation bias modification procedures are likely to improve (re)appraisal skills. In line with dual process views on mental health problems, many emotion regulation researchers have distinguished between relatively automatic, implicit emotion regulation and more effortful, explicit emotion regulation (Gyurak, Gross, & Etkin, 2011; Koole & Rothermund, 2011). Thus CBM techniques may prove crucial in improving implicit emotion regulation.

Unmotivated Participants: Where to Start?

As outlined previously, cognitive training paradigms have rather consistently demonstrated effectiveness in participants with some motivation to change (provided that the bias was indeed successfully changed). Through techniques like MI, motivation can be increased, but to participate in MI, there should be at least some level of motivation, to . . . participate in MI. What to do when this is not the case, an especially thorny problem with emerging substance use problems in youth? One obvious method is simply to pay for participation and hope that more intrinsic motivation will be activated during the following brief intervention. This may have some effect in adolescents (Kong et al., 2015), but not in students (Lindgren et al., 2015). Another strategy in adolescents and young adults is to seize the opportunity, when there is at least for some time some motivation to change, for example after an alcohol-related injury. In this context MI has been successfully applied (Monti et al., 1999), but we are not aware of interventions targeting more automatic cognitive processes in addition in this context. Short-lived effects on cognitive processes and behavior have been reported for samples (typically students) who were not motivated to change for some of the CBM interventions mentioned earlier, including selective inhibition (Allom et al., 2015), approach-bias modification (Wiers, Rinck, Kordts, Houben, & Strack, 2010), and using other techniques such as evaluative conditioning (Houben, Havermans, & Wiers, 2010), formation of implementation intentions (Sheeran et al., 2013; Veling et al., 2014), mindfulness meditation (Ostafin, Bauer, & Myxter, 2012), and physical exercise (Rensburg & Taylor, 2009). Although these paradigms may nudge people toward better health outcomes, we believe that for more enduring change, activation of goals incompatible with continuation of the unhealthy behavior is crucial (Kopetz et al., 2013; Wiers et al., 2016). Hence, from this perspective, for health interventions to be effective, a start with addressing impulsive affective processes may be helpful, and could be subjected to further investigation, but some cognitive restructuring appears to be a necessary additional ingredient for long-term change.

Substance Use as a Moderator in Health Behavior

Some final words follow about substance use and prevention from the present perspective. First, substance use can be considered as one of the possible outcomes in (dual) process models of health, but it is also an important moderator. There is ample evidence that the relative balance in decision-making shifts in favor of more impulsive processes as a result of intoxication, which affects also other health behaviors such as condom use (T. K. MacDonald et al., 2000) and snacking (Hofmann & Friese, 2008). In relation to dieting, alcohol has multiple effects: it may loosen dietary control and increase reactivity to attractive high-caloric foods, and adds many hidden calories by itself (Hofmann, Förster, Stroebe, & Wiers, 2011). This shift in control appears to be related to both strengthening of impulsive processing and weakening of EC-processes (Field, Wiers, Christiansen, Fillmore, & Verster, 2010). Further, there is some evidence for an increase in impulsive personality traits as a result of binge-drinking in adolescents (White et al., 2011), which may in the long run also affect other health behaviors, as a consequence of increased impulsivity.

Prevention

Finally, from the present perspective, traditional prevention methods may be effective, to the extent that they activate goals incompatible with initiation of the health-endangering behavior. However, the danger of non-intended effects should not be underestimated (Krank et al., 2010), and effects of general school-based prevention efforts in the substance use area are often small at best (Tobler et al., 2000). Two alternatives deserve brief mentioning. First, in (young) children an alternative could be to stimulate a relatively reflective way of processing (Diamond, 2012), and self-control training in schoolchildren has been demonstrated to delay onset of alcohol and cigarette use years later (Lier, Huizink, & Crijnen, 2009). Second, Conrod and colleagues developed a personality-based targeted intervention approach in adolescents, where adolescents scoring high on personality traits related to increased risk for substance use and related problems (impulsivity, sensation seeking, anxiety sensitivity, and hopelessness) receive a brief group-based CBT program, which teaches them different ways to deal with their needs than alcohol and drug use (e.g., participate in exciting sports in sensation seekers). Long-term effects have been found across different samples (Conrod, Castellanos-Ryan, & Strang, 2015), with specific outcomes depending on the targeted personality type (e.g., strongest effects on binge-drinking in sensation seekers who are most prone to develop these behaviors).

CONCLUSION

In conclusion, although dual process models have been criticized, especially when equated with specific brain processes, we argue that at a psychological level they can still be useful, for example to understand challenges to the development of a healthy lifestyle and for the development of interventions. Affective processes can influence impulsive decision-making in health, but also reflective processes, when they concern affectively relevant goals. Cognitive training methods have shown some success in changing health-behaviors, but a critical variable for long-term success appears to be motivation to change. Ideally therefore, interventions should be developed that nudge people not motivated to change toward motivation to change and then help them (if necessary) to overcome cue-induced interfering processes with long-term healthy behaviors.

ACKNOWLEDGMENT

The authors wish to thank Will Cunningham, Jay van Bavel, Michael Frank, Ron Dahl, and Thomas Gladwin for comments on an earlier version of the chapter.

NOTE

1. Note that ego-depletion has been criticized recently and appears at least to some extent to be dependent on beliefs (Job, Walton, Bernecker, & Dweck, 2013).

REFERENCES

Ahadi, S. A., & Rothbart, M. K. (1994). Temperament, development, and the Big Five. *The Developing Structure of Temperament and Personality from Infancy to Adulthood, 189207.*

Allom, V., Mullan, B., & Hagger, M. (2015). Does inhibitory control training improve health behaviour? A meta-analysis. *Health Psychology Review, 7199* (June 2015), 1–38. http://doi.org/10.1080/17437199.2015.1051078

Anderson, K. G., & Briggs, K. E. L. (2016). Self-regulation and decision making. In S. A. Brown & R. A. Zucker (Eds.), *Oxford Handbook of Adolescent Substance Abuse.* NY: Oxford University Press. http://doi.org/10.1093/oxfordhb/9780199735662.013.021

Ashby, F. G., Alfonso-Reese, L. A., Turken, U., & Waldron, E. M. (1998). A neuropsychological theory of multiple systems in category learning. *Psychological Review, 105,* 442–481. http://doi.org/10.1037/0033-295X.105.3.442

Bechara, A. (2005). Decision making, impulse control and loss of willpower to resist drugs: A neurocognitive perspective. *Nature: Neuroscience, 8,* 1458–1463. http://doi.org/Doi 10.1038/Nn1584

Beevers, C. G. (2005). Cognitive vulnerability to depression: A dual process model. *Clinical Psychology Review, 25,* 975–1002. http://doi.org/10.1016/j.cpr.2005.03.003

Bickel, W. K., Yi, R., Landes, R. D., Hill, P. F., & Baxter, C. (2011). Remember the future: Working memory training decreases delay discounting among stimulant addicts. *Biological Psychiatry, 69,* 260–265. http://doi.org/10.1016/j.biopsych.2010.08.017

Boendermaker, W. J., Boffo, M., & Wiers, R. W. (2015). Exploring elements of fun to motivate youth to do cognitive bias modification. *Games for Health Journal, 4,* 434–443. http://doi.org/10.1089/g4h.2015.0053

Boendermaker, W. J., Prins, P. J. M., & Wiers, R. W. (2015). Cognitive bias modification for adolescents with substance use problems—Can serious games help? *Journal of Behavior Therapy and Experimental Psychiatry, 49,* 13–20. http://doi.org/10.1016/j.jbtep.2015.03.008

Boffo, M., Pronk, T., Wiers, R. W., & Mannarini, S. (2015). Combining cognitive bias modification training with motivational support in alcohol dependent outpatients: Study protocol for a randomised controlled trial. *Trials, 16,* 63. http://doi.org/10.1186/s13063-015-0576-6

Carver, C. S., Johnson, S. L., & Joormann, J. (2008). Serotonergic function, two-mode models of self-regulation, and vulnerability to depression: What depression has in common with impulsive aggression. *Psychological Bulletin, 134,* 912–943. http://doi.org/10.1037/a0013740

Carver, C. S., Johnson, S. L., & Joormann, J. (2013). Major depressive disorder and impulsive reactivity to emotion: Toward a dual-process view of depression. *British Journal of Clinical Psychology, 52,* 285–299. http://doi.org/10.1111/bjc.12014

Carver, C. S., Johnson, S. L., & Joormann, J. (2014). Dual process models and serotonergic functioning. In J. P. Forgas & E. Harmon-Jones (Eds.), *Motivation and its regulation: The control within* (Vol. 16, pp. 55–78). New York, NY: Psychology Press.

Caspi, A., Houts, R. M., Belsky, D. W., Goldman-Mellor, S. J., Harrington, H., Israel, S., . . . Moffitt, T. E. (2014). The p factor: One general psychopathology factor in the structure of psychiatric disorders? *Clinical Psychological Science, 2*, 119–137. http://doi.org/10.1177/2167702613497473

Christiansen, P., Schoenmakers, T. M., & Field, M. (2015). Less than meets the eye: Reappraising the clinical relevance of attentional bias in addiction. *Addictive Behaviors, 44*, 43–50. http://doi.org/10.1016/j.addbeh.2014.10.005

Collins, A. G. E., & Frank, M. J. (2013). Cognitive control over learning: Creating, clustering, and generalizing task-set structure. *Psychological Review, 120*, 190–229. http://doi.org/10.1037/a0030852

Conrod, P. J., Castellanos-Ryan, N., & Strang, J. (2015). Brief, personality-targeted coping skills interventions and survival as a non–drug user over a 2-year period during adolescence. *Archives of General Psychiatry, 67*, 85–93.

Cristea, I. A., Kok, R. N., & Cuijpers, P. (2015). Efficacy of cognitive bias modification interventions in anxiety and depression: Meta-analysis. *British Journal of Psychiatry, 206*, 7–16. http://doi.org/10.1192/bjp.bp.114.146761

Crone, E. A., & Dahl, R. E. (2012). Understanding adolescence as a period of social-affective engagement and goal flexibility. *Nature Reviews. Neuroscience, 13*, 636–650. http://doi.org/10.1038/nrn3313

Cunningham, W. A., & Zelazo, P. D. (2007). Attitudes and evaluations: A social cognitive neuroscience perspective. *Trends in Cognitive Sciences, 11*, 97–104. http://doi.org/10.1016/j.tics.2006.12.005

Daw, N. D., Niv, Y., & Dayan, P. (2005). Uncertainty-based competition between prefrontal and dorsolateral striatal systems for behavioral control. *Nature Neuroscience, 8*, 1704–1711. http://doi.org/10.1038/nn1560

de Voogd, L. E., Wiers, R. W., Zwitser, R. J., & Salemink, E. (2016). Emotional working memory training as an online intervention for adolescent anxiety and depression: A randomised controlled trial. *Australian Journal of Psychology, 68*, 228–238.

Deutsch, R., Gawronski, B., & Strack, F. (2006). At the boundaries of automaticity: Negation as reflective operation. *Journal of Personality and Social Psychology, 91*, 385–405. http://doi.org/10.1037/0022-3514.91.3.385

Diamond, A. (2012). *Executive functions*. http://doi.org/10.1146/annurev-psych-113011-143750

Dovis, S., Van Der Oord, S., Wiers, R. W., & Prins, P. J. M. (2015). Improving executive functioning in children with ADHD: Training multiple executive functions within the context of a computer game. A randomized double-blind placebo controlled trial. *PLoS ONE, 10*, 1–30. http://doi.org/10.1371/journal.pone.0121651

Eberl, C., Wiers, R. W., Pawelczack, S., Rinck, M., Becker, E. S., & Lindenmeyer, J. (2013). Approach bias modification in alcohol dependence: Do clinical effects replicate and for whom does it work best? *Developmental Cognitive Neuroscience, 4*, 38–51. http://doi.org/10.1016/j.dcn.2012.11.002

Eberl, C., Wiers, R. W., Pawelczack, S., Rinck, M., Becker, E. S., & Lindenmeyer, J. (2014). Implementation of approach bias re-training in alcoholism—How many sessions are needed? *Alcoholism, Clinical and Experimental Research, 38*, 587–594. http://doi.org/10.1111/acer.12281

Eisenberg, N., Edwards, A., Spinrad, T. L., Sallquist, J., Eggum, N. D., & Reiser, M. (2013). Are effortful and reactive control unique constructs in young children? *Developmental Psychology, 49,* 2082.

Eisenberg, N., Smith, C. L., & Spinrad, T. L. (2010). Effortful control: Relations with emotion regulation, adjustment, and socialization in childhood. In K. D. Vohs & R. F. Baumeister (Eds.), *Handbook of self-regulation: Research, theory, and applications* (2nd ed., pp. 265–282). New York, NY: Guilford.

Elfeddali, I., de Vries, H., Bolman, C., Pronk, T., & Wiers, R. W. (2016). A randomized controlled trial of web-based attentional bias modification to help smokers quit. *Health Psychology: Official Journal of the Division of Health Psychology, American Psychological Association, 35,* 870–880. http://doi.org/10.1037/hea0000346

Ernst, M., Pine, D. S., & Hardin, M. (2006). Triadic model of the neurobiology of motivated behavior in adolescence. *Psychological Medicine, 36* (September 2005), 299–312. http://doi.org/10.1017/S0033291705005891

Evans, J. S. B. T. (2008). Dual-processing accounts of reasoning, judgment, and social cognition. *Annual Review of Psychology, 59,* 255–278. http://doi.org/10.1146/annurev.psych.59.103006.093629

Evans, J. S. B. T., & Stanovich, K. E. (2013). Dual-process theories of higher cognition: Advancing the debate. *Perspectives on Psychological Science, 8,* 223–241. http://doi.org/10.1177/1745691612460685

Field, M., Wiers, R. W., Christiansen, P., Fillmore, M. T., & Verster, J. C. (2010). Acute alcohol effects on inhibitory control and implicit cognition: Implications for loss of control over drinking. *Alcoholism: Clinical and Experimental Research, 34,* 1–7. http://doi.org/10.1111/j.1530-0277.2010.01218.x

Frank, M. J., Cohen, M. X., & Sanfey, A. G. (2009). Multiple systems in decision making: A neurocomputational perspective. *Current Directions in Psychological Science, 18,* 73–77. http://doi.org/10.1111/j.1467-8721.2009.01612.x

Friese, M., Hofmann, W., & Wiers, R. W. (2011). On taming horses and strengthening riders: Recent developments in research on interventions to improve self-control in health behaviors. http://doi.org/10.1080/15298868.2010.536417

Galvan, A. (2013). The teenage brain sensitivity to rewards. *Current Directions in Psychological Science, 22,* 88–93.

Gawronski, B., & Bodenhausen, G. V. (2006). Associative and propositional processes in evaluation: Conceptual, empirical, and metatheoretical issues: Reply to Albarracín, Hart, and McCulloch (2006), Kruglanski and Dechesne (2006), and Petty and Briñol (2006). *Psychological Bulletin, 132,* 745–750. http://doi.org/10.1037/0033-2909.132.5.745

Gladwin, T. E., Figner, B., Crone, E. A, & Wiers, R. W. (2011). Addiction, adolescence, and the integration of control and motivation. *Developmental Cognitive Neuroscience, 1,* 364–376. http://doi.org/10.1016/j.dcn.2011.06.008

Grafton, B., Macleod, C., Rudaizky, D., Holmes, E., Salemink, E., Fox, E., & Notebaert, L. (2017). Confusing procedures with process when appraising the impact of Cognitive Bias Modification (CBM) on emotional vulnerability: A response to Cristea et al. *British Journal of Psychiatry, 211,* 266–271. doi:10.1192/bjp.115.176123

Gray, J. A. (1994). Framework for a taxonomy of psychiatric disorder. In S. H. M. van Goozen, N. E. Van de Poll, & J. A. Sergeant (Eds.), *Emotions: Essays on emotion theory* (pp. 29–59). Hillsdale, NJ: Erlbaum.

Grenard, J. L., Ames, S. L., Wiers, R. W., Thush, C., Sussman, S., & Stacy, A. W. (2008). Working memory capacity moderates the predictive effects of drug-related associations on substance use. *Psychology of Addictive Behaviors: Journal of the Society of Psychologists in Addictive Behaviors, 22*, 426–432. http://doi.org/10.1037/0893-164X.22.3.426

Gross, J. J., & Thompson, R. A. (2007). Emotion regulation: Conceptual foundations. In J. J. Gross (Ed.), *Handbook of emotion regulation* (pp. 3–26). New York, NY: Guilford.

Gyurak, A., Gross, J. J., & Etkin, A. (2011). Explicit and implicit emotion regulation: A dual-process framework. *Cognition and Emotion, 25*, 400–412.

Hazy, T. E., Frank, M. J., & O'Reilly, R. C. (2007). Towards an executive without a homunculus: Computational models of the prefrontal cortex/basal ganglia system. *Philosophical Transactions of the Royal Society of London. Series B, Biological Sciences, 362*, 1601–1613. http://doi.org/10.1098/rstb.2007.2055

Heatherton, T. F., & Wagner, D. D. (2011). Cognitive neuroscience of self-regulation failure. *Trends in Cognitive Sciences, 15*, 132–139. http://doi.org/10.1016/j.tics.2010.12.005

Hirsch, C. R., Meeten, F., Krahé, C., & Reeder, C. (2016). Resolving ambiguity in emotional disorders: The nature and role of interpretation biases. *Annual Review of Clinical Psychology, 12*, 281–305.

Hofmann, W., Förster, G., Stroebe, W., & Wiers, R. W. (2011). The great disinhibitor: Alcohol, food cues, and eating behavior. In V. R. Preedy, R. R. Watson, & C. R. Martin (Eds.), *Handbook of behavior, food and nutrition* (pp. 2977–2991). New York, NY: Springer.

Hofmann, W., & Friese, M. (2008). Impulses got the better of me: Alcohol moderates the influence of implicit attitudes toward food cues on eating behavior. *Journal of Abnormal Psychology, 117*, 420–427. http://doi.org/10.1037/0021-843X.117.2.420

Hofmann, W., Friese, M., & Strack, F. (2009). Impulse and self-control from a dual-systems perspective. *Perspectives on Psychological Science, 4*, 1–15. http://doi.org/10.1111/j.1745-6924.2009.01116.x

Hofmann, W., Friese, M., & Wiers, R. W. (2008). Impulsive versus reflective influences on health behavior: A theoretical framework and empirical review. *Health Psychology Review, 2*, 111–137. http://doi.org/10.1080/17437190802617668

Hofmann, W., Friese, M., & Wiers, R. W. (2011). Impulsive processes in the self-regulation of health behaviour: Theoretical and methodological considerations in response to commentaries. *Health Psychology Review, 5*, 162–171. http://doi.org/10.1080/17437199.2011.565593

Hofmann, W., Gschwendner, T., Friese, M., Wiers, R. W., & Schmitt, M. (2008). Working memory capacity and self-regulatory behavior: Toward an individual differences perspective on behavior determination by automatic versus controlled processes. *Journal of Personality and Social Psychology, 95*, 962–977. http://doi.org/10.1037/a0012705

Hommel, B., & Wiers, R. W. (2017). Towards a Unitary Approach to Human Action Control. *TICS (Trends in Cognitive Sciences)*, *21*(12), 940–949. http://dx.doi.org/10.1016/j.tics.2017.09.009

Hoorelbeke, K., Koster, E. H. W., Vanderhasselt, M.-A., Callewaert, S., & Demeyer, I. (2015). The influence of cognitive control training on stress reactivity and rumination in response to a lab stressor and naturalistic stress. *Behaviour Research and Therapy*, *69*, 1–10. http://doi.org/10.1016/j.brat.2015.03.010

Houben, K., Havermans, R. C., Nederkoorn, C., & Jansen, A. (2012). Beer à no-go: Learning to stop responding to alcohol cues reduces alcohol intake via reduced affective associations rather than increased response inhibition. *Addiction*, *107*, 1280–1287. http://doi.org/10.1111/j.1360-0443.2012.03827.x

Houben, K., Havermans, R. C., & Wiers, R. W. (2010). Learning to dislike alcohol: Conditioning negative implicit attitudes toward alcohol and its effect on drinking behavior. *Psychopharmacology*, *211*, 79–86. http://doi.org/10.1007/s00213-010-1872-1

Houben, K., Nederkoorn, C., Wiers, R. W., & Jansen, A. (2011). Resisting temptation: Decreasing alcohol-related affect and drinking behavior by training response inhibition. *Drug and Alcohol Dependence, 116*, 132–136. http://doi.org/10.1016/j.drugalcdep.2010.12.011

Houben, K., Wiers, R. W., & Jansen, A. (2011). Getting a grip on drinking behavior: Training working memory to reduce alcohol abuse. *Psychological Science*, *22*, 968–975. http://doi.org/10.1177/0956797611412392

Janssen, T., Larsen, H., Vollebergh, W. A. M., & Wiers, R. W. (2015). Longitudinal relations between cognitive bias and adolescent alcohol use. *Addictive Behaviors*, *44*, 51–57. http://doi.org/10.1016/j.addbeh.2014.11.018

Job, V., Walton, G. M., Bernecker, K., & Dweck, C. S. (2013). Beliefs about willpower determine the impact of glucose on self-control, *110*, 14837–14842. http://doi.org/10.1073/pnas.1313475110

Kagan, J. (2013). Temperamental contributions to inhibited and uninhibited profiles. In P. D. Zelazo (Ed.), *The oxford handbook of developmental psychology* (Vol. 2) (pp. 142–165). New York, NY: Oxford.

Keren, G. (2013). A tale of two systems: A scientific advance or a theoretical stone soup? commentary on Evans & Stanovich (2013). *Perspectives on Psychological Science*, *8*, 257–262. http://doi.org/10.1177/1745691613483474

Keren, G., & Schul, Y. (2009). Two is not always better than one: A critical evaluation of two-system theories. *Perspectives on Psychological Science*, *4*, 533–550. http://doi.org/10.1111/j.1745-6924.2009.01164.x

Kerst, W. F., & Waters, A. J. (2014). Attentional retraining administered in the field reduces smokers' attentional bias and craving. *Health Psychology*, *33*, 1232–1240. http://doi.org/http://dx.doi.org/10.1037/a0035708

Kievit, R. A., Romeijn, J.-W., Waldorp, L. J., Wicherts, J. M., Scholte, H. S., & Borsboom, D. (2011). Mind the gap: A psychometric approach to the reduction problem. *Psychological Inquiry*, *22*, 67–87. http://doi.org/10.1080/1047840X.2011.550181

Klingberg, T. (2010). Training and plasticity of working memory. *Trends in Cognitive Sciences*, *14*, 317–324. http://doi.org/10.1016/j.tics.2010.05.002

Kong, G., Larsen, H., Cavallo, D. A., Becker, D., Cousijn, J., Salemink, E., . . . Krishnan-Sarin, S. (2015). Re-training automatic action tendencies to approach cigarettes among adolescent smokers: A pilot study. *American Journal of Drug and Alcohol Abuse, 41*, 425–432. http://doi.org/10.3109/00952990.2015.1049492

Koole, S. L., & Rothermund, K. (2011). "I feel better but I don't know why": The psychology of implicit emotion regulation. *Cognition and Emotion, 25*, 389–399.

Kopetz, C. E., Lejuez, C. W., Wiers, R. W., & Kruglanski, A. W. (2013). Motivation and self-regulation in addiction: A call for convergence. *Perspectives on Psychological Science, 8*, 3–24. http://doi.org/10.1177/1745691612457575

Kopetz, C. E., & Orehek, E. (2015). When the end justifies the means: Self-defeating behaviors as "rational" and "successful" self-regulation. *Current Directions in Psychological Science, 24*, 386–391. http://doi.org/10.1177/0963721415589329

Kounios, J., & Beeman, M. (2014). The cognitive neuroscience of insight. *Annual Review of Psychology, 65*, 71–93. http://doi.org/10.1146/annurev-psych-010213-115154

Krank, M. D., Ames, S. L., Grenard, J. L., Schoenfeld, T., & Stacy, A. W. (2010). Paradoxical effects of alcohol information on alcohol outcome expectancies. *Alcoholism: Clinical and Experimental Research, 34*, 1193–1200. http://doi.org/10.1111/j.1530-0277.2010.01196.x

Kriete, T., Noelle, D. C., Cohen, J. D., & O'Reilly, R. C. (2013). Indirection and symbol-like processing in the prefrontal cortex and basal ganglia. *Proceedings of the National Academy of Sciences, 110*, 16390–16395. http://doi.org/10.1073/pnas.1303547110

Lier, P. A. C. Van, Huizink, A., & Crijnen, A. (2009). Impact of a preventive intervention targeting childhood disruptive behavior problems on tobacco and alcohol initiation from age 10 to 13 years, *Drug and Alcohol Dependence, 100*, 228–233. http://doi.org/10.1016/j.drugalcdep.2008.10.004

Lindgren, K. P., Wiers, R. W., Teachman, B. A., Gasser, M. L., Westgate, E. C., Cousijn, J., . . . Neighbors, C. (2015). Attempted training of alcohol approach and drinking identity associations in us undergraduate drinkers: Null results from two studies. *PLoS ONE, 10*, 1–21. http://doi.org/10.1371/journal.pone.0134642

Luna, B., Paulsen, D. J., Padmanabhan, A., & Geier, C. (2013). The teenage brain cognitive control and motivation. *Current Directions in Psychological Science, 22*, 94–100.

MacDonald, K. B. (2008). Effortful control, explicit processing, and the regulation of human evolved predispositions. *Psychological Review, 115*, 1012–1031. http://doi.org/10.1037/a0013327

MacDonald, T. K., Fong, G. T., Zanna, M. P., Martineau, A. M., Ebel, A., Ellice, J., . . . Terp-, J. (2000). Alcohol myopia and condom use: Can alcohol intoxication be associated with more prudent behavior? *Journal of Personality and Social Psychology, 78*, 605–619. http://doi.org/10.1037//0022-3514.78.4.605

Macleod, C., & Clarke, P. J. F. (2015). The attentional bias modification approach to anxiety intervention. *Clinical Psychological Science*, 3, 58–78. http://doi.org/10.1177/2167702614560749

MacLeod, C., & Grafton, B. (2014). Regulation of emotion through modification of attention. In J. J. Gross (Ed.), *Handbook of emotion regulation* (2nd ed., pp. 508–528). New York, NY: Guilford.

Maddox, W. T., Gorlick, M. A., Koslov, S., McGeary, J. E., Knopik, V. S., & Beevers, C. G. (2015). Serotonin transporter genetic variation is differentially associated with reflexive- and reflective-optimal learning. *Cerebral Cortex*, bhv309. http://doi.org/10.1093/cercor/bhv309

Miller, W. R., & Rollnick, G. A. (2013). *Motivational interviewing: Helping people change.* New York, NY: Guilford.

Mischel, W., Shoda, Y., & Rodriguez, M. L. (1989). Delay of gratification in children. *Science, 244*, 933–938.

Moffitt, T. E., Arseneault, L., Belsky, D., Dickson, N., Hancox, R. J., Harrington, H., . . . Caspi, A. (2011). A gradient of childhood self-control predicts health, wealth, and public safety. *Proceedings of the National Academy of Sciences of the United States of America, 108*, 2693–2698. http://doi.org/10.1073/pnas.1010076108

Monti, P. M., Colby, S. M., Barnett, N. P., Spirito, A., Rohsenow, D. J., Myers, M., . . . Lewander, W. (1999). Brief intervention for harm reduction with alcohol-positive older adolescents in a hospital emergency department. *Journal of Consulting and Clinical Psychology, 67*, 989.

Nigg, J. T. (2000). On inhibition/disinhibition in developmental psychopathology: Views from cognitive and personality psychology and a working inhibition taxonomy. *Psychological Bulletin, 126*, 220.

Nigg, J. T. (2006). Temperament and developmental psychopathology. *Journal of Child Psychology and Psychiatry and Allied Disciplines, 47*, 395–422. http://doi.org/10.1111/j.1469-7610.2006.01612.x

Ostafin, B. D., Bauer, C., & Myxter, P. (2012). Mindfulness decouples the relation between automatic alcohol motivation and heavy drinking. *Journal of Social and Clinical Psychology, 31*, 729–745.

Ostafin, B. D., Marlatt, G. A., & Greenwald, A. G. (2008). Drinking without thinking: An implicit measure of alcohol motivation predicts failure to control alcohol use. *Behaviour Research and Therapy, 46*, 1210–1219. http://doi.org/10.1016/j.brat.2008.08.003

Ouimet, A. J., Gawronski, B., & Dozois, D. J. A. (2009). Cognitive vulnerability to anxiety: A review and an integrative model. *Clinical Psychology Review, 29*, 459–470. http://doi.org/10.1016/j.cpr.2009.05.004

Paus, T., Keshavan, M., & Giedd, J. N. (2008). Why do many psychiatric disorders emerge during adolescence? *Nature Reviews. Neuroscience, 9*, 947–957. http://doi.org/10.1038/nrn2513

Peeters, M., Monshouwer, K., van de Schoot, R. A. G. J., Janssen, T., Vollebergh, W. A. M., & Wiers, R. W. (2013). Automatic processes and the drinking behavior in early adolescence: A prospective study. *Alcoholism: Clinical and Experimental Research, 37*, 1737–1744. http://doi.org/10.1111/acer.12156

Peeters, M., Wiers, R. W., Monshouwer, K., van de Schoot, R., Janssen, T., & Vollebergh, W. A. M. (2012). Automatic processes in at-risk adolescents: The role of alcohol-approach tendencies and response inhibition in drinking behavior. *Addiction (Abingdon, England), 107*, 1939–1946. http://doi.org/10.1111/j.1360-0443.2012.03948.x

Peper, J. S., Koolschijn, P. C. M. P., & Crone, E. A. (2013). Development of risk taking: Contributions from adolescent testosterone and the orbito-frontal cortex. *Journal of Cognitive Neuroscience, 25*, 2141–2150.

Pessoa, L. (2008). On the relationship between emotion and cognition. *Nature Reviews. Neuroscience, 9*, 148–158. http://doi.org/10.1038/nrn2317

Posner, M. I., Rothbart, M. K., Sheese, B. E., & Voelker, P. (2014). Developing attention: Behavioral and brain mechanisms. *Advances in Neuroscience, 2014.*

Pronk, T., van Deursen, D. S., Beraha, E. M., Larsen, H., & Wiers, R. W. (2015). Validation of the Amsterdam Beverage Picture Set: A controlled picture set for cognitive bias measurement and modification paradigms. *Alcoholism: Clinical and Experimental Research, 39*, 2047–2055. http://doi.org/10.1111/acer.12853

Quevedo, K. M., Benning, S. D., Gunnar, M. R., & Dahl, R. E. (2009). The onset of puberty: Effects on the psychophysiology of defensive and appetitive motivation. *Development and Psychopathology, 21*, 27–45. http://doi.org/10.1017/S0954579409000030

Rensburg, K. J. Van, & Taylor, A. (2009). Acute exercise modulates cigarette cravings and brain activation in response to smoking-related images: An fMRI study. *Psychopharmacology, 203*, 589–598. http://doi.org/10.1007/s00213-008-1405-3

Rothbart, M. K., & Posner, M. I. (2011). Developing mechanisms of self-regulation in early life. *Emotion Review, 3*, 207–213. http://doi.org/10.1177/1754073910387943. Developing

Salemink, E., Friese, M., Drake, E., Mackintosh, B., & Hoppitt, L. (2013). Indicators of implicit and explicit social anxiety influence threat-related interpretive bias as a function of working memory capacity. *Frontiers in Human Neuroscience, 7*(May), 220. http://doi.org/10.3389/fnhum.2013.00220

Salemink, E., & Wiers, R. W. (2012). Adolescent threat-related interpretive bias and its modification: The moderating role of regulatory control. *Behaviour Research and Therapy, 50*, 40–6. http://doi.org/10.1016/j.brat.2011.10.006

Satpute, A. B., & Lieberman, M. D. (2006). Integrating automatic and controlled processes into neurocognitive models of social cognition. *Brain Research, 1079*, 86–97. http://doi.org/10.1016/j.brainres.2006.01.005

Schoenmakers, T. M., de Bruin, M., Lux, I. F. M., Goertz, A. G., Van Kerkhof, D. H. a T., & Wiers, R. W. (2010). Clinical effectiveness of attentional bias modification training in abstinent alcoholic patients. *Drug and Alcohol Dependence, 109*(1–3), 30–36. http://doi.org/10.1016/j.drugalcdep.2009.11.022

Schweizer, S., Grahn, J., Hampshire, A., Mobbs, D., & Dalgleish, T. (2013). Training the emotional brain: Improving affective control through emotional working memory training. *Journal of Neuroscience, 33*, 5301–5311.

Schweizer, S., Hampshire, A., & Dalgleish, T. (2011). Extending brain-training to the affective domain: Increasing cognitive and affective executive control through emotional working memory training. *PLoS ONE, 6*. http://doi.org/10.1371/journal.pone.0024372

Sheeran, P., Gollwitzer, P. M., & Bargh, J. A. (2013). Nonconscious processes and health. *Health Psychology, 32 VN-r*, 460. http://doi.org/10.1037/a0029203

Smith, E. R., & DeCoster, J. (2000). Dual-process models in social and cognitive psychology: Conceptual integration and links to underlying memory systems. *Personality and Social Psychology Review, 4*, 108–131. http://doi.org/10.1207/S15327957PSPR0402_01

Steinberg, L. (2010). A dual systems model of adolescent risk-taking. *Developmental Psychobiology, 52*, 216–224. http://doi.org/10.1002/dev.20445

Strack, F., & Deutsch, R. (2004). Reflective and impulsive determinants of social behavior. *Personality and Social Psychology Review*, *8*, 220–247. http://doi.org/10.1207/s15327957pspr0803_1

Thush, C., Wiers, R. W., Ames, S. L., Grenard, J. L., Sussman, S., & Stacy, A. W. (2008). Interactions between implicit and explicit cognition and working memory capacity in the prediction of alcohol use in at-risk adolescents. *Drug and Alcohol Dependence*, *94*(1–3), 116–124. http://doi.org/10.1016/j.drugalcdep.2007.10.019

Tobler, N. S., Roona, M. R., Ochshorn, P., Marshall, D. G., Streke, A. V, & Stackpole, K. M. (2000). School-based adolescent drug prevention programs: 1998 meta-analysis. *Journal of Primary Prevention*, *20*, 275–336.

Todd, R. M., Cunningham, W. A., Anderson, A. K., & Thompson, E. (2012). Affect-biased attention as emotion regulation. *Trends in Cognitive Sciences*, *16*, 365–372.

Van Bockstaele, B., Verschuere, B., Tibboel, H., De Houwer, J., Crombez, G., & Koster, E. H. W. (2014). A review of current evidence for the causal impact of attentional bias on fear and anxiety. *Psychological Bulletin*, *140*, 682.

van Deursen, D. S., Salemink, E., Boendermaker, W. J., Pronk, T., Hofmann, W., & Wiers, R. W. (2015). Executive functions and motivation as moderators of the relationship between automatic associations and alcohol use in problem drinkers seeking online help. *Alcoholism: Clinical and Experimental Research*, *39*, 1788–1796. http://doi.org/10.1111/acer.12822

Van Duijvenvoorde, A. C. K., & Crone, E. A. (2013). The teenage brain: A neuroeconomic approach to adolescent decision making. *Current Directions in Psychological Science*, *22*, 108–113.

Veling, H., Koningsbruggen, G. M. Van, Aarts, H., & Stroebe, W. (2014). Targeting impulsive processes of eating behavior via the Internet: Effects on body weight. *Appetite*, *78*, 102–109. http://doi.org/10.1016/j.appet.2014.03.014

White, H. R., Marmorstein, N. R., Crews, F. T., Bates, M. E., Mun, E. Y., & Loeber, R. (2011). Associations between heavy drinking and changes in impulsive behavior among adolescent boys. *Alcoholism: Clinical and Experimental Research*, *35*, 295–303. http://doi.org/10.1111/j.1530-0277.2010.01345.x

Whiteside, S. P., & Lynam, D. R. (2003). Understanding the role of impulsivity and externalizing psychopathology in alcohol abuse: Application of the UPPS impulsive behavior scale. *Experimental and Clinical Psychopharmacology*, *11*, 210.

Wiers, R. W., Bartholow, B. D., van den Wildenberg, E., Thush, C., Engels, R. C. M. E., Sher, K. J., . . . Stacy, A. W. (2007). Automatic and controlled processes and the development of addictive behaviors in adolescents: A review and a model. *Pharmacology, Biochemistry, and Behavior*, *86*, 263–283. http://doi.org/10.1016/j.pbb.2006.09.021

Wiers, R. W., Becker, D., Holland, R., Moggi, F., Lejuez, C. W., & Yield, A. (2016). Cognitive motivational processes underlying addiction treatment. In C. E. Kopetz & C. W. Lejuez (Eds.), *Addictions: A social psychological perspective* (pp. 201–236). New York, NY: Routledge.

Wiers, R. W., Beckers, L., Houben, K., & Hofmann, W. (2009). A short fuse after alcohol: Implicit power associations predict aggressiveness after alcohol consumption in young heavy drinkers with limited executive control. *Pharmacology, Biochemistry, and Behavior*, *93*, 300–305. http://doi.org/10.1016/j.pbb.2009.02.003

Wiers, R. W., Boelema, S. R., Nikolaou, K., & Gladwin, T. E. (2015). On the development of implicit and control processes in relation to substance use in adolescence. *Current Addiction Reports, 2*, 141–155. http://doi.org/10.1007/s40429-015-0053-z

Wiers, R. W., Eberl, C., Rinck, M., Becker, E. S., & Lindenmeyer, J. (2011). Retraining automatic action tendencies changes alcoholic patients' approach bias for alcohol and improves treatment outcome. *Psychological Science, 22*, 490–497. http://doi.org/10.1177/0956797611400615

Wiers, R. W., Boffo, M, & Field, M. (in press). What's in a Trial? On the Importance of Distinguishing between Experimental Lab-Studies and Randomized Controlled Trials; the Case of Cognitive Bias Modification and Alcohol Use Disorders. *Journal of Studies on Alcohol and Drugs.*

Wiers, R. W., & Gladwin, T. E. (2017). Reflective and impulsive processes in addiction and the role of motivation. In R. Deutsch, B. Gawronski, & W. Hofmann (Eds.), *Reflective and Impulsive Determinants of Human Behavior* (pp. 173–188). Psychology Press.

Wiers, R. W., Gladwin, T. E., Hofmann, W., Salemink, E., & Ridderinkhof, K. R. (2013). Cognitive bias modification and cognitive control training in addiction and related psychopathology: Mechanisms, clinical perspectives, and ways forward. *Clinical Psychological Science, 1*, 192–212. http://doi.org/10.1177/2167702612466547

Wiers, R. W., Houben, K., Fadardi, J. S., van Beek, P., Rhemtulla, M., & Cox, W. M. (2015). Alcohol cognitive bias modification training for problem drinkers over the web. *Addictive Behaviors, 40*, 21–26. http://doi.org/10.1016/j.addbeh.2014.08.010

Wiers, R. W., Rinck, M., Kordts, R., Houben, K., & Strack, F. (2010). Retraining automatic action-tendencies to approach alcohol in hazardous drinkers. *Addiction (Abingdon, England), 105*, 279–287. http://doi.org/10.1111/j.1360-0443.2009.02775.x

Wiers, R. W., & Stacy, A. (2006). Implicit cognition and addiction. *Current Directions in Psychological Science, 15*, 292–296. Retrieved from http://cdp.sagepub.com/content/15/6/292.short

9

The Behavioral Affective Associations Model

MARC T. KIVINIEMI AND LYNNE B. KLASKO-FOSTER

INTRODUCTION

Young adults are often embarrassed when they purchase condoms or bring up their use with a prospective sexual partner (Leary, Tchividijian, & Kraxberger, 1994). Individuals who decide not to undergo a colonoscopy screening sometimes attribute their failure to screen to a feeling of disgust when considering the procedure (Consedine, Ladwig, Reddig, & Broadbent, 2011; Kiviniemi, Jandorf, & Erwin, 2014). Feeling enthusiastic and energetic while exercising can positively influence the frequency of exercise, while feelings of fatigue during exercise can decrease the desire to commit to regular physical activity (Kwan & Bryan, 2010).

Each of these examples has a common underlying characteristic—in each, a health behavior (condom purchase/use, cancer screening, physical activity) the person is engaging in or considering engaging in is directly associated with a positively or negatively valenced emotional/affective state. Also, in each the affective state plays an important role in determining whether or not the behavior is enacted—young adults may avoid condoms to avoid the associated feelings of embarrassment, noncompliant screeners do not screen because they are experiencing disgust, and exercisers can continue to engage in the behavior in order to experience the positive affective state or avoid the behavior to evade negative feelings (Kwan, Stevens, & Bryan, in press).

In this chapter, we provide a conceptual overview and a summary of the research evidence concerning the role of these affective associations with behaviors in behavioral self-regulation, in the context of the *behavioral affective associations model* (Kiviniemi, Voss-Humke, & Seifert, 2007). We explore the nature of affective associations with behaviors, when and how they operate to influence behavioral outcomes, their relations to and interplay with social cognitive factors as determinants of behavioral practices, and ways to use affective associations as targets in intervention approaches to change behaviors.

Affective Associations with Behaviors—A Brief Overview

Each of the examples described previously—embarrassment and condom use, disgust and colonoscopy screening, positive mood and exercise—are exemplars of *affective associations with behaviors.* We use the term "affective associations" to describe a connection between an individual's mental conceptualization of a given behavioral practice and an affective/emotional state. Such a definition of affective association encompasses concepts from the attitudes, decision-making, and health behavior literatures such as affective components of attitudes, anticipated affect, and others (for an integrative review of these constructs see Williams & Evans, 2014). The defining feature is that an affective association is a feeling state (either a specific emotion such as disgust, excitement, fear, or happiness or a more diffuse positive or negative affect) associated with a specific behavior.

The idea that individuals associate affective/emotional states with behaviors is not unique to the behavioral affective associations model.

Indeed, the idea that attitudes toward particular attitude objects, including behaviors, can have affective components is a central tenet of the classic tripartite model of attitudes (Katz, 1959; Rosenberg, Hovland, McGuire, Abelson, & Brehm, 1960) and has been empirically demonstrated (Breckler, 1984; Breckler & Wiggins, 1989; Crites, Fabrigar, & Petty, 1994). In the health domain, affective components of attitudes about health behaviors have been demonstrated for health behaviors including drug use (Simons & Carey, 1998), food purchases (Dean, Raats, & Shepherd, 2008), physical activity (French et al., 2005), and other leisure time activities (Ajzen & Driver, 1992; for an integrative review of this literature, see McEachan et al., 2016). Studies examining multiple health behaviors have found consistent evidence for the role of affective associations as predictors of behavior (e.g., Conner, McEachan, Lawton, & Gardner, 2016; Conner, McEachan, Taylor, O'Hara, & Lawton, 2015; Lawton, Conner, & McEachan, 2009).

At the level of more specific emotional states, disgust has been shown to be associated with a variety of health-related behaviors, including novel dietary behaviors (Rozin, 1996), organ donation (O'Carroll, Foster, McGeechan, Sandford, & Ferguson, 2011), and colorectal cancer screening (Chapple, Ziebland, Hewitson, & McPherson, 2008; Denberg et al., 2005). The disgust elicited by consideration of a potential behavior is associated with failing to engage in that behavior, given that disgust plays an important role in signaling that one should keep a safe distance from an object, situation, or event (Rozin, Haidt, & McCauley, 2008). The degree of disgust can directly affect behavioral decision-making. For example, greater feelings of disgust when considering organ donation predicts potential donors failing to register (O'Carroll et al., 2011).

Behavioral Affective Associations Model

Although affective associations are well documented and frequently noted in health domains, most current theoretical models of decision-making primarily focus on cognitive processes to explain health behavior (for an exception, see Rhodes & Conner, 2010). Many current models primarily focus on consequentialist, expected utility constructs (for discussion see Loewenstein, Weber, Hsee, & Welch, 2001) in which behavior is determined through a cost/benefit analysis that weighs cognitive beliefs (such as benefits or barriers as a function of perceived vulnerability and severity in the health belief model). Although such models do predict and explain variance in health-related behaviors, they are limited in their focus on cognition to the exclusion of other factors, including affective factors.

The behavioral affective associations model (Kiviniemi et al., 2007) incorporates the concept of affective associations, or feelings associated with a specific health behavior, as a driver of health decision-making. The model takes seriously the role of cognitive beliefs, such as the constructs in most health decision-making models, but explicitly considers how those beliefs act in concert with affective associations to guide behavior.

The behavioral affective associations model is based on three main principles: (1) affective associations influence behavior; (2) affective associations mediate the impact of social cognitive beliefs on behavior; and (3) affective associations can influence behavior in two ways—both by serving as a mediator of the more distal effects of social cognitive factors and as a direct influence on behavior independent of cognitive factors (Kiviniemi & Bevins, 2008). Evidence for these tenets has been shown across multiple health behavior domains, including eating behaviors (Jun & Arendt, 2016; Kiviniemi & Duangdao, 2009; Walsh & Kiviniemi, 2014), smoking (Lawton, Conner, & Parker, 2007), physical activity (Helfer, Elhai, & Geers, 2015; Kiviniemi et al., 2007; Lawton et al., 2009), cancer screening (Brown-Kramer & Kiviniemi, 2015; Kiviniemi et al., 2014; Zhao & Nan, 2016), sunscreen use (Kiviniemi & Ellis, 2014), donating biospecimens for research (Kiviniemi et al., 2013), and condom use (Ellis, Homish, Parks, Collins, & Kiviniemi, 2015).

Affective Associations Influence Behavior

First, the model posits that affective associations are a direct motivator of behavior. Behavior is more likely to occur when associated with positive affective associations and less likely to occur when associated with negative affective associations. Affective associations, in this framework, are seen as serving a "signaling" role, indicating the relative favorability of behavioral actions (for more elucidation of this signaling role, see Bechara, Damasio, & Damasio, 1997; Damasio, 1994; Kiviniemi & Bevins, 2007; Kiviniemi et al., 2007).

Evidence for this tenet has been found in both observational (Brown-Kramer & Kiviniemi, 2015; Kiviniemi & Duangdao, 2009; Kiviniemi et al., 2014; Kiviniemi et al., 2007) and experimental studies (Ellis et al., 2015; Ellis, Kiviniemi, & Cook-Cottone, 2014; Walsh & Kiviniemi, 2014) testing the behavioral affective associations model. In particular, in the experimental studies we have shown that experimental manipulations of affective associations change behavior without any concomitant change in cognitive beliefs (see also Catellier & Yang, 2013). In addition to evidence from the behavioral affective associations studies cited previously, other labs have demonstrated direct relations of affective associations to a number of health behaviors and an effect of such associations over and above that of cognitive beliefs (Conner, Rhodes, Morris, McEachan, & Lawton, 2011; Jun & Arendt, 2016; Lawton et al., 2009).

Affective Associations Mediate the Influence of Cognitive Beliefs on Behavior

The second tenet of the behavioral affective associations model concerns the integrative interplay of cognitive beliefs and affective associations as influences on behavior. The model posits that affective associations serve as the proximal influence on behavior and that cognitive beliefs have an influence that is indirect and mediated through affective associations. Consistent with the notion of affect playing a signaling role for behavioral action, the model posits that cognitive beliefs "inform" the valence and content of the affective association, with cognitive beliefs favoring the behavior (e.g., high perceived benefits, favorable social norms) leading to more positive affective associations.

Consistent with this mediational tenet, affective associations have been shown to mediate the relation of constructs from both the health belief model and the theory of planned behavior and physical activity behavior (Kiviniemi et al., 2007), expected utility beliefs and dietary behavior (Kiviniemi & Duangdao, 2009) and colonoscopy screening (Kiviniemi et al., 2014), a number of social cognitive constructs and condom use (Ellis et al., 2015), and self-exam behaviors (Brown-Kramer & Kiviniemi, 2015). By and large, the cognitive beliefs constructs are fully mediated by affective associations (i.e., they have no direct effect on behavior after the mediational role of affective associations is modeled).

Although the bulk of this work has been done examining cognitive beliefs about and affective associations with health behaviors, there have been interesting extensions of the behavioral affective associations model to the relation of risk perception and behavior. For both the relation of perceived risk for skin cancer and sunscreen use (Kiviniemi & Ellis, 2014) and the relation of perceived cervical cancer risk and pap smear screening use (Zhao & Nan, 2016), the relation between cognitively based risk components (e.g., absolute and comparative risk) and behavior was mediated by affectively based risk components (e.g., feelings of worry about the health problem).

Affective Associations Influence Behavior Independent of Their Role as Mediators of Cognitive Beliefs

Finally, affective associations influence behaviors in two key ways. One effect of affective associations is the one covered already, that affective associations mediate the cognition-behavior relation for a number of constructs. Over and above this influence, in which one causal factor in determining an individual's affective associations with a behavior is the individual's cognitive beliefs about a behavior, there are portions of affective associations that are independent of this relation to cognitive beliefs. These independent components can influence behavior separately and distinctly from the cognitive-affective mediational pathway. Even after one accounts for the variance in affective associations explained by their association with cognitive beliefs, the remaining variance in affective associations is still systematically predictive of behavior (Kiviniemi & Duangdao, 2009; Kiviniemi et al., 2007). In other words, one determinant of affective associations is the content of one's cognitive beliefs about the behavior, but there are also meaningful sources and portions of affective associations over and above the cognitive beliefs route.

Changing Affective Associations

Given the evidence for the central role of affective associations as determinants of health behaviors, there is potential for changing affective associations to serve as important intervention targets—to the extent that an intervention can shape the positivity or negativity of an affective association with a behavior, it might effectively increase desired behaviors (by developing associations between the behavior and more positive affect) or decrease undesired ones (by developing new negative affective associations).

This possibility has been explored in a set of laboratory studies examining the ability to experimentally manipulate affective associations in the laboratory setting and the effects of those manipulations on subsequent behavior. In the first of these studies, participants were randomly assigned to receive positive, negative, or neutral affective primes associated with fruits (Walsh & Kiviniemi, 2014). Subsequent to this manipulation of affective associations, participants were given a snack selection task. Those participants primed with positive affective associations were more likely to select fruit as a snack (over granola bars). In a second study, a similar priming manipulation associating positive or neutral affective associations with condom use resulted in increased numbers of condoms taken in a subsequent condom selection task (Ellis et al., 2015). Moreover, this effect of the experimental manipulation on behavior was partially mediated by the changes in participants' affective associations with the behavior and occurred without any concomitant change in participants' cognitive beliefs about condoms. As posited by the behavioral affective associations model, these results suggest that at least part of the increased protective behavior (more condoms taken) functioned by way of the manipulated change in positive affective associations toward condom use.

There are also intervention techniques targeting affective associations that are feasible to incorporate in "real world" health behavior interventions. As one example, affective associations with exercise were manipulated by presenting participants with positive or neutral messages about postexercise feelings prior to a light exercise task (Helfer et al., 2015). Participants in the positive affect condition reported greater positive exercise intentions regardless of their preexisting physical activity level. Similarly, for inactive youth, an intervention using affectively driven text messages (for example, "Physical activity can make you feel cheerful") was more effective in increasing exercise uptake than more instrumental messages (for example, "Physical activity can help you maintain a healthy weight") (Sirriyeh, Lawton, & Ward, 2010; see Carfora, Caso, & Conner, 2016, for similar results for fruit and vegetable consumption).

Ferrer and colleagues incorporated an affective educational component into a social cognitive intervention to increase condom use among college students. In the interventions, video-based messaging argued that condom use could be associated with positive feelings (e.g., love, confidence, sexual arousal) and also delivered messages reducing the possible impact of negative emotions (e.g., guilt). Compared to a condition that only included a traditional social-cognitive intervention, those who received the social cognitive + the emotional intervention reported greater condom use 6 months later (Ferrer, Fisher, Buck, & Amico, 2011).

Affective associations can also be shifted by interventions without being directly, overtly targeted by the intervention technique. In a test of an educational intervention designed to increase participation by African Americans in epidemiological biobanking research, intervention components highlighting the importance of such research to understanding the causes of cancer in minority communities and framing participation as a social and community benefit significantly reduced the negativity of participants' affective associations with participation, which, in turn, predicted taking part in the biobanking recruitment process (Erwin et al., 2013; Kiviniemi et al., 2013).

Wrapping It All Together: Remaining Questions and New Directions for Research

While evidence exists for affective associations as proximal drivers of behavioral decision-making, interactions between affect and other elements of behavioral self-regulation are less understood. The final section of this chapter will present a cohesive summary of the research evidence described above, touch on some of the unexplored aspects of affect in relation to behavior change, and present implications of the behavioral affective association model for intervention development.

Summary of Research Evidence

As we have described earlier, to date there is converging evidence from both observational and experimental studies demonstrating that affective associations serve as proximal, seemingly direct determinants of behavior and that affective associations mediate the influence of a variety of social-cognitive influences on behavior. These findings and their integration into the tenets of the behavioral affective associations model shift thinking about the nature and operation of both cognitive and affective decision-making inputs from their traditional conceptualization in formal health decision-making theories.

Moreover, there is a newer but growing body of evidence suggesting that targeting affective associations in interventions designed to change health behaviors can be effective—a program of laboratory studies demonstrates that it is possible to create short-term change in an affective association and that such change effectively changes subsequent behaviors. More importantly from an intervention perspective, there is also evidence that affectively based intervention strategies that are feasible to implement in "real world" settings (like group educational sessions and video-based messages) can change behavior in ways that have impact over measurement periods ranging from a few days or weeks (in the case of the time required to complete a biobanking questionnaire process and blood draw, Kiviniemi et al., 2013) to up to 6 months (follow-up period for assessing condom use in Ferrer et al., 2011).

New Directions for Understanding the Mechanisms of Behavior Regulation

Although the research summarized previously has answered a number of questions about affective associations and behaviors, it also raises a number of equally (if not more!) interesting questions about how, when, and why affective associations influence behavior. In this section we raise a few of the most interesting of these questions. In the next section, we take a similar approach to addressing implications for interventions.

One area for consideration for new directions involves the intersection of affective associations and other facets of mood, affect, and emotion. There is both classical and contemporary work suggesting that mood has a substantial influence on decision-making. Not only do affective factors influence behavior directly (as in the behavioral affective associations model) but also affective factors moderate information processing. Demonstrations of these effects on decision-making processes have primarily explored how pieces of information (e.g., information about potential benefits and barriers) are processed and integrated to make a decision, and have shown that individuals interact with and process information differently when they are in positive moods than when they are in negative moods (Aspinwall, 1998; Isen, 2001; Peters, Lipkus, & Diefenbach, 2006).

Given the evidence for the role of affective associations and their interplay with cognitive beliefs, the question of whether positive versus negative moods would moderate the ways in which affective associations influence behavioral decision-making is an interesting but unanswered question. To the extent that we assume that one function of affective associations is to signal the types of feelings that one might experience if one were to engage in the behavior (e.g., expectancies about positive mood following exercise, the belief that one would be embarrassed if one were to recommend condom use), one might expect some congruence. When a person is in a bad mood, and is deciding whether or not to engage in a behavior or deciding between different possible courses of action, it may well be the case that positive affective associations would compel action. A person will then be likely to select the behavior that they believe is most optimally likely to increase their mood, that is, the one for which the affective associations are most positive. By contrast, when a person is in a positive mood and therefore presumably motivated to maintain that mood, one might avoid behaviors that have negative affective associations, even if one's beliefs about the behaviors are predominately positive. Although this hypothesis is intuitively plausible, direct empirical tests remain to be done.

A second unresolved question and area for future research is to probe at the nuances of affective associations. At the beginning we described a variety of differences between different types of constructs that are falling under the umbrella of affective associations. The question of whether these distinctions between constructs are precious and can be considered as a common umbrella of affective associations, or whether there are meaningful differences in the decision-making operation of these constructs remains an unanswered question. For example, is actual affect (which has an arousal component) in anticipatory affect different from the affective component of an attitude, which is typically conceived as a non-arousal-based association between the affect label and the attitude object? Similarly, is a diffuse affective state that is positively or negatively associated with a health behavior different from a specific emotion (for an example of how specific emotions differently signal different actions, see Lerner & Keltner, 2001)?

In addition, the nuances of relations to other constructs remain an interesting and important unanswered question. In the behavioral affective associations model, we look at cognitive beliefs as a set of constructs and affective associations as a set of constructs and examine mediational pathways between them. In each case where multiple constructs have been examined (Kiviniemi & Duangdao, 2009; Kiviniemi et al., 2007) the overall finding that the relation between cognitive factors and behavior is mediated by affective factors has been consistent across a range of different cognitive (e.g., attitudes, social norms, utility beliefs) and affective (global affective states, specific emotions) constructs. Our lab and others have demonstrated that a similar mediational relationship is seen for the interplay of affective and cognitive components of perceived risk—risk feelings (e.g., fear, worry) mediate the relation between risk cognitions (perceived absolute risk, social comparisons about risk) and behavior

(Chapman & Coups, 2006; Kiviniemi & Ellis, 2014; Zhao & Nan, 2016). Although there is demonstrated consistency in the nature of the mediational relations, a worthwhile question is whether there are meaningful differences in the constructs that should be explored. Although both fall under the general category of "cognitions," an expected utility construct such as perceived benefits and barriers is different from an effort justification construct like self-efficacy or an explicitly social construct like social norms. An open question is whether and how those differences across cognitive constructs might affect how they intersect with affective associations to influence decision-making.

This question of the consistency versus uniqueness of mechanisms for different "flavors" of social cognitive constructs intersects with a broader and tremendously important question—what is the mechanism by which an individual's cognitions about a behavior or a health risk come to shape one's affective associations about the behavior or risk? This question remains largely unexplored and has important implications for how we both understand the nature of behavior regulation and develop intervention strategies to change those behaviors.

Finally, an important question for the broader field of affective influences on behavior and behavioral decision-making is to consider the variety of constructs that have the label "affect" and to consider their similarities and differences and how those similarities and differences are implicated in understanding the variety of ways in which affect relates to and causes behavior. To provide just a few examples—is an affective association with a behavior in and of itself (as we have defined affective associations here) the same as or different from an affective association with an expected outcome of the behavioral decision (as in anticipated regret, e.g., Abraham & Sheeran, 2003; Sandberg & Conner, 2008). Is actually experiencing the affective state when considering a behavioral option (as in anticipatory affect, e.g., Loewenstein et al., 2001) associated with different outcomes or different mechanisms for behavioral regulation than is a mental representation of affect that may not involve actual arousal or physiological experience? More questions such as this could be generated, given the wide spectrum of "affect" constructs in the literature. The key point here is that, to fully understand the mechanisms through which affective associations (and other affective constructs) influence behavioral outcomes, we need to have a better understanding of which constructs share common features and act through common mechanisms and which do not.

Implications for Intervention Development

As with the implications for understanding behavioral regulation, there are a variety of questions raised for development of effective interventions to change health-related behaviors. Here, we focus on how the three tenets of the behavioral affective associations model may translate into effective intervention approaches.

The first and most basic implication is that the centrality of affective associations as an influence on behavior strongly suggests that interventions to change behavior will be more effective when they include a component targeting affective associations (for empirical evidence supporting this, see Ferrer et al., 2011). The evidence for the efficacy of traditional social-cognitive interventions to change behavior is decidedly mixed (Noar, 2008; Prestwich et al., 2014; Webb & Sheeran, 2006) and the effects of even well-designed interventions are moderate at best. Inclusion of affective intervention components has the potential to strengthen the effect of interventions on behavioral outcomes, ultimately leading to healthier behavioral patterns.

Second, the mediational pathway between cognitive beliefs and affective associations raises a set of interesting intervention development questions. Following from the point about including affective components, should interventions include both an affective and a cognitive component, or given the more proximal nature of affective associations is an affective component alone equally effective? Although there is evidence that affective associations can change behavior without any cognitive intervention strategy (Ellis et al., 2015; Walsh & Kiviniemi, 2014) and that affect + cognition is more effective than cognition alone (Ferrer et al., 2011), there is not, to our knowledge, evidence to address the question of whether affect + cognition is more effective than affect alone. In our minds, this question might be particularly important to understanding the distinction between behavioral initiation and behavioral maintenance (e.g., Rothman, 2000). Because affective processes are generally assumed to occur automatically, one might posit that long-term behavioral maintenance might be more effectively encouraged by an intervention that targets affective constructs given that, once changed, affective constructs can continue to influence behavior without active effort on the part of the individual.

With respect to the distinction between affective associations arising from the cognitive-affective mediation pathway versus those derived outside of the pathway, the question of other influences on affective associations and how to most effectively change those influences in intervention settings becomes important. Are the effective techniques for shifting associations the same for different facets of the affective associations construct? If not, how does one identify effective techniques for optimizing the change in affective associations necessary for an intervention strategy to be effective?

Last, but certainly not least, it is one thing to effectively change affective associations in a way that changes behavior and another to do so using techniques that are going to be amenable to implementation in the "real world" and particularly to implementation at scale for broad-based, population level reach (Frieden, 2010; Glasgow, McKay, Piette, & Reynolds, 2001; Jilcott, Ammerman, Sommers, & Glasgow, 2007). Successfully using the findings from our program of research and others on the behavioral affective associations model will require developing translatable intervention strategies for changing affective associations.

CONCLUSION

The dual goals of the science of health decision-making and the practice of health behavior change are to better understand the basic human psychology of how individuals make their decisions about health-related behaviors and more broadly, how they regulate engagement in those behaviors, and to then use that knowledge to develop optimally effective intervention techniques which use that knowledge of mechanisms to effectively change behaviors (for further articulation of these dual goals, see, e.g., Baranowski, 2006; Glanz, Rimer, & Viswanath, 2008; Kiviniemi & Rothman, 2010). With respect to both of these goals, the evidence summarized here as well as this volume as a whole highlights the critical role of affect. Affect is known to play a critical role in areas relevant to health, including signaling of risk and reward (e.g., Damasio, 1994), innate, evolutionary-based influences on behavior (e.g., Rozin & Fallon, 1987), and guidance of social relationships (e.g., Bagozzi, 2009). This centrality appears to extend to affective associations. One cannot fully understand behavior regulation and decision-making without affective associations—they are a central feature of the decision-making process and are intertwined in their influence with other known decision-making influences. Continued exploration of both affective associations and other affective influences on decision-making can only strengthen both the basic science and the public health intervention goals articulated previously.

REFERENCES

Abraham, C., & Sheeran, P. (2003). Acting on intentions: The role of anticipated regret. *British Journal of Social Psychology*, *42*, 495–511.

Ajzen, I., & Driver, B. L. (1992). Application of the theory of planned behavior to leisure choice. *Journal of Leisure Research*, *24*, 207–224.

Aspinwall, L. G. (1998). Rethinking the role of positive affect in self-regulation. *Motivation and Emotion*, *22*, 1–32.

Bagozzi, R. P., Verbeke, W., & Belschak, F. (2009). Self-conscious emotions as emotional systems: The role of culture in shame and pride systems. In R. S. Wyer, Chiu, C.-Y., Hong, Y.-Y. (Eds.), *Understanding culture: Theory, research, and application* (pp. 394–409). New York, NY: Psychology Press.

Baranowski, T. (2006). Advances in basic behavioral research will make the most important contributions to effective dietary change programs at this time. *Journal of the American Dietetic Association*, *106*, 808–811.

Bechara, A., Damasio, H. T. D., & Damasio, A. R. (1997). Deciding advantageously before knowing the advantageous strategy. *Science*, *275*, 1293–1295.

Breckler, S. J. (1984). Empirical validation of affect, behavior, and cognition as distinct components of attitude. *Journal of Personality and Social Psychology*, *47*, 1191–1205.

Breckler, S. J., & Wiggins, E. C. (1989). Affect versus evaluation in the structure of attitudes. *Journal of Experimental Social Psychology, 25*, 253–271.

Brown-Kramer, C. R., & Kiviniemi, M. T. (2015). Affective associations and cognitive beliefs relate to individuals' decisions to perform testicular or breast self-exams. *Journal of Behavioral Medicine, 38*, 664–672. doi:10.1007/s10865-015-9641-6

Carfora, V., Caso, D., & Conner, M. (2016). Randomized controlled trial of a messaging intervention to increase fruit and vegetable intake in adolescents: Affective versus instrumental messages. *British Journal of Health Psychology, 21*, 937–955. doi:10.1111/bjhp.12208

Catellier, J. R. A., & Yang, Z. J. (2013). The role of affect in the decision to exercise: Does being happy lead to a more active lifestyle? *Psychology of Sport and Exercise, 14*, 275–282. doi:10.1016/j.psychsport.2012.11.006

Chapman, G. B., & Coups, E. J. (2006). Emotions and preventive health behavior: Worry, regret, and influenza vaccination. *Health Psychology, 25*, 82–90.

Chapple, A., Ziebland, S., Hewitson, P., & McPherson, A. (2008). What affects the uptake of screening for bowel cancer using a faecal occult blood test (FOBt): A qualitative study. *Social Science and Medicine, 66*, 2425–2435.

Conner, M., McEachan, R., Lawton, R., & Gardner, P. (2016). Basis of intentions as a moderator of the intention-health behavior relationship. *Health Psychology, 35*, 219–227. doi:10.1037/hea0000261

Conner, M., McEachan, R., Taylor, N., O'Hara, J., & Lawton, R. (2015). Role of affective attitudes and anticipated affective reactions in predicting health behaviors. *Health Psychology, 34*, 642–652. doi:10.1037/hea0000143

Conner, M., Rhodes, R. E., Morris, B., McEachan, R., & Lawton, R. (2011). Changing exercise through targeting affective or cognitive attitudes. *Psychology and Health, 26*, 133–149. doi:10.1080/08870446.2011.531570

Consedine, N. S., Ladwig, I., Reddig, M. K., & Broadbent, E. A. (2011). The many faeces of colorectal cancer screening embarrassment: Preliminary psychometric development and links to screening outcome. *British Journal of Health Psychology, 16*, 559–579. doi:10.1348/135910710X530942

Crites, S. L., Fabrigar, L. R., & Petty, R. E. (1994). Measuring the affective and cognitive properties of attitudes: Conceptual and methodological issues. *Personality and Social Psychology Bulletin, 20*, 619–634.

Damasio, A. R. (1994). *Descartes' error: Emotion, reason and the human brain*. New York, NY: Putnam.

Dean, M., Raats, M. M., & Shepherd, R. (2008). Moral concerns and consumer choice of fresh and processed organic foods. *Journal of Applied Social Psychology, 38*, 2088–2107. doi:10.1111/j.1559-1816.2008.00382.x

Denberg, T. D., Melhado, T. V., Coombes, J. M., Beaty, B. L., Berman, K., Byers, T. E., . . . Ahnen, D. J. (2005). Predictors of nonadherence to screening colonoscopy. *Journal of General Internal Medicine, 20*, 989–995.

Ellis, E. M., Homish, G. G., Parks, K. A., Collins, R. L., & Kiviniemi, M. T. (2015). Increasing condom use by changing people's feelings about them: An experimental study. *Health Psychology, 34*, 941–950.

Ellis, E. M., Kiviniemi, M. T., & Cook-Cottone, C. (2014). Implicit affective associations predict snack choice for those with low, but not high levels of eating disorder symptomatology. *Appetite, 77*, 124–132. doi:http://dx.doi.org/10.1016/j.appet.2014.03.003

Erwin, D. O., Moysich, K., Kiviniemi, M. T., Saad-Harfouche, F. G., Davis, W., Clark-Hargrave, N., . . . Walker, C. (2013). Community-based partnership to identify keys to biospecimen research participation. *Journal of Cancer Education, 28*, 43–51. doi:10.1007/s13187-012-0421-5

Ferrer, R. A., Fisher, J. D., Buck, R., & Amico, K. R. (2011). Pilot test of an emotional education intervention component for sexual risk reduction. *Health Psychology, 30*, 656–660. doi:10.1037/a0023438

French, D. P., Sutton, S., Hennings, S. J., Mitchell, J., Wareham, N. J., Griffin, S., . . . Kinmonth, A. L. (2005). The importance of affective beliefs and attitudes in the theory of planned behavior: Predicting intention to increase physical activity. *Journal of Applied Social Psychology, 35*, 1824–1848.

Frieden, T. R. (2010). A framework for public health action: the health impact pyramid. *American Journal of Public Health, 100*, 590–595.

Glanz, K., Rimer, B. K., & Viswanath, K. (2008). Theory, research, and practice in health behavior and health education. In K. Glanz, B. K. Rimer, & K. Viswanath (Eds.), *Health behavior and health education: Theory, research, and practice* (4th ed., pp. 23–40). San Francisco, CA: Jossey-Bass.

Glasgow, R. E., McKay, H. G., Piette, J. D., & Reynolds, K. D. (2001). The RE-AIM framework for evaluating interventions: What can it tell us about approaches to chronic illness management? *Patient Education and Counseling, 44*, 119–127.

Helfer, S. G., Elhai, J. D., & Geers, A. L. (2015). Affect and exercise: Positive affective expectations can increase post-exercise mood and exercise intentions. *Annals of Behavioral Medicine, 49*, 269–279. doi:10.1007/s12160-014-9656-1

Isen, A. M. (2001). An influence of positive affect on decision making in complex situations: Theoretical issues with practical implications. *Journal of Consumer Psychology, 11*, 75–85.

Jilcott, S., Ammerman, A., Sommers, J., & Glasgow, R. E. (2007). Applying the RE-AIM framework to assess the public health impact of policy change. *Annals of Behavioral Medicine, 34*, 105–114. doi:10.1007/bf02872666

Jun, J., & Arendt, S. W. (2016). Understanding healthy eating behaviors at casual dining restaurants using the extended theory of planned behavior. *International Journal of Hospitality Management, 53*, 106–115. doi:10.1016/j.ijhm.2015.12.002

Katz, D., & Stotland, E. (1959). A preliminary statement to a theory of attitude structure and change. In S. Koch (Ed.), *Psychology: A Study of a Science*, Vol. 3: *Formulations of the person and the social context* (pp. 423–475). New York, NY: McGraw-Hill.

Kiviniemi, M. T., & Bevins, R. (2007). Affect-behavior associations in motivated behavioral choice: Potential transdisciplinary links. In P. R. Zelick (Ed.), *Issues in the psychology of motivation* (pp. 65–80). Hauppage, NY: Nova.

Kiviniemi, M. T., & Bevins, R. (2008). Role of affective associations in the planning and habit systems of decision making related to addiction. *Behavioral and Brain Sciences, 31*, 450–451.

Kiviniemi, M. T., & Duangdao, K. M. (2009). Affective associations mediate the influence of cost-benefit beliefs on fruit and vegetable consumption. *Appetite*, *52*, 771–775.

Kiviniemi, M. T., & Ellis, E. M. (2014). Worry about skin cancer mediates the relation of perceived cancer risk and sunscreen use. *Journal of Behavioral Medicine*, *37*, 1069–1074.

Kiviniemi, M. T., Jandorf, L., & Erwin, D. O. (2014). Disgusted, embarrassed, afraid: Affective associations relate to uptake of colonoscopy screening in an urban, African American population. *Annals of Behavioral Medicine*, *48*, 112–119.

Kiviniemi, M. T., & Rothman, A. J. (2010). Specifying the determinants of people's health beliefs and health behavior: How a social psychological perspective can inform initiatives to promote health. In J. M. Suls, K. W. Davidson, & R. M. Kaplan (Eds.), *Handbook of health psychology*. New York, NY: Guilford.

Kiviniemi, M. T., Saad-Harfouche, F. G., Ciupak, G. L., Davis, W., Moysich, K., Hargrave, N. C., . . . Erwin, D. O. (2013). Pilot intervention outcomes of an educational program for biospecimen research participation. *Journal of Cancer Education*, *28*, 52–59. doi:10.1007/s13187-012-0434-0

Kiviniemi, M. T., Voss-Humke, A. M., & Seifert, A. L. (2007). How do i feel about the behavior? The interplay of affective associations with behaviors and cognitive beliefs as influences on physical activity behavior. *Health Psychology*, *26*, 152–158.

Kwan, B. M., & Bryan, A. (2010). In-task and post-task affective response to exercise: Translating exercise intentions into behaviour. *British Journal of Health Psychology*, *15*(Pt 1), 115–131. doi:10.1348/135910709X433267

Kwan, B. M., Stevens, C. J., & Bryan, A. D. (in press). What to expect when you're exercising: An experimental test of the anticipated affect–exercise relationship. *Health Psychology*. doi:10.1037/hea0000453

Lawton, R., Conner, M., & McEachan, R. (2009). Desire or reason: Predicting health behaviors from affective and cognitive attitudes. *Health Psychology*, *28*, 56–65.

Lawton, R., Conner, M., & Parker, D. (2007). Beyond cognition: Predicting health risk behaviors from instrumental and affective beliefs. *Health Psychology*, *26*, 259–267.

Leary, M. R., Tchividijian, L. R., & Kraxberger, B. E. (1994). Self-presentation can be hazardous to your health: Impression management and health risk. *Health Psychology*, *13*, 461–470.

Lerner, J. S., & Keltner, D. (2001). Fear, anger, and risk. *Journal of Personality and Social Psychology*, *81*, 146–159. doi:10.1037//0022-3514.81.1.146

Loewenstein, G. F., Weber, E. U., Hsee, C. K., & Welch, N. (2001). Risk as feelings. *Psychological Bulletin*, *127*, 267–286.

McEachan, R., Taylor, N., Harrison, R., Lawton, R., Gardner, P., & Conner, M. (2016). Meta-analysis of the reasoned action approach (RAA) to understanding health behaviors. *Annals of Behavioral Medicine*, *50*, 592–612. doi:10.1007/s12160-016-9798-4

Noar, S. M. (2008). Behavioral interventions to reduce HIV-related sexual risk behavior: Review and synthesis of meta-analytic evidence. *AIDS and Behavior*, *12*, 335–353. doi:10.1007/s10461-007-9313-9

O'Carroll, R. E., Foster, C., McGeechan, G., Sandford, K., & Ferguson, E. (2011). The "ick" factor, anticipated regret, and willingness to become an organ donor. *Health Psychology*, *30*, 236–245. doi:10.1037/a0022379

Peters, E., Lipkus, I., & Diefenbach, M. A. (2006). The functions of affect in health communications and in the construction of health preferences. *Journal of Communication, 56*, S140–S162.

Prestwich, A., Sniehotta, F. F., Whittington, C., Dombrowski, S. U., Rogers, L., & Michie, S. (2014). Does theory influence the effectiveness of health behavior interventions? Meta-analysis. *Health Psychology, 33*, 465–474. doi:10.1037/a0032853

Rhodes, R. E., Conner, M. (2010). Comparison of behavioral belief structures in the physical activity domain. *Journal of Applied Social Psychology, 40*, 2105–2120.

Rosenberg, M. J., Hovland, C. I., McGuire, W. J., Abelson, R. P., & Brehm, J. W. (1960). *Attitude organization and change: An analysis of consistency among attitude components*. Yale Studies in Attitude and Communication. Vol. III. Oxford, UK: Yale University Press.

Rothman, A. J. (2000). Toward a theory-based analysis of behavioral maintenance. *Health Psychology, 19*(1 Suppl), 64–69.

Rozin, P. (1996). Towards a psychology of food and eating: From motivation to module to model to marker, morality, meaning, and metaphor. *Current Directions in Psychological Science, 5*, 18–24.

Rozin, P., & Fallon, A. E. (1987). A perspective on disgust. *Psychological Review, 94*, 23–41.

Rozin, P., Haidt, J., & McCauley, C. R. (2008). Disgust. In M. Lewis, J. M. Haviland-Jones, & L. F. Barrett (Eds.), *Handbook of emotions* (3rd ed., pp. 757–776). New York, NY: Guilford.

Sachs, M. L. (1991). Running—A psychosocial phenomenon. In L. Diamant (Ed.), *Psychology of sports, exercise, and fitness: Social and personal issues*. (pp. 237–247). New York, NY: Hemisphere.

Sandberg, T., & Conner, M. (2008). Anticipated regret as an additional predictor in the theory of planned behaviour: A meta-analysis. *British Journal of Social Psychology, 47*, 589–606.

Simons, J., & Carey, K. B. (1998). A structural analysis of attitudes toward alcohol and marijuana use. *Personality and Social Psychology Bulletin, 24*, 727–735.

Sirriyeh, R., Lawton, R., & Ward, J. (2010). Physical activity and adolescents: An exploratory randomized controlled trial investigating the influence of affective and instrumental text messages. *British Journal of Health Psychology, 15*, 825–840. doi:10.1348/135910710x486889

Walsh, E. M., & Kiviniemi, M. T. (2014). Changing how i feel about the food: Experimentally manipulated affective associations with fruits change fruit choice behaviors. *Journal of Behavioral Medicine, 37*, 322–331.

Webb, T. L., & Sheeran, P. (2006). Does changing behavioral intentions engender behavior change? A meta-analysis of the experimental evidence. *Psychological Bulletin, 132*, 249–268.

Williams, D. M., & Evans, D. R. (2014). Current emotion research in health behavior science. *Emotion Review, 6*, 277–287.

Zhao, X., & Nan, X. (2016). The influence of absolute and comparative risk perceptions on cervical cancer screening and the mediating role of cancer worry. *Journal of Health Communication, 21*, 100–108. doi:10.1080/10810730.2015.1033114

10

Psychological Hedonism, Hedonic Motivation, and Health Behavior

DAVID M. WILLIAMS

INTRODUCTION

Eating calorie-dense foods, smoking cigarettes, using psychoactive drugs, and engaging in promiscuous sex typically lead to immediate pleasure or relief from displeasure. As a result, people are often motivated to engage in these behaviors despite their association with negative health outcomes. Conversely, engaging in vigorous exercise, using condoms, and obtaining flu vaccines and cancer screenings typically lead to immediate displeasure or reduced pleasure; thus, people are often motivated to avoid these behaviors despite their association with positive health outcomes.

This intuitive explanation for health-related behavior is consistent with the ancient principle of psychological hedonism (PH), the idea that human motivation is a function of the pursuit of pleasure and avoidance of displeasure. Framing health-related behavior in terms of PH may seem obvious to some readers. But to others it may seem inadequate, if not patently false. Indeed, traditional formulations of PH have been criticized as either too broad and thus scientifically untestable, or too narrow and thus implausible. Moreover, the mechanism of PH—the way in which pleasures and displeasures influence behavior—has never been adequately specified.

This chapter offers a new way of thinking about PH, grounded, still, in the ancient and intuitive idea that humans tend to pursue pleasure and avoid displeasure, but updated based on recent theory and research in affective neuroscience (i.e., incentive salience theory) and psychology (i.e., dual-processing theory). To provide context, a prototypical formulation of PH is first presented along with the conceptual problems that have been levied against it. The reformulated version of PH is then discussed, including its potential as an overarching framework for health behavior science (see also Williams, forthcoming).

PSYCHOLOGICAL HEDONISM

Psychological hedonism dates back at least as far as Democritus and Epicurus (Moen, 2015) and was famously recast in the writings of Hobbes (1668/1994), Bentham (1780/2007), and Mill (1863/2012). A recent version of PH—one that is used herein as a prototype—was outlined by Sober and Wilson (1998) in their influential book, *Unto Others*: "[Psychological] Hedonism says that the only ultimate desires that people have are the desires to obtain pleasure and avoid pain. All other desires are purely instrumental with respect to these two ends" (p. 224).[1] They go on to clarify that "pain," as used here, includes "all aversive sensations." Similarly, "pleasure" is equated with all pleasant sensations.[2]

Psychological hedonism is a *descriptive* (or explanatory) rather than a *prescriptive* (or ethical) theory. This means that PH is about why people are motivated to behave as they do, rather than about how people *should* be motivated, with the latter referred to as ethical hedonism.[3] Additionally, PH should be distinguished from the burgeoning literature on human well-being in which well-being (i.e., feeling generally good versus bad), rather than motivation or behavior, is the target outcome (e.g., Lyubomirsky, King, & Diener, 2005; Ryan & Deci, 2000).

Sober and Wilson's PH is a type of *motivational hedonism* because it attempts to explain the sources of human motivation in terms of pleasure and displeasure. This allows that the motivation that is the output of psychological hedonism will sometimes fail to determine behavior either because of factors that are outside of one's control or because of what philosophers refer to as *weakness of will* (Moore, 2013). Likewise, PH does not attempt to account for whether a person will be successful in achieving any intended *goal* of their behavior. For example, PH may be applied to understand one's motivation to go into a burning building to save his neighbor, but it does not account for whether he will be successful in saving his neighbor. Nonetheless, Sober and Wilson's statement that "*All* other desires are purely instrumental" (emphasis added) makes PH a universal theory of motivation, meaning that, according to the psychological hedonist, *all* human motivations are *ultimately* a function of pleasure and displeasure. For example, one may have a desire to help another person with his groceries, but this desire is instrumental with respect to her ultimate hedonic desire to feel better about herself.[4]

CRITICISMS OF PSYCHOLOGICAL HEDONISM

The previous description of PH is intuitively appealing. But there are conceptual problems with PH that have been pointed out so many times in the philosophical literature that it is now considered a position of naiveté—one taken by first year undergraduate students who have not yet learned to think critically. The way in which the critiques have been formulated vary considerably (for a review see Moore, 2013), but in general the problems come down to three issues: (1) the ubiquity of counterexamples, (2) the inability to test the theory, and (3) the lack of a plausible mechanism.

The Counterexample Problem

Much of the writing on PH relates to its contrast with altruism, which can be defined as the desire to help others independent of any hedonic desire (Sober & Wilson, 1998). Consistent with the theme of this book, this chapter focuses on self-control over health-related behavior, rather than helping behavior, as the context for PH. As noted earlier, people eat calorie-dense foods, engage in promiscuous sex, drink alcohol, use drugs, and smoke cigarettes because of the pleasure (or relief from displeasure) that those behaviors bring; and people avoid exercise, cancer screenings, flu vaccines, and condoms because of the displeasure (or reduced pleasure) those behaviors bring.[5] This is hardly controversial. The conundrum for the psychological hedonist is that people are also often motivated to perform healthy behaviors that result in less pleasure or more displeasure than the unhealthy behavioral option. Every day people successfully resist the pleasure of tasty foods, alcohol, drug use, and promiscuous sex, and tolerate the pain and displeasure of vigorous exercise, cancer screenings, and flu vaccines. Thus, successful self-control—like the human tendency to help others in the absence of obvious personal benefit—appears to be directly at odds with PH (Atkins, 2015).

These counterexamples, however, are only a problem for a *narrow version* of PH in which people are posited to be motivated by the pleasure and displeasure experienced *immediately* in response to the target behavior. The counterexample criticism is not a problem, however, for a *broad version* of PH in which motivation is a function of the pleasure and displeasure that may occur as a more temporally distal result of the target behavior—that is, ultimate motivations. For example, one could argue that the apparently selfless act of helping someone with his groceries is ultimately motivated by the desire to feel good about oneself or to avoid the guilt that would come with simply walking away. Similarly, successful self-control, it could be argued, is still consistent with PH, because it often involves what is referred to in psychology as delayed gratification—foregoing immediate pleasure or enduring immediate displeasure in order to obtain *even more pleasure* or *even less displeasure* in the future (Mischel, Shoda, & Rodriguez, 1989). Thus, one could argue that the motivation to help others, forego immediate pleasure, or endure immediate displeasure are ultimately motivated by the pursuit of pleasure and the avoidance of displeasure.

The Untestable Problem

While a broad version of PH may solve the counterexample problem, it raises the *untestable problem*. Specifically, without some parameters around what counts as a pursuable pleasure or avoidable displeasure, one is bound to find some future pleasure or displeasure that could be motivating the target behavior. That is, choose any behavior that appears to refute PH—letting someone go in traffic, resisting a piece of chocolate cake, or going to the dentist for a root canal—and it is possible to conjure up any number of expected hedonic benefits that may ultimately be motivating those behaviors: for example, expected self-satisfaction, avoidance of guilt or worry, and so forth. Thus, for any case of apparent altruism or successful self-control, a psychological hedonist can always argue that there was an ultimate hedonic desire that was unaccounted for and was actually driving what appeared to be altruistic or self-controlled behavior. The upshot is that while a broad version of PH can be used to explain a behavior that has already occurred, it is not useful for *predicting* which course of action someone will be motivated to pursue. This leaves the psychological hedonist stuck between two problems. The counterexample problem refutes a narrow version of PH, and a broad theory of PH is untestable.

The Mechanism Problem

A third problem with traditional formulations of PH is that they often are not explicit about exactly *how* people become motivated to pursue pleasure and avoid displeasure. Previous pleasures have typically long since dissipated by the next time the behaviors that produced them are once again available. That is, by the time someone has another opportunity to indulge in chocolate cake, his pleasure from previous cake-eating has long since subsided. So how does the previous pleasure of cake-eating lead to his present motivation to eat the cake?

It is often implied that the mechanism of PH is the *expectation* of future pleasure or displeasure (Troland, 1928). According to this hedonism-of-the-future formulation, the desire to eat the chocolate cake is a function of the conscious and deliberate expectation of the pleasure one will experience from eating the cake. Such expected pleasures (and displeasures) are a form of affective outcome expectancies, which have been posited as key determinants of health-related behavior and are consistent with expectancy-value theories prevalent in contemporary psychology (Conner, this volume).

However, it seems implausible that human desires are always determined by conscious and deliberate thinking about future pleasure or displeasure. Indeed, nearly 300 years ago Bishop Butler argued that PH must be false because desires can occur in the absence of expected pleasure (Stewart, 1992). The visceral desire for the chocolate cake occurs automatically, without having to think about the future pleasure that will result from eating it. Thus, while deliberate expectations of pleasure and displeasure may sometimes constitute the source of human motivation, it is unlikely that such deliberate expectations can explain all motivation.

FOUNDATIONS FOR A REFORMULATED THEORY OF PSYCHOLOGICAL HEDONISM

Advances in affective neuroscience and psychology provide the foundations for a reformulated theory of PH that can overcome the criticisms of past versions of the theory.

'Liking' and 'wanting'

One such scientific advance is the elucidation of the neurobiological underpinnings of reward. Like PH, reward has traditionally been conceptualized in terms of pleasure, with little clarity on what connects pleasurable responses to a reward to future pursuit of the reward. However, a more sophisticated understanding of reward is provided by *incentive salience theory*, in which reward is parsed into the separable components of 'liking' and 'wanting', as well as the incentive learning process that connects previous 'liking' to future 'wanting' (Berridge, 2007; Berridge & Robinson, 1998, 2003).

'Liking' refers to the neurobiological underpinnings of the immediate pleasurable response to a stimulus, such as the taste of food. 'Wanting' refers to the neurobiological underpinnings of *incentive salience*—a specific kind of motivation that is mediated by the mesolimbic dopaminergic system and is automatically triggered upon presentation of a relevant behavioral cue, such as the sight or smell of available food. Because 'liking' and 'wanting' are conceptualized as core neurobiological processes, they include single quotation marks to distinguish them from the colloquial terms *liking* and *wanting* (without quotation marks).

Generally speaking, previous 'liking' of a stimulus leads to future 'wanting' of that stimulus the next time it is cued, although there are some instances in which 'liking' and 'wanting' can become dissociated, thus demonstrating their independence (Berridge, 2007; Berridge & Robinson, 1998, 2003). In addition to its distinction from 'liking', the mesolimbic dopaminergic pathway that underpins 'wanting' is also distinct from the higher cortical processing that undergirds expectations of future pleasure (Berridge, 2012; Dickinson & Balleine, 2010). Thus, with 'wanting', no prediction, expectation, or declarative memory regarding future or previous pleasure is necessary. Instead, organisms *automatically* 'want' certain things upon presentation of a relevant environmental cue.

Finally, according to incentive salience theory, the polar opposites of 'liking' and 'wanting' are 'disliking' and 'dread', respectively, with 'dread' a function of, but also distinct from, previous 'disliking' (Berridge, 1999).

Hedonic Response and Hedonic Motivation

Incentive salience theory provides the foundation for a reformulation of PH—referred to hereafter as the theory of hedonic motivation (THM). In the THM 'liking' and 'disliking' represent the neurobiological underpinnings of *hedonic response*—an organism's *automatic* and *immediate* pleasure versus displeasure (i.e., affective valence; Russell, 1980) in response to a behavior or immediate behavioral outcome. 'Wanting' and 'dread' represent the neurobiological underpinnings of *hedonic motivation*—a neurobiological process that is automatically triggered by a stimulus and manifests in a felt *hedonic desire* to produce an immediate behavioral outcome that has previously brought immediate pleasure (or relief from displeasure) or a felt *hedonic dread* of producing an immediate behavioral outcome that has previously brought immediate displeasure (or reduced pleasure).

Consistent with incentive salience theory, in the THM hedonic motivation is positioned as the proximal mechanism through which *previous* hedonic responses influence future behavior. This formulation represents a hedonism-of-the-past as an alternative to the hedonism-of-the-future in which deliberate *expectations* of future pleasure serve as the mechanism of PH (cf. Morillo, 1995; Seligman, Railton, Baumeister, & Sripada, 2013; Troland, 1928). Moreover, hedonic motivation, like 'wanting' and 'dread' in incentive salience theory, is triggered *automatically* upon encountering a relevant behavioral cue. This explains the psychological experience of desiring a piece of chocolate cake, a beer, a cigarette, or a sexual encounter *without the need for deliberate expectations of the pleasure that these rewards will bring*. That is, one need not first consider how good the chocolate cake will taste in order to "decide" that she wants it. She just hedonically desires the cake, regardless of whether or not she has considered how good it will taste. This is not to deny that people do sometimes *expect* pleasure in response to a behavior or behavioral outcome. However, such expectations of pleasure are neurobiologically and experientially distinct from hedonic motivation, and, in the present formulation, are not posited to be a mechanism of PH.

Also consistent with incentive salience theory, in the THM hedonic response is limited to the *immediate* affective response to a behavior or immediate outcome of the behavior, thus limiting the range of pleasures and displeasures that are posited to determine hedonic motivation and, in turn, behavior. This resolves the untestable problem by narrowing the scope of the theory and thus eliminating the distal-hedonic-consequence-loophole that allows one to save the theory from otherwise contrary data.

Dual Processing

The second scientific development that provides the basis for a reformulated theory of PH is the distinction between automatic and controlled cognitive processing as explicated in dual-processing theories in psychology (e.g., Gawronski & Bodenhausen, 2006; Kahneman, 2011; Sloman, 1996; Smith & DeCoster, 2000; Strack & Deutsch, 2004). Automatic processing is phylogenetically primitive, intuitive, and based on associative learning, and occurs quickly and outside full conscious awareness except for the final output of the processing. Controlled processing, on the other hand, is more phylogenetically recent, deliberative, based on if-then reasoning, and occurs more slowly, with the subject conscious of the processing that leads to the final output (Evans, 2008).

Dual-processing theory can be applied to the *cognitive processing of affective experiences*, and provides a causal connection between previous affective experiences and future motivations (Williams & Evans, 2014; see also Wiers et al., this volume). *Automatic processing of affect* involves the learning of *associations* between environmental stimuli and affective responses. These associations are then automatically triggered when a relevant stimulus or cue is encountered. *Reflective processing of affect* is, on the other hand, a function of *consciously and deliberately formulated* if-then expectancies that may involve anticipated affective responses to the target behavior. Such anticipated affective responses may include *expectations* of immediate pleasure or displeasure in response to a behavior or behavioral outcome—that is, expected hedonic responses—as well as expectations of more distal affective consequences of behavior.

Hedonic and Reflective Motivation

In the THM, it is posited that there are two distinct types of motivation that stem from separate automatic and controlled processing inputs. *Hedonic motivation*, as defined earlier, is based on automatic associations between behavioral cues and previous hedonic responses. *Reflective motivation* is akin to, but not identical to, behavioral intentions, with the latter a causal consequence of the former and further characterized by a *decision* to perform a behavior. Unlike hedonic motivation, reflective motivation is a function of a broad range of controlled processing inputs, including, but not limited to, *expected* pleasures and displeasures, as well as nonaffective outcome expectancies. Accordingly, relative to hedonic motivation, which is a function of relatively discrete and consistent processes emanating from the mesolimbic dopaminergic system, the brain structures that underlie reflective motivation include broad and diverse regions of the cerebral cortex (Reflective motivation as described herein is similar to what K. Berridge refers to as *cognitive wanting*; personal communication, April 28, 2017).

According to the THM, behavior is a function of both hedonic and reflective motivation. By acknowledging that there are multiple types of motivation, the THM overcomes the counterexample problem, as there will be many situations—counterexamples—in which people's actions are a function of reflective rather than hedonic motivation. That is, there will be instances in which reflective motivation outweighs hedonic motivation, leading us to choose the fruit salad instead of the chocolate cake, dutifully perform our often painful workout, and resist the temptation of smoking, drinking, and drugs. Thus, rather than being a universal theory of behavior, the THM allows for a synthesis of the ancient and intuitive notion of PH, as manifest in hedonic motivation, with the predominant sociocognitive emphasis in psychology in which motivation is driven by deliberate thought, as manifest in reflective motivation.

HEDONIC MOTIVATION

The focus in the remainder of this chapter is on the concept of hedonic motivation. Hedonic motivation is distinct from both hedonic response (i.e., pleasure and displeasure) and reflective motivation (i.e., see previous section) and is positioned herein as the mechanism of PH. Hedonic motivation encompasses the neurobiological concept of "wanting," but also emphasizes the psychological experience of hedonic motivation as a manifestation of its neurobiological underpinnings (cf., Panksepp, 2011).[6]

Just as the neurobiological underpinnings of hedonic response and hedonic motivation (i.e., 'liking' versus 'wanting') are distinct, so are their experiential manifestations. The pleasure of biting into a piece of chocolate cake and the discomfort of vigorous exercise are different experiences than the hedonic desire to eat the chocolate cake and the hedonic dread of exercising. Besides the fact that, in these examples, pleasure or displeasure occurs *while* eating or running, and desire or dread occurs *before* the behavior, the experiences of hedonic response and hedonic motivation *feel* different. While the pleasure of eating chocolate cake may lead to future hedonic desire for chocolate cake, the experience of pleasure has no necessary motivational quality in its own right. Conversely, hedonic motivation has no necessary affective quality to it. Hedonic motivation may sometimes be associated with pleasure, particularly when the object of hedonic motivation is within reach, or with displeasure, when the object of hedonic motivation is likely to go unfulfilled. But these affective qualities (pleasure or displeasure) that *may be associated* with hedonic motivation are not *defining qualities* of the experience of hedonic motivation.

Likewise, the experience of hedonic motivation is distinct from the experience of reflective motivation. Hedonic motivation manifests as an experiential feeling ranging from hedonic desire to hedonic dread. Reflective motivation, on the other hand, lacks the experiential feeling of desire or dread. Hedonic motivation has an affective quality of urgency, whereas reflective motivation is affectively "dry." This characterization of the experience of hedonic versus reflective motivation is consistent with Davis's (1982) distinction between appetitive and volative desires (see also Schueler, 1995; for a slightly different view see Schroeder, 2004). Davis (1982) says:

> In one sense, "desire" is synonymous with *want, wish,* and *would like* . . . I refer to desire in this sense as *volative desire*. . . . In its second sense, "desire" has the near synonyms *appetite, hungering, craving, yearning, longing,* and *urge* . . . I refer to desire in this sense as *appetitive desire*. (pp. 181–182, emphasis in original)

Hedonic motivation, like appetitive desires, is experienced as an "appetite, hungering, craving, yearning, longing, [or] urge" whereas reflective motivation, like volative desires, lacks these experiential qualities and is instead more cold and calculated. Hedonic motivation occurs automatically, without any conscious and deliberate thought processes about the sources of one's motivation, whether it is logical, or whether one *should be* so motivated. Conversely, the experience of reflective motivation necessarily involves conscious deliberation about the pros and cons of a given action or the outcomes of that action. Additionally, reflective motivation may be characterized as *ego syntonic*, or emanating from the self, whereas hedonic motivation is *ego dystonic*, or coming from outside the self. As a result, it is possible to have higher order reflective motivations about hedonic motivations: for example, "I wish I didn't *want* to drink so much" or "I want to *want* to exercise." Likewise, we typically do not have *reasons* for our hedonic desires or at least not reasons for which we are acutely aware (Davis, 1982). As a result, it would seem peculiar and perhaps off-putting to ask someone why they are experiencing a hedonic desire, such as a desire for a beer: "Why do you want a beer?" On the other hand, it makes perfect sense and would be appropriate to ask someone who has just turned down a beer: "Why *don't* you want a beer?" This is presumably because we recognize that the desire for a beer is a hedonic desire (even if we do not use that terminology) and that there are no *reasons* for such hedonic desires, whereas the desire to *not* have a beer is (or at least is more likely to be) a reflective desire that has reasons, such as needing to drive home soon, having to get up early the next morning, and so forth.

Targets of Hedonic Motivation

Hedonic motivation is a desire to produce (or dread of producing) an immediate behavioral outcome. However, many behavioral outcomes are so consistently tied to a particular behavior that the distinction between the behavior and the target outcome may become blurred. For example, the *taste* of chocolate, a cigarette, or a beer, and the *sensation* of sex or heroin use are behavioral outcomes that are intimately tied to the behaviors of eating chocolate, smoking a cigarette, drinking beer, having sex, and using heroin. Because of the tight contingency between these behaviors and their outcomes, the behaviors themselves may become a target of hedonic motivation. Of note, many of the behaviors that tend to become the direct target of hedonic motivation are in some way related to health—for example, eating, exercise, sex, smoking, alcohol and drug use.

Importantly, *pleasure and displeasure themselves are not the targets of hedonic motivation*. We do not hedonically desire pleasure or hedonically dread displeasure; we hedonically desire chocolate, cigarettes, beer, sex, and heroin, and hedonically dread exercise and colonoscopies. The fact that the behavior or behavioral outcome is the target of hedonic motivation rather than the hedonic response that it elicits is consistent with Butler's observation that people do not desire pleasure but instead desire the things that bring pleasure (Stewart, 1992).

Sources of Hedonic Motivation

Consistent with incentive salience theory, hedonic motivation varies in direction ('wanting' versus 'dread') and intensity based on between-person differences in learning history. This includes previous contingencies between environmental cues and behavioral outcomes that trigger immediate hedonic responses, and previous direction ('liking' versus 'disliking') and strength of hedonic responses to behavioral outcomes in the presence of the cue. Through incentive learning[7] hedonic desire or dread is triggered in response to an environmental cue that has consistently been present during previous experiences of pleasure or displeasure. Often the environmental cue is the sight, sound, or smell of an object that is the *source* of the taste or tactile feeling that has previously induced the hedonic response. For example, through incentive learning, the sight of chocolate cake can trigger hedonic motivation to eat the chocolate cake. Other times the environmental cue is simply a stimulus that signals the *availability* of a behavioral outcome that has previously resulted in pleasure or displeasure. For example, the sight of a local bar may trigger the hedonic desire for a beer. Hedonic motivation may, at least in humans, also be triggered by *imagined cues*, and cues may generalize to some extent such that, for example, the sight of any bar or pub—not only those experienced previously—may trigger a hedonic desire for beer.

Additionally, the occurrence, direction, and intensity of hedonic response is also a function of within-person differences in the biological context of the environmental cue, such as the person's state of hunger versus satiation (Berridge, 2012; Zhang et al., 2009). For example, one may experience a strong hedonic desire for chocolate cake, an absence of hedonic motivation, or even hedonic dread or aversion to the cake depending on whether or not they are hungry and how much chocolate cake they have already consumed.

Hedonic Motivation and Extant Motivation Concepts

Hedonic motivation is similar in many ways to recent conceptualizations of *desire* that have also emphasized the concept of 'wanting' (i.e., incentive salience) as well as desire's causal connection to pleasure and displeasure (Hofmann & Van Dillen, 2012; Kavanagh, Andrade, & May, 2005). Particularly relevant is Hofmann and Nordgren's (2015) conceptualization in which they explicitly distinguish desire from cognitively derived goals—a position that directly maps on to the distinction herein between hedonic and reflective motivation, respectively. Nonetheless, the word "desire" is still ambiguous with respect to the distinction between hedonic and reflective motivation. Use of the "hedonic" qualifier in the term "hedonic desire" provides a level of specificity not present in the unqualified term "desire." That is, hedonic desire is less likely to be confused or confounded with cognitively determined desires (i.e., goals or intentions).

Likewise, the concepts of craving and urge as used in addiction and eating research (e.g., Wilson & Sayette, 2015) closely map on to the meaning of hedonic motivation. Moreover, the colloquial terms "craving" and "urge" are, unlike the words "wanting" and "desire," unlikely to be confounded with reflective motivation. That is, people are unlikely to think of cravings or urges as a function of deliberate reflection on the potential pros and cons of a behavior. In this way craving and urge are very much akin to hedonic desire, the positive pole of hedonic motivation. Indeed, the only difference between craving and hedonic desire is that the latter is broader and can be used in behavioral contexts in which craving does not make sense, such as sex. The term "urge," however, makes sense for a broader range of behaviors, including nonconsumption behaviors, like sex. Thus, further research on hedonic motivation should draw on the existing scientific literature on craving and urge.

The concept of hedonic motivation is in some ways similar to the concept of intrinsic motivation, which is most commonly associated with self-determination theory (Ryan & Deci, 2000). Intrinsic motivation is, like hedonic motivation, tied to pleasure and contrasted with extrinsic motivation, which in many ways maps on to the present concept of reflective motivation. There are, however, clear differences between intrinsic motivation and hedonic motivation as defined herein. Intrinsic motivation has been defined in terms of how one feels in response to the behavior or about the behavior: "Intrinsic motivation will occur only for activities that hold intrinsic interest for an individual—those that have the appeal of novelty, challenge, or aesthetic value for that individual" (p. 60); and, "intrinsically motivated activities . . . are experienced as fun and enjoyable" (Ryan, Williams, Patrick, & Deci, 2009, p. 109). Thus, the concept of intrinsic motivation seems better suited to retrospectively characterize a hypothetical motivational state after a behavior has been performed—and can be judged as having been enjoyable or not—rather than to predict a behavior based on a preexisting motivational state. Alternatively, hedonic motivation, unlike intrinsic motivation, is defined as a neurobiological process and corresponding experiential state that can clearly be distinguished from both the behavior it is hypothesized to determine and the affective consequences of the behavior.

Finally, hedonic motivation should not be confused with colloquial use of the word "motivation," which may refer to a characteristic that involves will-power, mental fortitude, and the tendency to work hard. One who is "motivated" in the colloquial sense is the opposite of lazy. Hedonic motivation, on the other hand, is a dynamic psychobiological phenomenon that occurs at the time of the behavioral opportunity. It is defined by automatically triggered desires and dreads—not by the reasonableness or nobility of those desires and dreads; that is, hedonic motivation is value free. For example, the hedonic desire to smoke is a fundamental cause of smoking even for the person whose habit is maintained by constant stressors and addiction to nicotine. The hedonic desire to eat fast food is a fundamental cause of eating fast food even for the person who has limited access to affordable healthier foods and limited time to prepare such foods. The hedonic dread of exercise is a fundamental cause of avoidance of exercise even for the single parent who has limited leisure time in which to exercise. Hypothesizing hedonic motivation as a determinant of unhealthy behavior entails no moral judgment.

Assessment of Hedonic Motivation

The concept of hedonic motivation—as distinct from pleasure and displeasure, and reflective motivation—is intuitive and based on a solid and growing foundation of theory and research in affective neuroscience and psychology. While the concept is theoretically viable, further research is needed to develop valid assessments of hedonic motivation.

When considering how best to assess hedonic motivation it makes sense, as a starting point, to consider existing measures of 'wanting' as used in (mostly laboratory) research on incentive salience (for a review see Pool, Sennwald, Delplanque, Brosch, & Sander, 2016). Such research has employed neurobiological, behavioral, and implicit measures of 'wanting.' All these types of measures are useful for their basic science purposes, but have weaknesses that detract from their use in more applied settings. Specifically, assessment of the neurobiological underpinnings of hedonic motivation (i.e., 'wanting'), while crucial for theory testing and refinement, is not as useful for applied field-based research. Likewise, behavioral measures of 'wanting,' such as amount of or willingness to work for the behavioral outcome that is the target of hedonic motivation (Pool et al., 2016), while indispensable in research that attempts to dissociate 'liking' and 'wanting,' are not as useful for research in which behavior is the dependent variable because they confound hedonic motivation with behavior. Finally, assessment of hedonic motivation via reaction-time-type measures similar to those used to assess other automatic or implicit concepts (Greenwald, McGhee, & Schwartz, 1998), while consistent with the conceptualization of hedonic motivation, are cumbersome and unlikely to be highly predictive of behavior (Conner, Prestwich, & Ayres, 2011).

What is needed for research in which the goal is to predict and understand behavior, including applied field-based research, is development of a valid self-report measure(s) of the experiential aspect of hedonic motivation that is distinct from reflective motivation. Such a measure could be used in research on the psychological experience and self-report of hedonic desire (and dread) to mirror research on the psychological experience and self-report of pleasure (and displeasure). The development of a self-report measure of hedonic motivation will be difficult though because of the apparent absence of colloquial terms that distinguish between hedonic and reflective motivation.

In previous laboratory research among humans, self-reported 'wanting' (i.e., incentive salience) has been assessed by simply asking people to rate on numerical scales "How much do you want to eat this item right now?" (Born et al., 2011), "How much do you want to eat it?" (Bushman, Moeller, & Crocker, 2011), or, "I want to eat the food very much" versus "I don't want to eat the food at all" (Jiang et al., 2008). The problem with such measures is that responses may tap either hedonic or reflective motivation, or both. Someone may, for example, *want* a piece of chocolate cake, but, at the same time, *want* to resist the cake and instead eat the fruit salad. Thus, the word "want" is ambiguous. As a result of this ambiguity, simply asking participants whether they want something is likely not enough to parse hedonic motivation from reflective motivation.

Relative to the word "want," colloquial use of the word "desire" may better map on to hedonic motivation. That is, colloquially, one is more likely to say that she *desires* a beer, chocolate cake, a cigarette, or sex with an attractive acquaintance (i.e., typically hedonic desires), than to say that she *desires* to be able to go to work in the morning, to stick to her diet, to quit smoking, or to remain faithful to her partner (i.e., typically reflective desires). Hofmann, Baumeister Förster, and Vohs (2012) and Bagozzi, Dholakia, and Basuroy (2003) have assessed self-reported desire in field-based research using ecological momentary assessment and traditional questionnaires, respectively. Moreover, Perugini and Bagozzi (2004) have shown that a questionnaire assessment of "desire" is empirically distinguishable from assessment of "intention" (see also Perugini & Conner, 2000). Thus, self-reported "desire" may be a better indicator of hedonic motivation than self-reported "wanting." Nonetheless, while perhaps less ambiguous than self-reported "wanting", assessments of self-reported "desire" may still be conflated with intentions, goals, and other aspects of reflective motivation, as indicated by previous conceptual parsing of desire subtypes (Davis, 1982; Schroeder, 2004; Schueler, 1995).

One possible approach for distinguishing between hedonic and reflective motivation is to provide the respondent with vignettes illustrating the distinction prior to sequential or parallel assessment of the two constructs. Such an approach has been somewhat successful in disentangling self-efficacy from behavioral intention (Rhodes, Williams, & Mistry, 2016).

Clearly, more work is needed to empirically distinguishing between self-reported experiences of hedonic and reflective motivation. Until more refined measures of hedonic motivation can be developed, the Theory of Hedonic Motivation can be tested using methods to assess self-reported "craving" (when relevant), "urge", or "desire", keeping in mind the caveats noted previously regarding the need to disentangle hedonic from reflective motivation.

HEDONIC MOTIVATION AND HEALTH BEHAVIOR

According to the THM, people are hedonically motivated to perform behaviors that have previously resulted in immediate pleasure and to avoid behaviors that have previously resulted in displeasure. In the context of health behavior, this means that people are typically hedonically motivated to engage in unhealthy behaviors, such as eating calorie-dense foods, smoking cigarettes, drinking alcohol, and using drugs, and to avoid healthy behaviors such as vigorous exercise, colonoscopies, and use of condoms. However, people do not always act in accordance with their hedonic motivation. That is, hedonic motivation is a probabilistic rather than a universal cause of behavior. The triggering of hedonic motivation increases the likelihood that the behavior will be performed. Other factors that contribute to the determination of behavior are the environmental context and one's reflective motivation for the behavior.

The environment moderates the effects of hedonic motivation on behavior by providing the opportunity or lack thereof to perform the behavior (Rhodes, Blanchard, & Matheson, 2006). For example, even if someone has a strong hedonic desire for a beer, he cannot have one if he has no way to get one. In addition to the moderating effects of the environment on behavior, reflective motivation has independent effects on behavior. Reflective motivation often operates in unison with hedonic motivation. For example, one's hedonic motivation to skip an exercise session because it has been aversive in the past may be bolstered by her reflective motivation to skip the exercise upon remembering that she had better spend the evening preparing for an important meeting the next day. However, reflective motivation is often at odds with hedonic motivation, particularly for health behaviors. For example, someone may be hedonically motivated to skip tonight's run, but reflectively motivated to go for the run because she knows exercise is good for her.

When hedonic and reflective motivation are at odds, behavior is ultimately a function of the relative strength of hedonic and reflective motivation, as well as situational factors that may give either hedonic or reflective motivation more influence over our actions. The interaction between competing motivations in the context of health behavior has been a focus of recent dual-processing theories of self-control for which the THM is complementary (see particularly Hofmann, Friese, & Wiers, 2008). What the THM adds to this dual-processing formulation is a more precise conceptualization of the hedonic and reflective motivations that compete in self-control situations, as the well as the situating of hedonic motivation in terms of the ancient and intuitive theory of PH.

Hedonic Motivation, Evolution, and Evolutionary Mismatch

The THM is grounded in basic principles of evolutionary biology. First, the existence of PH in humans, including the psychological mechanisms of hedonic response and hedonic motivation, is a function of evolutionary processes (Cabanac, 1996; Spencer, 1851). Psychological hedonism is a *domain-general* mechanism through which environmental stimuli lead organisms to engage in behaviors that lead to adaptive outcomes and avoid behaviors that lead to maladaptive outcomes. Second, evolution has shaped the *domain-specific* content that fills the domain-general structure of PH. That is, evolution shapes the specific stimuli—including behavioral outcomes—that trigger hedonic responses under certain conditions. The stimuli that innately produce pleasure or displeasure differ across species depending on which stimuli tended to be adaptive or maladaptive for that species at the time that the innate stimulus-hedonic response contingency evolved. For example, among humans, the taste of sweet foods, except when sated, is pleasurable (Cota, Tschop, Horvath, & Levine, 2006). Conversely, while nearly everyone feels good *after* exercise, humans have an evolved tendency to experience increasing discomfort and displeasure *during* physical exertion that exceeds the anaerobic threshold (Ekkekakis, 2003). These innate hedonic responses to specific stimuli serve as a starting point for the development of a broad array of stimulus-hedonic response associations that develop through the life course based on associative learning processes, and thus create *within-species* variability in the complete set of stimulus-hedonic response associations on which PH operates.

This raises the question: If humans are genetically predisposed to respond with pleasure to behavioral outcomes that are adaptive and with displeasure to behavioral outcomes that are maladaptive, then why is unhealthy behavior such a big public health problem? The answer is that modern environments are "mismatched" to the environments in which our evolutionary ancestors evolved, such that some of the stimuli that were once adaptive—and for which we evolved an innate pleasurable response to—are now maladaptive. This "mismatch" problem (Gluckman & Hanson, 2006) lies at the heart of the emerging field of evolutionary medicine, which focuses on etiology and potential treatments for human disease in the context of evolutionary processes (Stearns & Koella, 2008; G. Williams & Nesse, 2012).

Hedonic response tendencies and their influence on hedonic motivation and behavior are an extension of our evolved biology and thus also a function of evolutionary processes (Dawkins, 1982). Thus, when adopting an evolutionary perspective to understand the health behaviors that are responsible for morbidity and mortality in modern times (Eaton et al., 2002; Tybur, Bryan, & Hooper, 2012), the focus should be squarely on the mismatch between our modern environments and our genetically predisposed hedonic and motivational tendencies. It is our evolutionary history that results in the tendency among modern humans to take greater pleasure in eating the chocolate cake instead of the fruit salad (King, 2013; Stice, Figlewicz, Gosnell, Levine, & Pratt, 2013; van den Bos & de Ridder, 2006) and to react with immediate displeasure to vigorous physical exertion (Lee, Emerson, & Williams, 2016; Lieberman, 2015). And the coopting of these innate tendencies leads many of us to take pleasure in smoking cigarettes, and consuming alcohol and drugs (Panksepp, Knutson, & Burgdorf, 2002).

It is no coincidence that many, perhaps nearly all of the stimuli that innately produce pleasure or displeasure are outcomes of what are considered health-related behaviors, including the pleasure of eating, drinking, and sex, and the displeasure of unnecessary energy expenditure and tissue damage. This is because health is intimately tied to survival and reproduction, which is the currency of natural selection. Thus, the use of the THM to understand health-related behavior is not arbitrary.

POTENTIAL LIMITATIONS

The THM is for the most part descriptive and integrative rather than creative. It is descriptive in the sense that it limits the scope of traditional PH by saying, "instead of referring to instances of X *and* Y as psychological hedonism, we should only refer to instances of X as psychological hedonism," with X representing pursuit of pleasure based on hedonic motivation and Y representing pursuit of pleasure based on expected pleasure (the latter an aspect of reflective motivation). The THM is integrative in the sense that it synthesizes relatively new theory and research in affective neuroscience and psychology with the ancient theory of PH in order to overcome the conceptual problems with the latter. Although the incentive salience and dual processing theories from which the THM borrows are not without controversy (e.g., Berridge & O'Doherty, 2014; Evans & Stanovich, 2013), they may certainly be characterized as mainstream. Moreover, the major points of controversy with these theories—whether the mesolimbic dopaminergic pathway also mediates reward prediction errors, and whether there are more than just two types of cognitive processing—do not affect the major tenets of the THM.

Some readers may argue that the THM is not a *version of* PH because PH is *defined* with respect to expected pleasures and displeasures. These readers are invited to, instead, think of the THM as a new theory that is distinct from, rather than a version of, PH. On the other hand, because the THM represents an integration of previous theory and research, some readers may say that rechristening these ideas as a "new theory" is unnecessary. These readers are invited to think of the THM as merely an updated version of PH. Indeed, in a bid to mitigate these criticisms from either side, a middle road was taken by referring to the present formulation as a reformulated version of PH in order to acknowledge its roots in existing theory, but also giving it a new name (i.e., THM) in order to differentiate it from traditional versions of PH.

IMPLICATIONS AND CONCLUSIONS

Psychological hedonism tells us that we, as humans, are often strongly motivated to pursue actions that lead to immediate pleasure and to avoid actions that lead to immediate displeasure. Contemporary affective neuroscience and psychology tells us that the traditional unitary concept of motivation, as well as related notions of wanting and desire, are no longer viable. Instead, the traditional concept of motivation can be divided into two distinct concepts of hedonic motivation and reflective motivation. Hedonic motivation is automatically triggered by environmental cues, is based on previous immediate pleasures and displeasures that have resulted from a target behavior, is a function of an evolutionarily primitive and uniform reward processing system, and manifests in the felt experience of hedonic desire or dread. Reflective motivation, on the other hand, is deliberately produced through conscious if-then reasoning based on numerous factors both temporally distal and proximal, is a function of an evolutionarily recent and complex cognitive processing system, and manifests in cognized behavioral intentions or goals. The fact that these two types of motivation are so clearly distinct in terms of both neurobiology and psychological experience suggests that use of the unqualified words "motivation," "desire," or "want," in a scientific context should be considered ambiguous and obsolete.

As a contemporary version of PH, the THM posits hedonic motivation as the mechanism through which previous pleasures and displeasures influence future behavior. Importantly, hedonic motivation is automatically triggered upon presentation of an associated cue, without the need for reflection on expected pleasure or displeasure that may result from a particular course of action. Although hedonic motivation does not always determine behavior, behavioral scientists must account for the fact that people will have strong hedonic motivation to behave in ways that will produce immediately pleasurable outcomes and reduce or avoid immediately displeasurable outcomes. Indeed, in order for the field of health behavior science to move forward, PH must be the explicit starting point in all frameworks, theories, and models of human behavior and in all attempts to predict and understand human behavior.

In addition to the theoretical implications, there are clear implications of the THM for health behavior interventions. Behavioral interventions have tended to emphasize bolstering of reflective motivation to overcome our automatic hedonic tendencies. However, human hedonic tendencies are strong, and may be difficult to overcome. With this point always in focus, interventionists should seek to (1) reshape the environment to limit access to unhealthy behaviors that elicit immediate pleasure and "nudge" people toward healthy behaviors that elicit immediate displeasure (Thaler & Sustein, 2009; Wong et al., 2015) and (2) provide immediate extrinsic rewards to increase pleasurable outcomes for performing behaviors that are healthy but naturally elicit immediate displeasure and for avoiding behaviors that are unhealthy but naturally elicit immediate pleasure (e.g., contingency management; e.g., Burns et al., 2012; Galarraga, Genberg, Martin, Barton Laws, & Wilson, 2013; Prendergast, Podus, Finney, Greenwell, & Roll, 2006; Strohacker, Galárraga, & Williams, 2014). When these are not possible, attempts may be made to reshape innate tendencies toward hedonic responses through conditioning procedures, such an evaluative conditioning (Hofmann, De Houwer, Perugini, Baeyens, & Crombez, 2010; Houben, Schoenmakers, & Wiers, 2010).

In closing, it is important to note that the THM is not an *alternative* to any of the approaches to affect-related determinants of health behavior espoused in this book, many of which emphasize expected affective consequences of behavior and reflective motivation. Nor is the THM an alternative to the still dominant sociocognitive paradigm that underpins the latter approaches. Instead the THM provides an integrative and overarching framework that encompasses both deliberate and automatic determinants of behavior, but with particular emphasis on the hedonic processes that drive our evolutionarily primitive yet extremely powerful hedonic motivations. In doing so, the THM shifts the emphasis back toward the human hedonistic tendencies that, for good reason, have been a focus of attempts to understand human behavior for thousands of years.

ACKNOWLEDGMENTS

I thank Kent Berridge, Mark Conner, Ryan Rhodes, and Michael Ruse for their comments on an earlier version of this chapter.

NOTES

1. It should be noted that Sloan and Wilson (1998) present PH for the purposes of critiquing it, with a particular emphasis on altruistic behavior as a refutation of PH.
2. Hereafter the term "pleasure" is used to refer to any positively valenced affect and "displeasure" is used to refer to any negatively valenced affect.
3. Some of the most famous psychological hedonists were also ethical hedonists (Epicurus, Bentham, Mill), but the two doctrines are nonetheless distinct.
4. Additional contemporary versions of PH can be found in philosophy (Brandt, 1979/1998; Mees & Schmitt, 2008; Morillo, 1995; Silverstein, 2000; Sobel, 2002, pp. 245–248; Stich, 2006) and behavioral science (Cabanac, 2009/2003; Johnston, 1999; Kahneman et al., 1997; Panksepp, 2013).
5. The desire to avoid displeasure may manifest as motivation to avoid behaviors that typically result in displeasure (e.g., vigorous exercise, flossing) or to engage in behaviors that allow one to relieve displeasure or avoid the displeasurable consequences of nonaction (e.g., smoking, drinking, or using drugs to relieve or avoid withdrawal symptoms).
6. Additional relevant works include Damasio (2010), Gottfried (2011), Kringelbach and Berridge (2010), LeDoux (2012), and Rolls (2014). For excellent reviews of the development of ideas that form the basis of the concept of hedonic motivation see Berridge (2004) and Marks (2011). For a divergent philosophical account of desire and motivation based on Berridge's distinction between "liking" and "wanting" see Schroeder (2004).
7. Confusingly, the term "incentive learning" is also used to describe deliberate rule-based learning that leads to expected pleasure (i.e., Balleine, 2011).

REFERENCES

Atkins, R. K. (2015). Peirce's critique of PH. *British Journal for the History of Philosophy, 23*, 349–367. doi: 10.1080/09608788.2015.1005569

Bagozzi, R. P., Dholakia, U. M., & Basuroy, S. (2003). How effortful decisions get enacted: The motivating role of decision processes, desires, and anticicpated emotions. *Journal of Behavioral Decision Making, 16*, 273–295. doi: 10.1002/bdm.446

Balleine, B. W. (2011). Sensation, incentive learning, and the motivational control of goal-directed action. In J. A. Gottfried (Ed.), *Neurobiology of sensation and reward* (pp. 287–310). Boca Raton, FL: Taylor and Francis.

Bentham, J. (1780/2007). *An introduction to the principles of morals and legislation*. Mineola, NY: Dover Publications.

Berridge, K. C. (1999). Pleasure, pain, desire, and dread: Hidden core processes of emotion. In D. Kahneman, E. Diener & N. Schwarz (Eds.), *Well-being: The foundations of hedonic psychology* (pp. 525–557). New York, NY: Russell Sage Foundation.

Berridge, K. C. (2004). Motivation concepts in behavioral neuroscience. *Physiology and Behavior, 81*, 179–209. doi: 10.1016/j.physbeh.2004.02.004

Berridge, K. C. (2007). The debate over dopamine's role in reward: The case for incentive salience. *Psychopharmacology (Berl), 191*, 391–431. doi: 10.1007/s00213-006-0578-x

Berridge, K. C. (2012). From prediction error to incentive salience: Mesolimbic computation of reward motivation. *European Journal of Neuroscience, 35*, 1124–1143. doi: 10.1111/j.1460-9568.2012.07990.x

Berridge, K. C., & O'Doherty, J. P. (2014). From experienced utility to decision utility. In P. W. Glimcher & E. Fehr (Eds.), *Neuroeconomics: Decision making and the brain* (2nd ed., pp. 335–351). Tokyo: Academic Press. doi: 10.1016/B978-0-12-416008-8.00018-8

Berridge, K. C., & Robinson, T. E. (1998). What is the role of dopamine in reward: Hedonic impact, reward learning, or incentive salience? *Brain Research Reviews, 28*, 309–369. doi: 10.1016/S0165-0173(98)00019-8

Berridge, K. C., & Robinson, T. E. (2003). Parsing reward. *Trends in Neuroscience, 26*, 507–513. doi: 10.1016/S0166-2236(03)00233-9

Born, J. M., Lemmens, S. G., Martens, M. J., Formisano, E., Goebel, R., & Westerterp-Plantenga, M. S. (2011). Differences between liking and wanting signals in the human brain and relations with cognitive dietary restraint andbody mass index. *American Journal of Clinical Nutrition, 94*, 392–403.

Brandt, R. B. (1979/1998). *A theory of the good and the right*. Amherst, NY: Prometheus.

Burns, R. J., Donovan, A. S., Ackermann, R. T., Finch, E. A., Rothman, A. J., & Jeffery, R. W. (2012). A theoretically grounded systematic review of material incentives for weight loss: implications for interventions. *Annals of Behavioral Medicine, 44*, 375–388. doi: 10.1007/s12160-012-9403-4

Bushman, B. J., Moeller, S. J., & Crocker, J. (2011). Sweets, sex, or self-esteem? Comparing the value of self-esteem boosts with other pleasant rewards. *Journal of Personality, 79*, 993–1012.

Cabanac, M. (1996). On the origin of consciousness, a postulate and its corollary. *Neuroscience and Biobehavioral Reviews, 20*, 33–40. doi: 0149-7634(95)00032-A

Cabanac, M. (2009/2003). *The fifth influence: Or, the dialectics of pleasure*. Bloomington, IN: iUniverse.

Conner, M., Prestwich, A., & Ayres, K. (2011). Using explicit affective attitudes to tap influences on health behaviour: A commentary on Homann et al. (2008). *Health Psychology Review, 5*, 145–149. doi: 10.1080/17437199.2010.539969

Cota, D., Tschop, M. H., Horvath, T. L., & Levine, A. S. (2006). Cannabinoids, opioids and eating behavior: The molecular face of hedonism? *Brain Research Reviews, 51*, 85–107. doi: 10.1016/j.brainresrev.2005.10.004

Damasio, A. R. (2010). *Self comes to mind: Constructing the conscious brain*. New York, NY: Pantheon.

Davis, W. A. (1982). The two senses of desire. *Philosophical Studies, 45*, 181–195. doi: 10.1007/BF00372477

Dawkins, R. (1982). *The extended phenotype*. New York: Oxford.

Dickinson, A., & Balleine, B. W. (2010). Hedonics: The cognitive-motivational interface. In M. L. Kringelbach & K. C. Berridge (Eds.), *Pleasures of the brain* (pp. 74–84). New York, NY: Oxford.

Eaton, S. B., Strassman, B. I., Nesse, R. M., Neel, J. V., Ewald, P. W., Williams, G. C., . . . Cordain, L. (2002). Evolutionary health promotion. *Preventive Medicine, 34*, 109–118. doi: 10.1006/pmed.2001.0876

Ekkekakis, P. (2003). Pleasure and displeasure from the body: Perspectives from exercise. *Cognition and Emotion, 17*, 213–239. doi: 10.1080/02699930302292

Evans, J. S. (2008). Dual-processing accounts of reasoning, judgment, and social cognition. *Annual Review of Psychology, 59*, 255–278. doi: 10.1146/annurev.psych.59.103006.093629

Evans, J. S., & Stanovich, K. E. (2013). Dual-process theories of higher cognition: Advancing the debate. *Perspectives on Psychological Science, 8*, 223–241. doi: 10.1177/1745691612460685

Galarraga, O., Genberg, B. L., Martin, R. A., Barton Laws, M., & Wilson, I. B. (2013). Conditional economic incentives to improve HIV treatment adherence: Literature review and theoretical considerations. *AIDS and Behavior*. doi: 10.1007/s10461-013-0415-2

Gawronski, B., & Bodenhausen, G. V. (2006). Associative and propositional processes in evaluation: An integrative review of implicit and explicit attitude change. *Psychological Bulletin, 132*, 692–731.

Gluckman, P., & Hanson, M. (2006). *Mismatch: The lifestyle diseases timebomb*. Oxford, UK: Oxford.

Gottfried, J. A. (Ed.). (2011). *Neurobiology of sensation and reward*. Boca Raton, FL: Taylor & Francis.

Greenwald, A. G., McGhee, D. E., & Schwartz, J. L. K. (1998). Measuring individual differences in implicit cognition: The implicit association test. *Journal of Personality and Social Psychology, 74*, 1464–1480. doi: 10.1037/0022-3514.74.6.1464

Hobbes, T. (1668/1994) *Leviathon*. Edited by E. Curley. Indianapolis, IN: Hackett.

Hofmann, W., Baumeister, R. F., Förster, G., & Vohs, K. D. (2012). Everyday temptations: An experience sampling study of desire, conflict, and self-control. *Journal of Personality and Social Psychology, 102*, 1318–1335. doi: 10.1037/a0026545

Hofmann, W., De Houwer, J., Perugini, M., Baeyens, F., & Crombez, G. (2010). Evaluative conditioning in humans: A meta-analysis. *Psychological Bulletin, 136*, 390–421. doi: 10.1037/a0018916

Hofmann, W., Friese, M., & Wiers, R. W. (2008). Impulsive versus reflective influences on health behavior: A theoretical framework and empirical review. *Health Psychology Review, 2*, 111–137. doi: 10.1080/17437190802617668

Hofmann, W., & Nordgren, L. F. (2015). Introduction. In W. Hofmann & L. F. Nordgren (Eds.), *The psychology of desire* (pp. 1–13). New York, NY: Guilford.

Hofmann, W., & Van Dillen, L. (2012). Desire: The new hot spot in self-control research. *Current Directions in Psychological Science, 21*, 317–322. doi: 10.1177/0963721412453587

Houben, K., Schoenmakers, T. M., & Wiers, R. W. (2010). I didn't feel like drinking but I don't know why: The effects of evaluative conditioning on alcohol-related attitudes, craving and behavior. *Addictive Behaviors, 35*, 1161–1163. doi: 10.1016/j.addbeh.2010.08.012

Jiang, T., Soussignan, R., Rigaud, D., Martin, S., Royet, J. P., Brondel, L., & Schaal, B. (2008). Alliesthesia to food cues: Heterogeneity across stimuli and sensory modalities. *Physiology and Behavior, 95*, 464–470.

Johnston, V. S. (1999). *Why we feel: The science of human emotions*. Reading, MA: Perseus Books.

Kahneman, D. (2011). *Thinking, fast and slow.* New York, NY: Farrar, Straus, and Giroux.

Kahneman, D., Wakker, P. P., & Sarin, R. (1997). Back to Bentham? Explorations of experienced utility. *Quarterly Journal of Economics, 112*, 375–405. doi: 10.1162/003355397555235

Kavanagh, D. J., Andrade, J., & May, J. (2005). Imaginary relish and exquisite torture: The elaborated intrusion theory of desire. *Psychological Review, 112*, 446–467. doi: 10.1037/0033-295X.112.2.446

King, B. M. (2013). The modern obesity epidemic, ancestral hunter-gatherers, and the sensory/reward control of food intake. *Am Psychol, 68*, 88–96. doi: 10.1037/a0030684

Kringelbach, M. L., & Berridge, K. C. (Eds.). (2010). *Pleasures of the brain*. New York, NY: Oxford University Press.

LeDoux, J. E. (2012). Evolution of human emotion: A view through fear. *Progress in Brain Research, 195*, 431–442. doi: 10.1016/B978-0-444-53860-4.00021-0

Lee, H. H., Emerson, J. A., & Williams, D. M. (2016). The exercise-affect-adherence pathway: An evolutionary perspective. *Frontiers in Psychology, 7*, 1285. doi: 10.3389/fpsyg.2016.01285

Lieberman, D. E. (2015). Is exercise really medicine? An evolutionary perspective. *Current Sports Medicine Reports, 14*, 313–319. doi: 10.1249/JSR.0000000000000168

Lyubomirsky, S., King, L., & Diener, E. (2005). The benefits of frequent positive affect: Does happiness lead to success? *Psychological Bulletin, 131*, 803–855. doi:10.1037/0033-2909.131.6.803

Marks, L. E. (2011). A brief history of sensation and reward. In J. A. Gottfried (Ed.), *Neurobiology of sensation and reward* (pp. 15–43). Boca Raton, FL: Taylor & Francis.

Mees, U., & Schmitt, A. (2008). Goals of action and emotional reasons for action: A modern version of the theory of ultimate PH. *Journal for the Theory of Social Behaviour, 38*, 157–178. doi: 10.1111/j.1468-5914.2008.00364.x

Mill, J. S. (1863/2012). *Utilitarianism*. New York, NY: Renaissance Classics.

Mischel, W., Shoda, Y., & Rodriguez, M. I. (1989). Delay of gratification in children. *Science, 244*, 933–938.

Moen, O. M. (2015). Hedonism before Bentham. *Journal of Bentham Studies, 17*, 1–18. http://discovery.ucl.ac.uk/1469354/

Moore, A. (2013). Hedonism. *The Stanford encyclopedia of philosophy* Winter 2013 Edition. Retrieved December 1, 2016, from http://plato.stanford.edu/archives/win2013/entries/hedonism/

Morillo, C. R. (1995). *Contingent creatures: A reward event theory of motivation and value*. Lanham, MD: Rowman & Littlefield.

Panksepp, J. (2011). Cross-species affective neuroscience decoding of the primal affective experiences of humans and related animals. *PLOS ONE, 6*, e21236. doi: 10.1371/journal.pone.0021236

Panksepp, J. (2013). Cross-species neuroaffective parsing of primal emotional desires and aversions in mammals. *Emotion Review, 5*, 235–240. doi: 10.1177/1754073913477515

Panksepp, J., Knutson, B., & Burgdorf, J. (2002). The role of brain emotional systems in addictions: A neuro-evolutionary perspective and new "self-report" animal model. *Addiction, 97*, 459–469.

Perugini, M., & Bagozzi, R. P. (2004). The distinction between desires and intentions. *European Journal of Social Psychology, 34*, 69–84. doi: 10.1002/ejsp.186

Perugini, M., & Conner, M. (2000). Predicting and understanding behavioral volitions: The interplay between goals and behaviors. *European Journal of Social Psychology, 30*, 705–731. doi: 10.1002/1099-0992(200009/10)30

Pool, E., Sennwald, V., Delplanque, S., Brosch, T., & Sander, D. (2016). Measuring wanting and liking from animals to humans: A systematic review. *Neuroscience and Biobehavioral Reviews, 63*, 124–142. doi: 1 0.1016/j.neubiorev.2016.01.006

Prendergast, M., Podus, D., Finney, J., Greenwell, L., & Roll, J. (2006). Contingency management for treatment of substance use disorders: A meta-analysis. *Addiction, 101*, 1546–1560. doi: 10.1111/j.1360-0443.2006.01581.x

Rhodes, R. E., Blanchard, C. M., & Matheson, D. H. (2006). A multicomponent model of the theory of planned behaviour. *British Journal of Health Psychology, 11*, 119–137. doi: doi: 10.1348/135910705X52633

Rhodes, R. E., Williams, D. M., & Mistry, C. (2016). Using short vignettes to disentangle perceived capability from motivation: A test using walking and resistance training behaviors. *Psychology, Health, and Medicine, 21*, 639–651. doi: 10.1080/13548506.2015.1074710

Rolls, E. T. (2014). *Emotion and decision-making explained*. Oxford, UK: Oxford University Press.

Ryan, R. M., & E. L. Deci (2000). Self-determination theory and the facilitation of intrinsic motivation, social development, and well-being. *American Psychologist, 55*, 68–78. doi: 10.1037/0003-066X.55.1.68

Ryan, R. M., Williams, G. C., Patrick, H., & Deci, E. L. (2009). Self-determination theory and physical activity: The dynamics of motivation in development and wellness. *Hellenic Journal of Psychology, 6*, 107–124.

Russell, J. A. (1980). A circumplex model of affect. *Journal of Personality and Social Psychology, 39*, 1161–1178. doi:10.1037/h0077714

Schroeder, T. (2004). *Three faces of desire*. New York, NY: Oxford University Press.

Schueler, G. F. (1995). *Desire: Its role in practical reason and the explanation of action*. Cambridge, MA: MIT.

Seligman, M. E., Railton, P., Baumeister, R. F., & Sripada, C. (2013). Navigating into the future or driven by the past. *Perspectives on Psychological Science, 8*, 119–141. doi: 10.1177/1745691612474317

Silverstein, M. (2000). In defense of happiness: A response to the experience machine. *Social Theory and Practice, 26*, 279–300.

Sloman, S. A. (1996). The empirical case for two systems of reasoning. *Psychological Bulletin, 119*, 3–22.

Smith, E. R., & J. DeCoster (2000). Dual-process models in social and cognitive psychology: Conceptual integration and links to underlying memory systems. *Personality and Social Psychology Review, 4*, 108–131.

Sobel, D. (2002). Varieties of hedonism. *Journal of Social Philosophy, 33*, 240–256. doi: 10.1111/0047-2786.00007

Sober, E., & Wilson, D. S. (1998). *Unto others: The evolution and psychology of unselfish behavior*. Cambridge, MA: Harvard.

Spencer, H. (1851). *Social statics: Or the conditions essential to human happiness specified, and the first of them developed.* London: Chapman.

Stearns, S. C., & Koella, J. C. (2008). *Evolution in health and disease* (2nd ed.). New York, NY: Oxford University Press.

Stewart, R. M. (1992). Butler's argument against PH. *Canadian Journal of Philosophy, 22*, 211–221. doi: 10.1080/00455091.1992.10717278

Stice, E., Figlewicz, D. P., Gosnell, B. A., Levine, A. S., & Pratt, W. E. (2013). The contribution of brain reward circuits to the obesity epidemic. *Neuroscience and Biobehavioral Reviews, 37*, 2047–2058. doi: 10.1016/j.neubiorev.2012.12.001

Stich, S. (2006). Evolution, altruism, and cognitive architecture: A critique of Sober and Wilson's argument for psychological altruism. *Biology and Philosophy, 22*, 267–281. doi: 10.1007/s10539-006-9030-1

Strack, F., & Deutsch, R. (2004). Reflective and impulsive determinants of social behavior. *Personality and Social Psychology Review, 8*, 220–247.

Strohacker, K., Galárraga, O., & Williams, D. M. (2014). The impact of incentives on exercise behavior: A systematic review of randomized controlled trials. *Annals of Behavioral Medicine, 48*, 92–99. doi: 10.1007/s12160-013-9577-4

Thaler, R. H., & Sustein, C. R. (2009/2008). *Nudge: Improving decisions about health, wealth, and happiness*. New York, NY: Penguin.

Troland, L. T. (1928). *The fundamentals of human motivation.* New York, NY: D. van Nostrand.

Tybur, J. M., Bryan, A. D., & Hooper, A. E. (2012). An evolutionary perspective on health psychology: New approaches and applications. *Evolutionary Psychology, 10*, 855–867.

van den Bos, R., & de Ridder, D. (2006). Evolved to satisfy our immediate needs: Self-control and the rewarding properties of food. *Appetite, 47*, 24–29. doi: 10.1016/j.appet.2006.02.008

Williams, D. M., & Evans, D. R. (2014). Current emotion research in health behavior science. *Emotion Review, 6*, 277–287. doi: 10.1177/1754073914523052

Williams, D. M., & Ruse, M. (forthcoming). *Darwinian hedonism and the epideimc of unhealthy behavior.* New York, NY: Cambridge University Press.

Williams, G., & Nesse, R. M. (2012). *Why we get sick: The new science of Darwinian medicine.* New York, NY: Vintage.

Wilson, S. J., & Sayette, M. A. (2015). Neuroimaging craving: Urge intensity matters. *Addiction, 110*, 195–203. doi: 10.1111/add.12676

Wong, M. S., Nau, C., Kharmats, A. Y., Vedovato, G. M., Cheskin, L. J., Gittelsohn, J., & Lee, B. Y. (2015). Using a computational model to quantify the potential impact of changing the placement of healthy beverages in stores as an intervention to "Nudge" adolescent behavior choice. *BMC Public Health, 15*, 1284. doi: 10.1186/s12889-015-2626-0

Zhang, J., Berridge, K. C., Tindell, A. J., Smith, K. S., & Aldridge, J. W. (2009) A neural computation model of incentive salience. *PLoS Computational Biology, 5*, e1000437. doi: 10.1371/journal.pcbi.1000437

PART 2

The Influence of Affect on Specific Health-Related Behaviors

11

Affect as a Potential Determinant of Physical Activity and Exercise

Critical Appraisal of an Emerging Research Field

PANTELEIMON EKKEKAKIS, ZACHARY ZENKO, MATTHEW A. LADWIG, AND MARK E. HARTMAN

Contemporary investigations examining the determinants of physical activity and exercise behavior are typically based on a small set of cognitivist theories, namely the theory of planned behavior (Ajzen & Manstead, 2007), social-cognitive theory (Bandura, 2004), the transtheoretical model (Prochaska & Marcus, 1994), and self-determination theory (Ryan, Williams, Patrick, & Deci, 2009). In the framework of these theories, human beings are modeled as rational thinkers who collect, evaluate, and act on information that is relevant to the mission of promoting their self-interest (i.e., staying alive, healthy, and happy). In turn, intervention methods based on these theoretical models follow a "rational-educational" approach; if individuals are given correct, complete, comprehensible, and engagingly presented information pertaining to, for example, anticipated benefits versus costs, the ability to carry out a behavior, or sources of support, the theories predict that individuals will change their behavior in the desired direction. For decades, campaigns to promote physical activity have adhered to this approach, focusing on building an informational basis (e.g., improving awareness, knowledge, beliefs, outcome expectations), from which a change in behavior was expected to result. According to the Lancet Physical Activity Series Working Group (the diplomatic qualifiers "to some extent" and "so far" notwithstanding), "the traditional public health approach based on evidence and exhortation has—to some extent—been unsuccessful so far" (Hallal et al., 2012, p. 254).

The aforementioned cognitivist theories are based on the assumptions that (1) despite occasional errors, humans behave to promote their self-interest, (2) the postulated algorithms comply with standards of rationality (i.e., follow rules of logic and probability), and (3) the human information-processing system is capable of the cognitive operations required for the algorithms to function as envisioned (i.e., possesses adequate speed and memory capacity). Research originating in behavioral economics has demonstrated that these assumptions are untenable. Humans commonly act against their self-interests (even when possessing knowledge about the detrimental consequences of their actions or inactions) and can be shown to reliably make decisions or choices that violate the assumption of rationality. These discoveries have had growing influence within psychology (Shafir & LeBoeuf, 2002) and the field of health behavior (Corrigan, Rüsch, Ben-Zeev, & Sher, 2014; Rice, 2013). Violations of rationality found in other contexts can also be demonstrated in the context of physical activity (Zenko, Ekkekakis, & Kavetsos, 2016).

Prompted by the realization that the portrayal of human beings in cognitivist theories was untenable, researchers from several behavioral-science fields have developed so-called dual-process theories. These theories are based on the premise that human behavior, besides following from the reflective, controlled, rational thought processes of the type postulated in cognitivist theories, may also emanate, in a more-or-less direct or impulsive manner, from alternate pathways that rely on nondeliberative processes, such as heuristics, previously established associations of stimuli with approach or avoidance tendencies, and affective responses (e.g., Strack & Deutsch, 2004). Dual-process conceptualizations have found application in the domain of health behavior (e.g., Hofmann, Friese, & Wiers, 2008), including physical activity (e.g., Ekkekakis & Zenko, 2016a; Williams & Evans, 2014).

THE AFFECTLESS HUMANOID ROBOT: THE LEGACY OF THE COGNITIVIST PARADIGM

Examined with a sense of perspective, the state of affairs in the line of research investigating the psychological processes leading to physical activity behavior change appears remarkably well aligned with what Kuhn (1962/1996) had written regarding scientific fields dominated by a paradigm. One of the characteristic signs of a field in the grip of a paradigm is the loss of diversity in conceptual perspectives. Kuhn (1962/1996) wrote of an "immense restriction of the scientist's vision" causing science to become "increasingly rigid" (p. 64).

Given the multifariousness of the problem of raising physical activity rates and the failure to make any appreciable progress toward addressing it, perhaps one would expect vigorous, diverse, and creative efforts at theorizing. What one finds instead is a fixation on the same few theories over the past 40 years. Inspection of the details of studies published even in the most prestigious and selective journals in health psychology and behavioral medicine offers clues on how the paradigm rewards continued investment in these theories. The typical study is still a correlational survey that can be carried out with relatively low cost. To use the theory of planned behavior as an example, the "principle of compatibility" (Ajzen, 2005) requires that all constructs (i.e., attitude, subjective norm, perceived behavioral control, intention) be defined in terms of the same elements, namely target, action, context, and time. Researchers have applied the principle of compatibility by wording question stems in identical or nearly identical terms. Parenthetically, similar requirements have been posited for measures of constructs from other theories (e.g., self-efficacy scales must describe the target behavior with great specificity). For example, instrumental attitude may be measured by the statement "*Exercising regularly over the next four weeks* would be . . ." (1 = "harmful"; 7 = "beneficial"), affective attitude may be measured by "*Exercising regularly over the next four weeks* would be . . ." (1 = "unpleasant"; 7 = "pleasant"), and so forth. Behavior may be measured by "In the *past four weeks, I have exercised regularly*" (1 = "never"; 7 = "always"). A typical result is that these variables are found to be intercorrelated and a typical conclusion is that follow-up experimental studies are needed.

As psychometricians would point out, repeating the phrase "exercise regularly over the next four weeks" in each item and using the same 7-point response format capitalize on common method bias to inflate the correlations between the variables, including the all-important correlations between theorized predictors and criteria. In most research fields, researchers are advised to "eliminate common scale properties" (e.g., the type of response scale, the number of scale points, scale polarity) in items used to measure different constructs (Podsakoff, MacKenzie, Lee, & Podsakoff, 2003, p. 888). Likewise, reviewers are instructed to expect "lack of overlap in items for different constructs" (Conway & Lance, 2010, p. 330). Some journal editors outright "desk-reject" all studies in which postulated predictors and criteria are measured by the same method, such as self-report (Chang, van Witteloostuijn, & Eden, 2010). The reasons why these guidelines are unheeded in studies investigating the factors underlying physical activity and exercise behavior are arguably more likely paradigmatic than substantive.

Kuhn (1962/1996) warned that there is bound to be "considerable resistance to paradigm change" (p. 64). Data and perspectives "that will not fit the box are often not seen at all" (p. 24). Scientists indoctrinated under the dominant paradigm "[do not] aim to invent new theories, and they are often intolerant of those invented by others" (p. 24). As an example, Sniehotta, Presseau, and Araújo-Soares (2014) published a compelling critique of the theory of planned behavior based on theoretical and empirical grounds, including its "exclusive focus on rational reasoning" and its neglect of "the role of emotions" (p. 2). They then urged researchers to adopt a "broader theoretical approach" (p. 4), including "dual process models" (p. 5). Although Sniehotta et al. (2014) identified specific alternatives that offer the type of expanded theoretical perspective they envisioned, commentators argued that "one is hard pressed to identify [the] formal successors" of the theory of planned behavior (Rhodes, 2015, p. 156) beyond "extended" versions of the same theory (Hagger, 2015; Rhodes, 2015). One extended version (Hagger & Chatzisarantis, 2014), described as an exemplar of the "next generation of physical activity models" (Rhodes, 2014, p. 43), represents "a blend of the theory of planned behavior and self-determination theory" (p. 43). Even in this "next generation" theory, there was "[no] consideration of the affective domain in physical activity behavior" (p. 43).

Kuhn (1962/1996) emphasized that the transition from an old to a new paradigm never depends solely on a mismatch between empirical data generated by the paradigm and the real world. According to Kuhn, when scientists are confronted by even severe and prolonged "anomalies" in the paradigm, "they may begin to lose faith and then to consider alternatives" but they "do not renounce the paradigm that has led them into crisis" (p. 77). Instead, defenders of the paradigm "will devise numerous articulations and ad hoc modifications of their theory in order to eliminate any apparent conflict" (p. 78).

To stay with the theory of planned behavior as the working example, Ajzen and Fishbein (2005) acknowledged that critics have questioned the reliance on the assumption of rationality that formed the basis of the reasoned action framework. In particular, they noted that the theory did not "take into account emotions, compulsions, and other noncognitive or irrational determinants of human behavior" (p. 203). They conceded that "much of the research conducted in the framework of the theories of reasoned action and planned behavior has devoted little attention to the role of emotion in the prediction of intentions and actions" (p. 203). However, they argued that "emotions can have a strong impact on intentions and behaviors, but like other background factors, this influence is assumed to be indirect" (p. 203). For example, "people in a positive mood tend to evaluate events more favorably and to judge favorable events as more likely than people in a negative mood" (p. 203). The thesis that emotions (and affective factors, in general) cannot influence behavior directly has since persisted as the standard response to critics on this point (Ajzen, 2011).

These maneuvers represent good examples of the "articulations and ad hoc modifications" that Kuhn (1962/1996) had predicted. Similar maneuvers can be found in the literatures pertaining to other cognitivist theories (see Ekkekakis & Zenko, 2016a). All these represent variations of the idea of "affect as information." According to this idea, at some point along the path of the information-processing system, a device converts affect to data (e.g., humans ask themselves "how do I feel about it?"). These data are then fed into the cognitive algorithm alongside other data (e.g., knowledge, beliefs, appraisals). By converting affect into data, the cognitivist paradigm can continue to model the mind as an information-processing system, without the need to discard, or even greatly alter, any of its theories. Elsewhere in this volume, readers will find assertions that constructs such as "affective attitudes" (e.g., Lawton, Conner, & McEachan, 2009), "affective judgments" (e.g., Rhodes, Fiala, & Conner, 2009), and "anticipated affective responses" (e.g., Conner, McEachan, Taylor, O'Hara, & Lawton, 2015) constitute "affective determinants of health behavior." Here, we explain that these are cognitive constructs; they may be cognitions *about affect* but that does not render them genuinely "affective."

Affect is a lived, embodied, experiential state: "a neurophysiological state consciously accessible as a simple primitive nonreflective feeling most evident in mood and emotion but always available to consciousness" (Russell & Feldman Barrett, 2009, p. 104). Russell (2003) emphasized that "as consciously experienced, core affect is mental but not cognitive or reflective" (p. 148). To decide whether "affective attitudes," "affective judgments," and "anticipated affective responses" are genuinely "affective," readers could apply a litmus test: are these constructs applicable to the hypothetical case of an individual who has never experienced physical activity or exercise? It should be apparent that nothing would preclude such an individual from having "affective attitudes," "affective judgments," and "anticipated affective responses" since all three could develop by simply providing this individual with information (e.g., about how she or he will probably feel or how other people usually feel). However, this individual would not be able to report her or his affective experiences since none would exist.

This point has important implications for the types of interventions that must be developed to improve the affective determinants of physical activity and exercise. If "affective attitudes," "affective judgments," and "anticipated affective responses" are "affective," then interventions could adequately address the element of affect by developing messaging strategies (e.g., on how individuals should expect to feel in response to physical activity and exercise). On the other hand, if one agrees that an intensely negative affective response to a bout of exercise would likely overpower and negate any prior positive messages, then one should concede that fully addressing the element of affect cannot be accomplished without also researching ways to improve the experience of exercise itself.

Are "Affective Attitudes" Affective?

Both affect and attitude have valence (positive vs. negative) as a defining element. However, while affect can only exist and can only be measured "in the moment," attitudes about an object can exist under different circumstances. For example, people can rate how "enjoyable" or "aversive" they believe exercise to be at any time, even while sitting at their sofa. However, they can only report their affective response to exercise when fully immersed in the experience. Recall that affect, by definition, is "not cognitive or reflective" (Russell, 2003, p. 148). As soon as a researcher asks people to reflect, such as asking them to average their affective experiences across several past instances, the response, although still technically about affect, becomes the result of extensive cognitive operations. These operations may include consideration of normative responses, social pressure and desirability, and after-the-fact theorizing on the part of respondents (Podsakoff et al., 2003). Study participants can readily devise boxes-and-arrows theories to explain their affective responses (e.g., attributing them to "perceptions of ability, immediate and anticipated outcomes, attentional focus and perceptions of control"; see Rose & Parfitt, 2010, p. 1). Such reflections, however, represent thinking about affect, not affect per se.

The social-psychological literature is replete with examples of researchers admitting that they "do not draw such sharp divisions" between constructs that researchers in affective psychology consider "apples and oranges," such as "evaluative reactions and emotions" (Larsen, McGraw, & Cacioppo, 2001, p. 687). For example, one may be inclined to believe that "*feelings* toward exercise" and "*feeling* pleasure while exercising" belong to the same conceptual category; they do not. Failure to recognize this difference has led to debates constructed entirely on the basis of assigning the term "affect" different meanings (Larsen et al., 2001; Russell & Feldman Barrett, 1999). Can people "feel" positive and negative "affect" at the same time? If by "affect" one means the cognitive evaluation of an object as positive or negative, then the answer is "yes." Fanatics of high-intensity exercise would probably evaluate exercise as simultaneously exhausting and enjoyable (presumably due to the interpretation of physical exhaustion as a sign of achievement). On the other hand, if one defines "affect" as it is defined in affective psychology (Russell & Feldman Barrett, 2009), then the answer is "no." Affect is bipolar because it would be an adaptational disaster for beings to experience both the "approach" signal of pleasure and the "avoid" signal of displeasure at the same time.

In the theory of planned behavior, attitudes result from beliefs (Ajzen, 1991). Beliefs are quintessential cognitions. Nothing would preclude a person with no personal experience of physical activity to hold beliefs and associated attitudes *about* physical activity. If a person is given information that physical activity will make one feel better, this person should develop the belief that physical activity will have this effect, in turn leading this person to form a positive attitude consistent with this belief. This attitude is labeled "affective," presumably only in reference to the nature of the outcome of this behavior (i.e., feeling good). This is essentially an identical scenario to this person being given information that physical activity will reduce the risk of heart disease; this person should develop a belief that this will indeed happen and, in turn, should form a positive attitude consistent with this belief. To keep the naming convention consistent, this type of attitude should have been labeled "health-related attitude" but, for reasons that are not readily apparent, it has been labeled "cognitive" attitude instead. Clearly, however, nothing renders the latter scenario any more "cognitive" than the former. Both are cognitive since both rest on information that led to the formation of beliefs. Ajzen (1991) conceded that evaluating something as "healthy" may not correlate with finding it "pleasant" but was not convinced of the need to distinguish between the two. In his thinking, what matters is whether one ultimately evaluates the behavior in question as positive or negative.

To illustrate, it is useful to consider how researchers have attempted to manipulate "cognitive" versus "affective" attitudes toward physical activity. Both are manipulated in the same manner, namely by providing individuals with information designed to influence their beliefs. In one example, to manipulate "affective" attitude, researchers told participants that "regular physical activity has been shown to reduce anxiety, depression and stress," reinforced the information with research data (e.g., "after only 20 min of moderate-to-vigorous physical activity, anxiety symptoms have been shown to decrease"), and provided supporting bibliographic references. To manipulate "cognitive" attitude, researchers told participants that physical activity "reduces the risk of developing colon and breast cancer," reinforced the information with research data (e.g., "the risk of getting a cardiovascular disease increases by 1.5 times in people who do not follow minimum physical activity recommendations"), and again provided supporting bibliographic references (Conner, Rhodes, Morris, McEachan, & Lawton, 2011). In another study (Morris, Lawton, McEachan, Hurling, & Conner, 2016), the messages designed to manipulate "affective" attitude referred to changes in the "mental sphere" more broadly, including cognitive benefits (e.g., "exercise can reduce muscular tension and enhance concentration"), whereas messages designed to manipulate "cognitive" attitude referred to the "physical sphere" (e.g., "exercise has been shown to bolster the immune system").

It should be clear that these experimental conditions are cognitive in the sense that both appeal to the prefrontal/executive parts of the brain and both target the same model of the mind (i.e., a deliberative, analytical, rational mind that seeks, stores, and evaluates information with the purpose of using it to make probabilistic predictions about future consequences). The difference is whether the information that is provided pertains to the benefits that physical activity or exercise have from the neck up (i.e., on mental health) versus from the neck down (i.e., on physical health). What an experiment of this sort demonstrates is not that manipulating "affect" is more effective than manipulating "cognition" for changing health behavior but rather that humans perhaps value their mental health (including their happiness, well-being, and cognitive function) more than their physical health (i.e., extending the duration of their lives). Alternatively, it may also be the case that promises of immediate benefits resonate more than promises of benefits that may occur (with a given probability) years or decades in the future.

Are "Affective Judgments" Affective?

The term "affective judgment" was used by Ajzen (1991) to describe "beliefs about positive or negative feelings derived from the activity" (p. 201). As implied by the term "judgment" and the fact that it referred to "beliefs," this construct was also meant as cognitive. What may complicate matters somewhat is that the term "affective judgments" was also used by Zajonc (1980) in his classic article on the primacy of affect as one of a rather large assortment of descriptors that also included, for example, "affective reactions" (e.g., I feel good vs. I feel bad) and "affective discriminations" (e.g., I like vs. I dislike). According to one statement illustrative of his essential thesis, Zajonc (1980) argued that "affective judgments," in contradistinction to "cognitive judgments," "may be fairly independent of, and precede in time, the sorts of perceptual and cognitive operations commonly assumed to be the basis of these affective judgments" (p. 151). Although Zajonc used "affective judgments" to refer to *precognitive* affective states, in articles in which the concept is considered as a possible determinant of physical activity, the use seems aligned with that of Ajzen rather than Zajonc. Specifically, Rhodes et al. (2009) defined affective judgments as "judgments about the overall pleasure/displeasure, enjoyment, and feeling states expected from enacting physical activity" (p. 181). This judgment of expectation is believed to be based on (1) information one is given about what is likely to occur and (2) information acquired "from reflection on past activity" (Nasuti & Rhodes, 2013, p. 358). According to Rhodes et al. (2009), affective judgments "presumably require some cognitive processing of affect in order to form the judgment" (p. 181). Therefore, although past affective experiences might have played a role in shaping these judgments, "affective judgments" refer to cognitions (beliefs, expectations) about affect rather than affect per se.

Are "Anticipated Affective Responses" Affective?

The term "anticipated affective responses" was introduced in investigations pertaining to physical activity, described variously as a "type of affective evaluation" (Conner, Godin, Sheeran, & Germain, 2013, p. 265), a "form of attitude" (p. 270), or a "feeling" (p. 271), making the exact nature of this variable somewhat enigmatic. To some readers, the term may be reminiscent of "affective forecasting," namely predictions about the affect that one may experience in response to future events (Wilson & Gilbert, 2003). It is important to emphasize that, as operationalized in the research literature, affective forecasts typically refer to the positive or negative valence of future affective experiences (i.e., "I will feel good" vs. "I will feel bad"), the specific emotions that one will likely experience (e.g., pride, disappointment), and the expected intensity and duration of these experiences. Thus, in studies examining the relationship of affective forecasts to physical activity, researchers have asked participants to indicate how much they expect to "enjoy" an upcoming exercise session on a scale from "not at all" to "very much" (Loehr & Baldwin, 2014; Ruby, Dunn, Perrino, Gillis, & Viel, 2011) or rate the extent to which they expect to experience pleasant (delighted, happy, fulfilled, calm) or unpleasant states (sad, dissatisfied, nervous, anxious) using a scale from "not at all" to "extremely" (Dunton & Vaughan, 2008). In experimental research, affective forecasts have been manipulated by telling participants that physical activity has been shown to induce "good moods, happiness, contentedness, feelings of personal satisfaction, and increases in self-esteem" (Helfer, Elhai, & Geers, 2015, p. 273), and the effect of this manipulation has been evaluated by asking respondents how they felt after a bout of exercise in terms of positive (e.g., happy, lively) and negative adjectives (e.g., miserable, nervous), using a scale from "do not feel" to "feel very strongly." In other words, although, by its very nature, a forecast depends on cognitive operations (using available data to make a prediction) and a person could form forecasts even in the absence of personal experience, affective forecasts are typically assessed in terms of what type and how much affect one expects to experience.

On the surface, this seems consistent with how "anticipated affective responses" were described by Ajzen and Sheikh (2013): "From the perspective of the [theory of planned behavior], anticipated regret and, more generally, anticipated affect are behavioral beliefs, i.e., beliefs about the likely affective consequences of performing a behavior" (p. 155). The phrase "beliefs about the likely affective consequences" may lead one to think that the object of these beliefs, as in affective forecasts, would be the "affective consequences." However, Ajzen and Sheikh (2013) did not ask respondents to evaluate the anticipated nature or intensity of affective experiences but rather asked them to give a rating of probability (i.e., how likely/unlikely or probable/improbable) it would be to feel certain affective states, albeit to an unspecified degree. This example has been emulated in studies linking "anticipated affective responses" to physical activity or exercise behavior. Respondents are asked to indicate the predicted probability that a certain state will occur at an unspecified level of intensity: "I will feel regret if I do not exercise over the next four weeks" ("definitely no" vs. "definitely yes"; Conner et al., 2015, p. 647). Thus, although any prediction about future affective responses relies on cognitive operations, this particular operationalization of "anticipated affective responses" may be characterized by even less affective "content saturation" than others. Imagine two individuals, one who reliably experiences mild and inconsequential levels of regret after each missed exercise session and another who reliably experiences intense regret, depression, self-loathing, and thoughts of self-harm. Both would probably occupy the same position on this continuum, rating regret as equally likely to occur, although their anticipated affective responses would be vastly different.

SUMMARY OF PRELIMINARY FINDINGS

The line of research investigating the relationship of affective responses to physical activity or exercise with physical activity is still at a nascent stage. Therefore, the search for best methodological practices is ongoing and the evidence base is fluid. This makes any attempt to draw conclusions perilous. Before interpreting any weak or inconsistent results as evidence of a null association or ineffectiveness of an intervention, it would be more sensible to subject the research methods to a critical evaluation.

Correlational Studies

Research has progressed in two main directions. One examines the association of naturally occurring oscillations in pleasant and unpleasant affect in daily life with physical activity behavior during the ensuing period (e.g., the next 30 minutes). The emerging finding is that periods of elevated pleasant affect, particularly when this is combined with high perceived activation (e.g., resulting in a sense of energy), tend to be followed by increased physical activity (Liao, Shonkoff, & Dunton, 2015). A strength of this line of research is that it increasingly uses technological tools that allow predictors and outcomes to be measured by different methods (e.g., smart phone applications for ecological momentary assessment of affect, accelerometers for physical activity). On the other hand, affect is often measured without a guiding theory, raising questions about how comprehensively this content domain is captured.

The second line of research examines the association of affective responses to bouts of physical activity or exercise with subsequent physical activity behavior. This research may stimulate the development of new advice about the types, doses, or settings of physical activity or exercise that may encourage participation and adherence. Reviews have shown associations between pleasant affective responses, especially during the activity, and higher physical activity, despite diverse methodologies (Ekkekakis & Dafermos, 2012; Rhodes & Kates, 2015).

For example, in a study of 146 low-active adults, the participants rated their pleasure or displeasure during and after a 10-minute treadmill walk at a moderate intensity (Williams, Dunsiger, Jennings, & Marcus, 2012). This assessment was conducted twice, 6 and 12 months into a lifestyle physical activity promotion trial. Physical activity of at least moderate intensity was measured by the 7-day recall method. The pleasure or displeasure reported during the walks was associated with physical activity, whereas ratings obtained after the walks were not. Specifically, in cross-sectional analyses at month 6, each 1-unit increase in an 11-point rating scale of pleasure-displeasure during the walk and cool-down was associated with 29 and 21 additional minutes of at-least moderate-intensity physical activity per week, respectively. In prospective analyses, during-walk ratings of pleasure-displeasure at month 6 were associated with 15 additional minutes of at-least moderate-intensity physical activity at month 12. Importantly, significant relationships have been found not only when physical activity was measured by self-report but also when it was measured by objective means, including accelerometers (Schneider, Dunn, & Cooper, 2009) and heart rate (Rizk et al., 2015).

Experimental Studies

Early results of experimental studies have been predictably inconsistent. Studies have examined manipulations of exercise intensity and, in particular, (1) allowing participants autonomy in regulating their exercise intensity and (2) affect-based exercise prescriptions.

Self-Selection of Exercise Intensity

In one study, 59 low-active and overweight or obese adults were randomly assigned to one of two 6-month experimental conditions (Williams et al., 2015, 2016). In one, participants were told to "walk at a pace that achieves a heart rate range" corresponding to 64%–76% of maximal heart rate (moderate intensity). In the other, participants were told that they should "select [their] own pace when walking for exercise" but were also told to not exceed 76% of maximal heart rate. Thus, both groups were given some autonomy to regulate their pace during unsupervised walking but one group was given both a lower and upper boundary of heart rate ("prescribed moderate intensity") whereas the other group was only given an upper boundary ("self-paced"). All participants were given handheld electronic diaries, which they used to complete ecological momentary assessments. Intensity recorded via heart rate monitors differed minimally between the groups ("prescribed": 62%; "self-paced": 58% of maximal heart rate). Nevertheless, on average, participants in the "self-paced" group reported approximately 26 additional minutes of walking per week. Importantly, there was some evidence that affective responses mediated the effects of the intervention on physical activity, with participants in the "self-paced" condition reporting more pleasant affect during sessions and, in turn, those reporting more pleasure also reported more activity (Williams et al., 2016).

Another study compared a condition of self-selected intensity to a condition of imposed intensity that was 10% higher than the individually determined ventilatory threshold and, therefore, likely to result in reduced pleasure (Freitas, 2014; Freitas et al., 2015). Fifty obese women participated in one of two 12-week supervised walking programs. Women in the self-selected intensity group were instructed to "choose a walking intensity of [their] preference," whereas women in the imposed-intensity group had their heart rate monitored and were given verbal feedback to maintain it at the prescribed level. The women in the self-selected intensity group gradually increased their heart rate during the program, whereas the women in the imposed-intensity group walked consistently at a higher intensity. Thus, women in the self-selected intensity group reported smaller declines in pleasure during the walks than women in the imposed-intensity group. Only 3 of 25 women dropped out of the self-selected intensity group (12%), whereas 13 of the 25 women dropped out of the imposed-intensity group (52%).

Affect-Based Exercise Prescriptions

In one study, 74 6th-grade students participated in two laboratory-based 30-minute bouts on a cycle ergometer (Schneider, 2014; Schneider, Schmalbach, & Godkin, 2017). For the first, resistance was set at 50% of the maximal work rate achieved during an earlier graded test, culminating at approximately 83% of maximal heart rate. For the second, participants could change the resistance every 3 minutes, to achieve a work rate that "felt good." This culminated at approximately 71% of maximal heart rate. The participants were then randomly assigned to two groups, both of which participated in 8 weeks of daily physical education. One was given a "traditional" exercise prescription consisting of a target heart rate zone extending from an upper boundary of 80% of the maximum heart rate achieved during the initial graded test to a lower boundary set at −20 beats per minute from the upper boundary. The other was given an individualized exercise prescription in which the target zone extended from an upper boundary set at +10 beats per minute from the heart rate that was achieved during the "feel-good" laboratory session to a lower boundary set at −20 beats per minute from the upper boundary. For both groups, the target zones were programmed into heart rate monitors that indicated whether the participants were below, above, or within their target zone. In other words, participants in both groups were given nearly identical intensity prescriptions (approximately 60%–80% of maximal heart rate), were asked to monitor their heart rate, and took part in the same physical education classes. Because participants were blinded to group allocation, those assigned to the "personalized" prescription group were not instructed to regulate their intensity to "feel good" and were unaware that the target they were given approximated the intensity they had selected as making them "feel good" during the cycle ergometer test. Since the groups received virtually identical treatments, the participants "did not undergo the affective experience that was intended" (Schneider et al., 2017, p. 9) and none of the outcome variables (e.g., intrinsic motivation, objectively measured physical activity) differed between the groups. Just as adults have been found to do in similar trials (Ekkekakis, 2009), the young participants in this trial disregarded their prescriptions, spending, on average, fewer than 10 of the 45 minutes of each class period within their target heart rate zone.

In another study, 67 low-active adults were randomly assigned to one of two month-long treatments (Baldwin et al., 2016). In one, participants were given a card with a target heart rate zone corresponding to "moderate" intensity (i.e., 64%–76% of maximal heart rate). In the other, participants were given a card with an 11-point bipolar rating scale, in which the midpoint (zero) was "I feel neutral," +5 was "I feel very good," and -5 was "I feel very bad." These participants were given the instruction to adjust their exercise intensity to ensure that they always felt "neutral" (i.e., zero) or better. Average heart rates (approximately 68% of maximal) and affect ratings (approximately +2.5) did not differ between groups. After the first week, based on a 7-day physical activity recall interview, participants in the affect-based prescription group reported more minutes of moderate-to-vigorous physical activity than those in the traditional prescription group (203 vs. 185, $d = 0.19$) but the difference did not reach statistical significance. Again, a critical appraisal of the methods must focus on the failure to alter the hypothesized mediator, namely the affective response. When respondents from Western cultures are asked "how they feel" at rest, they do not typically reply "I feel neutral" (i.e., zero) but rather "I feel good" (i.e., +3). Thus, even in response to strenuous exercise causing declines in pleasure, ratings on the 11-point rating scale are rarely below zero. Therefore, instructing participants to maintain their affect at zero or higher still allows for substantial declines from typical baseline scores. Therefore, an arguably more appropriate instruction would have been to ask participants to regulate their exercise intensity to feel at least "good" (i.e., +3 on the 11-point bipolar rating scale; see Parfitt, Alrumh, & Rowlands, 2012) or at least as "good" as they felt before starting the exercise.

RECOMMENDATIONS FOR FUTURE RESEARCH

Until recently, affective constructs had remained outside the scope of investigations on the determinants of physical activity and exercise behavior, presumably because they did not fit within the dominant cognitivist paradigm. In the last few years, this has started to change. While this is a positive development, the picture is complicated by the fact that most researchers jumping on the affect bandwagon come from a cognitivist background. However, the study of affect presents certain extraordinary challenges. There is no singular theory of affect, there is no singular authority on the subject whose writings can be used as a de facto guide, and there is no singular measure. Instead, the affective psychology literature is vast (its dawn predates cognitivism and extends to the beginnings of modern psychology in the 19th century), it interfaces minimally with the cognitivist literature but extensively with the neurophysiological and psychophysiological literatures, and is characterized by an overwhelming plurality of viewpoints. More than a century of experience shows that researchers seeking to quickly incorporate affective constructs into their studies will inevitably become confused.

To Study the Affective Determinants of Physical Activity, (1) Study Affect

A major source of confusion for researchers making their first foray into affective psychology is terminology. For example, newcomers are shocked to discover that "positive affect" does not mean pleasure or happiness and "negative affect" does not mean displeasure or sadness (Ekkekakis, 2013; Ekkekakis & Zenko, 2016b). Likewise, a common phenomenon is the obliteration of distinctions between affective constructs, such as affect and emotion. The new area of research examining affect as a possible determinant of physical activity will predictably grapple with definitional issues, such as what constitutes "affect." There are two options. One is for this line of research to allow itself to be infused by over a century of research and theorizing in affective psychology. The alternative is for this line of research to develop its own terminological conventions. Within this system, for example, constructs such as "enjoyment" and "excitement" could be labeled "emotions" (Lawton et al., 2009, p. 57; Conner et al., 2013,

p. 265; Conner et al., 2015, p. 643) despite these not being considered emotions in affective psychology. We propose that the former option is more advantageous than the latter. Taking advantage of the long experience of a research field dedicated to the study of affective phenomena will likely prevent wasteful detours, pointless debates, and frustrating dead-ends.

To Study the Affective Determinants of Physical Activity, (2) Study Physical Activity

In most studies investigating the "affective determinants" of physical activity or exercise, these behaviors are studied alongside similar questions about other health behaviors (e.g., eating fruits and vegetables, using sun screen, brushing and flossing teeth). The uniqueness of physical activity and exercise as gripping, whole-body experiences is overlooked. If this emerging line of research defines affect as a lived, embodied experience, this would also entail making the affective response to physical activity, when and where it occurs, its focal phenomenon of study. The salient experiences of pleasure or displeasure during physical activity or exercise must form the core of the cluster of variables considered the "affective determinants" of subsequent behavior. These affective determinants cannot be taught. They must be experienced, reliably over multiple instances, until positive associations are consolidated, linking physical activity or exercise to pleasure and approach tendencies. It is reasonable to assume, albeit untested, that efforts to associate physical activity or exercise with pleasure via messaging (e.g., Conner et al., 2011; Morris et al., 2016) or image-based conditioning (e.g., Antoniewicz & Brand, 2016) will be rendered powerless when confronted with repeated experiences of displeasure. Therefore, we concur that the most urgent agenda item is "experimental tests that attempt to manipulate the affective experience during exercise and its impact on sustained behavior change" (Rhodes & Kates, 2015, p. 728). To manipulate the affective experience and study the process by which it becomes an affective determinant of physical activity and exercise, researchers must embrace physical activity and exercise as inherently *psychobiological* phenomena. In particular, given how closely affective responses track changes in exercise intensity (Ekkekakis, Parfitt, & Petruzzello, 2011), the need to develop an understanding of the underlying physiological processes, as well as an appreciation for affect as an embodied phenomenon, should be considered paramount.

To Study the Affective Determinants of Physical Activity, (3) Study Affective Responses

Researchers may be inclined to represent the affective response during a session of physical activity by sampling affect several times and averaging them (e.g., Baldwin et al., 2016; Sala, Baldwin, & Williams, 2016). This approach, however, would be appropriate only if all ratings fell close to the average, without much change over time. In other cases, the average would offer a poor representation of the nature of the response (e.g., improvement or decline over time, linear or curvilinear change). In forming affective associations that determine future behavioral inclinations, the average affect may be inconsequential. Instead, the most influential elements appear to be (1) the affect experienced at the end of the episode, (2) the peak (pleasant or unpleasant) affect experienced during the episode, and (3) the slope of affective change during the episode (Ekkekakis & Dafermos, 2012; Hargreaves & Stych, 2013; Zenko, Ekkekakis, & Ariely, 2016). Moreover, due to the idiosyncratic use of rating scales, it may be more meaningful, rather than measuring affect in an absolute manner, to focus on how affective responses to physical activity compare to the manner in which a particular person responds to alternative options, such as sedentary behaviors (Varey & Kahneman, 1992).

REFERENCES

Ajzen, I. (1991). The theory of planned behavior. *Organizational Behavior and Human Decision Processes, 50*, 179–211.

Ajzen, I. (2005). *Attitudes, personality and behavior* (2nd ed.). New York, NY: Open University Press.

Ajzen, I. (2011). The theory of planned behaviour: Reactions and reflections. *Psychology and Health, 26*, 1113–1127.

Ajzen, I., & Fishbein, M. (2005). The influence of attitudes on behavior. In D. Albarracín, B. T. Johnson, & M. P. Zanna (Eds.), *The handbook of attitudes* (pp. 173–221). Mahwah, NJ: Erlbaum.

Ajzen, I., & Manstead, A. S. R. (2007). Changing health-related behaviours: An approach based on the theory of planned behaviour. In M. Hewstone, H. A.W. Schut, J. B. F. de Wit, K. van den Bos, & M. S. Stroebe (Eds.), *The scope of social psychology: Theory and applications* (pp. 43–63). East Sussex, UK: Psychology Press.

Ajzen, I., & Sheikh, S. (2013). Action versus inaction: Anticipated affect in the theory of planned behavior. *Journal of Applied Social Psychology, 43*, 155–162.

Antoniewicz, F., & Brand, R. (2016). Learning to like exercising: Evaluative conditioning changes automatic evaluations of exercising and influences subsequent exercising behavior. *Journal of Sport and Exercise Psychology, 38*, 138–148.

Baldwin, A. S., Kangas, J. L., Denman, D. C., Smits, J. A. J., Yamada, T., & Otto, M. W. (2016). Cardiorespiratory fitness moderates the effect of an affect-guided physical activity prescription: A pilot randomized controlled trial. *Cognitive Behaviour Therapy, 45*, 445–457.

Bandura, A. (2004). Health promotion by social cognitive means. *Health Education and Behavior, 31*, 143–164.

Chang, S.-J., van Witteloostuijn, A., & Eden, L. (2010). From the Editors: Common method variance in international business research. *Journal of International Business Studies, 41*, 178–184.

Conner, M., Godin, G., Sheeran, P., & Germain, M. (2013). Some feelings are more important: Cognitive attitudes, affective attitudes, anticipated affect, and blood donation. *Health Psychology, 32*, 264–272.

Conner, M., McEachan, R., Taylor, N., O'Hara, J., & Lawton, R. (2015). Role of affective attitudes and anticipated affective reactions in predicting health behaviors. *Health Psychology, 34*, 642–652.

Conner, M., Rhodes, R. E., Morris, B., McEachan, R., & Lawton, R. (2011). Changing exercise through targeting affective or cognitive attitudes. *Psychology and Health, 26*, 133–149.

Conway, J. M., & Lance, C. E. (2010). What reviewers should expect from authors regarding common method bias in organizational research. *Journal of Business and Psychology, 25*, 325–334.

Corrigan, P. W., Rüsch, N., Ben-Zeev, D., & Sher, T. (2014). The rational patient and beyond: Implications for treatment adherence in people with psychiatric disabilities. *Rehabilitation Psychology, 59*, 85–98.

Dunton, G. F., & Vaughan, E. (2008). Anticipated affective consequences of physical activity adoption and maintenance. *Health Psychology, 27*, 703–710.

Ekkekakis, P. (2009). Let them roam free? Physiological and psychological evidence for the potential of self-selected exercise intensity in public health. *Sports Medicine, 39*, 857–888.

Ekkekakis, P. (2013). *The measurement of affect, mood, and emotion: A guide for health-behavioral research.* New York, NY: Cambridge University Press.

Ekkekakis, P., & Dafermos, M. (2012). Exercise is a many-splendored thing but for some it does not feel so splendid: Staging a resurgence of hedonistic ideas in the quest to understand exercise behavior. In E.O. Acevedo (Ed.), *The Oxford handbook of exercise psychology* (pp. 295–333). New York, NY: Oxford University Press.

Ekkekakis, P., Parfitt, G., & Petruzzello, S. J. (2011). The pleasure and displeasure people feel when they exercise at different intensities: Decennial update and progress towards a tripartite rationale for exercise intensity prescription. *Sports Medicine, 41*, 641–671.

Ekkekakis, P., & Zenko, Z. (2016a). Escape from cognitivism: Exercise as hedonic experience. In M. Raab, P. Wylleman, R. Seiler, A. M. Elbe, & A. Hatzigeorgiadis (Eds.), *Sport and exercise psychology research from theory to practice* (pp. 389–414). London: Academic.

Ekkekakis, P., & Zenko, Z. (2016b). Measurement of affective responses to exercise: From "affectless arousal" to "the most well-characterized" relationship between the body and affect. In H. L. Meiselman (Ed.), *Emotion measurement* (pp. 299–321). Duxford, UK: Woodhead.

Freitas, L. A. (2014). *Efeito de um programa de atividades aeróbias em intensidades autosselecionada e imposta nas respostas fisiológicas, perceptuais e afetivas de mulheres obesas* (Unpublished doctoral dissertation). Universidade Federal do Paraná, Curitiba, Brazil.

Freitas, L. A., Ferreira, S. D. S., Freitas, R. Q., de Souza, C. H., Garcia, E. D. S. D. A., & da Silva, G. S. (2015). Effect of a 12-week aerobic training program on perceptual and affective responses in obese women. *Journal of Physical Therapy Science, 27*, 2221–2224.

Hagger, M. S. (2015). Retired or not, the theory of planned behaviour will always be with us. *Health Psychology Review, 9*, 125–130.

Hagger, M. S., & Chatzisarantis, N. L. D. (2014). An integrated behavior change model for physical activity. *Exercise and Sport Sciences Reviews, 42*, 62–69.

Hallal, P. C., Andersen, L. B., Bull, F. C., Guthold, R., Haskell, W., & Ekelund, U. (2012). Global physical activity levels: Surveillance progress, pitfalls, and prospects. *Lancet, 380*, 247–257.

Hargreaves, E. A., & Stych, K. (2013). Exploring the peak and end rule of past affective episodes within the exercise context. *Psychology of Sport and Exercise, 14*, 169–178.

Helfer, S. G., Elhai, J. D., & Geers, A. L. (2015). Affect and exercise: Positive affective expectations can increase post-exercise mood and exercise intentions. *Annals of Behavioral Medicine, 49*, 269–279.

Hofmann, W., Friese, M., & Wiers, R. W. (2008). Impulsive versus reflective influences on health behavior: A theoretical framework and empirical review. *Health Psychology Review, 2*, 111–137.

Kuhn, T. S. (1962/1996). *The structure of scientific revolutions.* Chicago: University of Chicago Press.

Larsen, J. T., McGraw, A. P., & Cacioppo, J. T. (2001). Can people feel happy and sad at the same time? *Journal of Personality and Social Psychology, 81*, 684–696.

Lawton, R., Conner, M., & McEachan, R. (2009). Desire or reason: Predicting health behaviors from affective and cognitive attitudes. *Health Psychology, 28*, 56–65.

Liao, Y., Shonkoff, E. T., & Dunton, G. F. (2015). The acute relationships between affect, physical feeling states, and physical activity in daily life: A review of current evidence. *Frontiers in Psychology, 6*, 1975.

Loehr, V. G., & Baldwin, A. S. (2014). Affective forecasting error in exercise: Differences between physically active and inactive individuals. *Sport, Exercise, and Performance Psychology, 3*, 177–183.

Morris, B., Lawton, R., McEachan, R., Hurling, R., & Conner, M. (2016). Changing self-reported physical activity using different types of affectively and cognitively framed health messages, in a student population. *Psychology, Health, and Medicine, 21*, 198–207.

Nasuti, G., & Rhodes, R. E. (2013). Affective judgment and physical activity in youth: Review and meta-analyses. *Annals of Behavioral Medicine, 45*, 357–376.

Parfitt, G., Alrumh, A., & Rowlands, A. V. (2012). Affect-regulated exercise intensity: Does training at an intensity that feels "good" improve physical health? *Journal of Science and Medicine in Sport, 15*, 548–553.

Podsakoff, P. M., MacKenzie, S. B., Lee, J.-Y., & Podsakoff, N. P. (2003). Common method biases in behavioral research: A critical review of the literature and recommended remedies. *Journal of Applied Psychology, 88*, 879–903.

Prochaska, J. O., & Marcus, B. H. (1994). The transtheoretical model: Applications to exercise. In R. K. Dishman (Ed.), *Advances in exercise adherence* (pp. 161–180). Champaign, IL: Human Kinetics.

Rhodes, R. E. (2014). Adding depth to the next generation of physical activity models. *Exercise and Sport Sciences Reviews, 42*, 43–44.

Rhodes, R. E. (2015). Will the new theories (and theoreticians!) please stand up? A commentary on Sniehotta, Presseau and Araújo-Soares. *Health Psychology Review, 9*, 156–159.

Rhodes, R. E., Fiala, B., & Conner, M. (2009). A review and meta-analysis of affective judgments and physical activity in adult populations. *Annals of Behavioral Medicine, 38*, 180–204.

Rhodes, R. E., & Kates, A. (2015). Can the affective response to exercise predict future motives and physical activity behavior? A systematic review of published evidence. *Annals of Behavioral Medicine, 49*, 715–731.

Rice, T. (2013). The behavioral economics of health and health care. *Annual Review of Public Health, 34*, 431–447.

Rizk, A. K., Wardini, R., Chan-Thim, E., Bacon, S. L., Lavoie, K. L., & Pepin, V. (2015). Acute responses to exercise training and relationship with exercise adherence in moderate chronic obstructive pulmonary disease. *Chronic Respiratory Disease, 12*, 329–339.

Rose, E. A., & Parfitt, G. (2010). Pleasant for some and unpleasant for others: A protocol analysis of the cognitive factors that influence affective responses to exercise. *International Journal of Behavioral Nutrition and Physical Activity, 7*, 15.

Ruby, M. B., Dunn, E. W., Perrino, A., Gillis, R., & Viel, S. (2011). The invisible benefits of exercise. *Health Psychology, 30*, 67–74.

Russell, J. A. (2003). Core affect and the psychological construction of emotion. *Psychological Review, 110*, 145–172.

Russell, J. A., & Feldman Barrett, L. (1999). Core affect, prototypical emotional episodes, and other things called emotion: Dissecting the elephant. *Journal of Personality and Social Psychology, 76*, 805–819.

Russell, J. A., & Feldman Barrett, L. (2009). Core affect. In D. Sander & K. R. Scherer (Eds.), *The Oxford companion to emotion and the affective sciences* (p. 104). New York, NY: Oxford University Press.

Ryan, R. M., Williams, G. C., Patrick, H., & Deci, E. L. (2009). Self-determination theory and physical activity: The dynamics of motivation in development and wellness. *Hellenic Journal of Psychology, 6*, 107–124.

Sala, M., Baldwin, A. S., & Williams, D. M. (2016). Affective and cognitive predictors of affective response to exercise: Examining unique and overlapping variance. *Psychology of Sport and Exercise, 27*, 1–8.

Schneider, M. (2014). Process evaluation and proximal impact of an affect-based exercise intervention among adolescents. *Translational Behavioral Medicine, 4*, 190–200.

Schneider, M., Dunn, A., & Cooper, D. (2009). Affect, exercise, and physical activity among healthy adolescents. *Journal of Sport and Exercise Psychology, 31*, 706–723.

Schneider, M., Schmalbach, P., & Godkin, S. (2017). Impact of a personalized versus moderate-intensity exercise prescription: A randomized controlled trial. *Journal of Behavioral Medicine, 40*, 239–248.

Shafir, E., & LeBoeuf, R. A. (2002). Rationality. *Annual Review of Psychology, 53*, 491–517.

Sniehotta, F. F., Presseau, J., & Araújo-Soares, V. (2014). Time to retire the theory of planned behaviour. *Health Psychology Review, 8*, 1–7.

Strack, F., & Deutsch, R. (2004). Reflective and impulsive determinants of social behavior. *Personality and Social Psychology Review, 8*, 220–247.

Varey, C., & Kahneman, D. (1992). Experiences extended across time: Evaluation of moments and episodes. *Journal of Behavioral Decision Making, 5*, 169–185.

Williams, D. M., & Evans, D. R. (2014). Current emotion research in health behavior science. *Emotion Review, 6*, 277–287.

Williams, D. M., Dunsiger, S., Emerson, J. A., Gwaltney, C. J., Monti, P. O. M., & Miranda, R., Jr. (2016). Self-paced exercise, affective response, and exercise adherence: A preliminary investigation using ecological momentary assessment. *Journal of Sport and Exercise Psychology, 38*, 282–291.

Williams, D. M., Dunsiger, S., Jennings, E. G., & Marcus, B. H. (2012). Does affective valence during and immediately following a 10-min walk predict concurrent and future physical activity? *Annals of Behavioral Medicine, 44*, 43–51.

Williams, D. M., Dunsiger, S., Miranda, R., Gwaltney, C. J., Emerson, J. A., Monti, P. M., & Parisi, A. F. (2015). Recommending self-paced exercise among overweight and obese adults: A randomized pilot study. *Annals of Behavioral Medicine, 49*, 280–285.

Wilson, T. D., & Gilbert, D. T. (2003). Affective forecasting. *Advances in Experimental Social Psychology, 35*, 345–411.

Zajonc, R. B. (1980). Feeling and thinking: Preferences need no inferences. *American Psychologist, 35*, 151–175.

Zenko, Z., Ekkekakis, P., & Ariely, D. (2016). Can you have your vigorous exercise and enjoy it too? Ramping intensity down increases postexercise, remembered, and forecasted pleasure. *Journal of Sport and Exercise Psychology*, *38*, 149–159.

Zenko, Z., Ekkekakis, P., & Kavetsos, G. (2016). Changing minds? Bounded rationality and heuristic processes in exercise-related judgments and choices. *Sport, Exercise, and Performance Psychology*, *5*, 337–351.

12

"Stressed Spelled Backward Is Desserts"

Affective Determinants of Eating Behavior

DENISE DE RIDDER AND CATHARINE EVERS

INTRODUCTION

Thinking about affect and eating, examples of negative emotions leading people to consume more than they want easily come to mind. Take Marcia, who just broke up with her boyfriend and is feeling very sad. To cope with these negative feelings, she consumes a big bag of crisps, only to feel even sadder afterward. Or take Mark, who was just turned down for a job he really liked. Mindlessly he empties the cookie jar, while ruminating about the reasons why he was not picked for the job. Or take Jessie, who feels bad about just having had a fight with her best friend. She reasons that she deserves a treat after this bad event and decides to buy her favorite chocolate bar. These and other examples of a phenomenon that has been coined "emotional eating" sound familiar because they are prominently present in the scientific literature and even in movies, popular books, and magazines: many people seem to agree that it is a proven fact that people overeat when they feel sad or angry or otherwise experience negative affect. The scientific literature on emotional eating has expanded in the past decades and focuses on laying out the conditions under which negative emotions lead to eating more than one wants to. The scientific literature also has witnessed several controversies such as whether only negative affect leads to overeating or that positive affect may influence eating behavior as well, or whether emotional eating is a phenomenon that is primarily observed in people who are concerned about their weight or have an otherwise problematic attitude toward eating.

In this chapter we review the literature on emotional eating and examine which emotions lead to (over)eating and the psychological underpinnings of this relation. In doing so, we pay particular attention to the type of affect (e.g., positive versus negative emotions; low arousal versus high arousal emotions) and the mechanisms that underlie the impact of affect on eating (e.g., coping, licensing). Before we turn to these classic topics in the literature on affect and eating, we take a slightly different angle and address questions that pertain to the relation between affect and eating from a different perspective, that is that eating is not only influenced by affect but also brings affect—either positive or negative. Indeed, complementing the abundant literature on negative emotions contributing to overeating, there is literature showing that eating (and even thinking about eating) has important consequences for how we feel. To better understand in what way negative or positive emotional states affect eating behavior, it is important to consider the flip side as well. After all, eating is a necessity and as such knowing more about how eating and affect influence each other bidirectionally may help to understand this complex relationship. For frequently repeated behaviors such as eating, which we all do on a daily basis, previous affective experiences with eating (affective consequences of eating) may have a direct impact on our affective expectations of eating (affective determinants). Thus, how we felt during previous eating occasions may in turn influence how these feelings determine subsequent behavior. Before we discuss the affective determinants of eating behavior in detail, we first review the literature on the affective consequences of eating behavior.

EATING BRINGS PLEASURE, OR DOESN'T IT?

To illustrate in what way affective determinants of eating are intertwined with its affective consequences, consider the following example. Many people nowadays experience considerable ambivalence when making food decisions, especially when these choices are about foods they like (which are unfortunately often unhealthy foods, containing large amounts of sugar, salt, and fat). Before even tasting the food, people anticipate how they will feel about eating the food. For most of us, eating decisions generate mixed feelings. On the one hand we expect to derive pleasure from eating while on the other hand we realize that we might feel guilty after indulging because of the negative consequences for health and weight. This anticipated conflict—enjoyment versus guilt—is rooted in previous affective experiences with eating, which are driven by both the biological rewarding properties of food and a social-cultural context that warns against eating too much.

Reward of Eating

One of the most pervasive accounts of overeating holds that people eat too much because of food's rewarding value. Eating is a biological function that is crucial for survival and as such our genes have prepared us to enjoy eating (Pinel, Assanand, & Lehman, 2000). In particular foods high in fat and sweet are related to release of endorphins and result in enhanced positive affect (Benton & Donohoe, 1999), mostly within several hours after ingestion (Smith, Leekam, Ralph, & McNeill, 1988). While the affective bonus from eating was adaptive in the old days when food was scarce, in our modern society with high caloric food available any time, any place, this inherent pleasure people derive from eating has made us vulnerable, especially as we seem to enjoy eating even more when it concerns palatable foods that contain large amounts of sugar, salt, and fat (Berridge, 2000). These hedonic reactions to food are a robust phenomenon and have a biological basis: because we like food so much we are motivated to put effort into getting it (Berridge, 2000). Simply looking at food can evoke immediate appetitive responses in terms of salivation, blood pressure, and gastric activity (Nederkoorn, Smulders, & Jansen, 2000). As a result, even in these modern times many of our daily desires center around food. In an experience sampling study of German adults it was reported that no less than one-third of our longings during the day relates to food (28.1%), which is considerably more than the wish for sleep (10.3%), leisure (7.2%), social contact (7.1%), sex (4.6%), or spending (2.2%) (Hofmann, Baumeister, Förster, & Vohs, 2012).

Moralization of Eating

While the rewarding function of food has been extensively documented in the literature (mostly in terms of its biological significance for survival), the positive consequences of eating in terms of immediate positive affect or overall psychological well-being have largely been neglected so far in eating research (Rozin, 1999). It has been speculated that ignoring the pleasure of eating in food research may be a consequence of our preoccupation with healthy food, initiated by health professionals who have documented the detrimental effects of unhealthy food on health and weight, and widely adopted by consumers who have come to realize that eating too much brings health risks. The literature on eating and health (unintentionally) suggests that eating healthy foods is incompatible with enjoying food, with the result that many people think that eating healthily is not a fun activity. The "moralization of pleasure" in food research (Askegaard et al., 2014) has made healthy eating a virtue that requires a great deal of self-regulation to the extent that people have to forego (unhealthy) foods they like in order to stay slim and healthy in the long run. Even worse, Askegaard and colleagues (2014) argue, enjoying foods seems to signal indulgence and failure of self-regulation, with the result that pleasure derived from eating is a vice typical for people who cannot restrain their impulses for immediate satisfaction of their low-level visceral urges and only strive for short-lived hedonic relief. In an attempt to create a more nuanced view of the role of pleasure in eating behavior, Cornil and Chandon (2016) recently proposed the concept of *Epicurean eating*, which they define as "the enduring pleasure derived from the aesthetic appreciation of the sensory and symbolic value of food." Different from the almost caricatural picture that enjoyment of eating is typical for people who indulge in big portions of fat food, they found that Epicurean eaters enjoy good food in small portions, slightly reminiscent of Paul Rozin's study of French consumers who eat small (rather than big) portions at the local McDonald's in Paris while having a good time with their friends (rather than worrying about their consumption) (Rozin, Kabnick, Pete, Fischler, & Shields, 2003). Exact numbers on the prevalence of Epicurean eating are lacking so far. It may well be that Epicurean eating, as proposed by Cornil and Chandon, is an atypical phenomenon that only applies to a small group of well-educated foodies who can afford to engage in what also has been labeled as mindful eating (Papies, Barsalou, & Custers, 2012). There are some indications, however, that Epicurean eating is a phenomenon that it is typical for food cultures that allow for the enjoyment of small bites, such as Mediterranean Europe (Rozin, 1999).

Culture and Pleasure of Food

Large cultural differences have been documented with regard to whether people primarily enjoy the experience of eating versus thinking about food in terms of health consequences (Rozin, Fischler, Imada, Sarubin, & Wrzesniewki, 1999). Americans tend to associate food most with health and the least with pleasure, while the opposite pattern is found in French and Belgian consumers (Rozin et al., 1999). Ironically, the Americans who do the most to alter their diet in the service of their health are the least likely to classify themselves as healthy eaters. Moreover, they tend to enjoy food the least while they eat the most. The most extreme differences in the Rozin et al. study were found between French male and American female students on typical items relating to food on the worry versus pleasure dimension, such as "Enjoying food is one of the most important pleasures of my life" with the American female students scoring substantially lower than the French men. These findings seem to suggest that primarily thinking about food in terms of health ruins the pleasure of eating (at least, to the extent that healthy food is regarded as incompatible with good taste, see what follows). The apparent contradiction that people who value health the most are in fact unhealthy eaters, while people who enjoy food and even eat more unhealthy foods are healthier, has been associated with the *French paradox*. This paradox is derived from the observation that mortality rates from coronary heart disease are substantially lower among the French than Americans, yet the French have a higher blood cholesterol level (Renaud & de Lorgeril, 1992). Several explanations for this paradox have been suggested, such as genetically based metabolic differences between the French and the Americans or the French having a lower BMI (even though their diet contains more fat) (Rozin et al., 2003). One of the most appealing accounts seems to be that "food life" in France is less stressful because people have a more positive attitude toward food and are less bothered by worries about the health consequences of consuming particular foods, which eventually results in eating less with more fun (Rozin, 1999; Rozin et al., 1999).

Dieting and Pleasure

Whereas France and the United States may represent the extremes of positive versus negative attitudes to food, it seems that only very few people have an uncomplicated way of thinking about food nowadays. In fact, it seems that many people are slightly obsessed by the potential negative consequences of food for their health and weight while still craving for (unhealthy) foods, resulting in mixed feelings and ambivalence rather than straightforward negative feelings about food. The prototypical example is a study of American undergraduate students, showing that especially female students very much enjoyed eating but at the same time reported serious worries about the impact of food on weight and health (Rozin, Bauer, & Catanese, 2003). The most illustrative items that were used in the survey reveal that many respondents associated chocolate cake with guilt rather than celebration and ice cream with fattening rather than delicious. Similar findings were reported in a large community survey in the Netherlands, that documented that many people—regardless their age, gender, and education—were not so much negative about food but nevertheless reported considerable concerns about the impact of food on their weight and health (De Ridder, Adriaanse, Evers, & Verhoeven, 2014). Interestingly, more than 60% of the participants qualified as a dieter according to the sex-specific norms of the Dutch Eating Behavior Questionnaire (Van Strien, Frijters, Bergers, & Defares, 1986), and it was dieting status that was most strongly associated with concerns about food without having any impact whatsoever on how much people actually ate (snack consumption reported in a 1-week diary).

These findings clearly reveal an intriguing phenomenon in our modern society. While we still enjoy food (or are at least not very negative about it), we are also well aware of the potential negative consequences of food for health, especially in terms of the risks of overweight. The obesogenic environment has generated much information about the health risks of overweight with the objective to warn people to restrain their food intake. Being aware of the negative consequences of overeating is important to change eating behavior, but a negative side effect of the exposure to the ubiquitous and complex information about the diet–health link (Rozin, 1999) is that we need to pay constant attention to what and how much we eat. Many people (up to about 65% of the population) call themselves a dieter these days (Andreyeva, Long, Henderson, & Grode, 2010; De Ridder et al., 2014), which may be the direct result of having been bombarded with information about the negative health consequences of overeating. It is now generally agreed that the self-proclaimed dieter status has not so much to do with how much people actually eat (De Ridder et al., 2014; Stice, Cooper, Schoeller, Tappe, & Lowe, 2007). Rather, considering oneself a dieter seems to be an expression of concerns about the consequences of food for weight and health (Adriaanse, De Ridder, & Evers, 2011). Dieting has therefore been labeled as "double trouble," because dieters do not eat less and still feel worse (De Witt Huberts, Evers, & De Ridder, 2013). The reason that there are so many dieters—that is, people who worry about their food intake without being able or willing to actually restrain it—may thus be a direct consequence of the public moralization of an unhealthy diet (Askegaard et al., 2014). Such moralization may instigate feelings of worry that serve as a means to decrease feelings of guilt about not having made sufficient effort to change one's eating behavior (De Ridder et al., 2014). Indeed, it has been reported that restraint status is associated with feelings of guilt that are unrelated to actual food intake but rather pertain to having transgressed one's personal standards (De Witt Huberts et al., 2013). Feelings of guilt about eating are incompatible with the enjoyment of food (Lindeman & Stark, 2000; Macht & Dettmer, 2006; Rozin, 1999), suggesting that restrained eating not only leads to a greater experience of guilt but also makes eating a less pleasurable experience.

Healthy Food and Taste

It thus seems that a greater emphasis on the potential negative consequences of food for health and weight has serious implications for the immediate experience of food in terms of pleasure. This is also manifest in studies that report on the influence of the labeling of food as "healthy" on sensory experiences in terms of taste. One study has shown that such labeling leads people to enjoy food less and even makes them hungry (Finkelstein & Fishbach, 2010). This study demonstrated that consumers who were asked to sample a food item framed as "healthy" later reported being hungrier and consumed more food than those who sampled the same item framed as tasty or those who did not eat at all (Finkelstein & Fishbach, 2010). Importantly, these effects of healthy eating depended on the consumer's perception that healthy eating was mandatory; only imposed healthy eating made consumers hungrier, whereas freely choosing to eat healthy did not increase hunger. Whereas this study suggests that healthy food is perceived as *less* rewarding, the opposite has also been demonstrated, namely that unhealthy (i.e., high caloric) food is considered to be *more* rewarding (Kroese, Evers, & De Ridder, 2013; Raghunathan,

Naylor, & Hoyer, 2006) in spite of being perceived as "more dangerous" in terms of health consequences (Macht, Gerer, & Ellgring, 2003). In a series of experiments Raghunathan and colleagues (Raghunathan et al., 2006) found evidence that the less healthy a food item was portrayed, the better its inferred taste, the more it was enjoyed during actual consumption, and the greater the preference for it in a subsequent food choice task. These findings speak to the intuition that healthy food has a negative appeal because it is consumed for its assumed positive consequences for health rather than for the immediate enjoyable experience of food.

However, there are some limitations to this intuition, depending on the extent to which healthy food actually is considered untasty (Werle, Trendel, & Ardito, 2013) or is considered as part of one's eating routines (Gillebaart, Schneider, & De Ridder, 2015). The typical association of healthy with untasty may only apply in a context where people perceive a conflict between their immediate need for palatable food and their wish for staying healthy and slim in the long term. This association has been observed in female American students who would like to diet and for whom fatty foods are a guilty pleasure. However, "healthy" and "tasty" are not inherently opposite to each other. In a French study, researchers found that unhealthy food (rather than healthy) was spontaneously associated with bad taste, whereas healthy food was linked to tastiness (Werle et al., 2013). This study also reported that the link between healthy food and tastiness was weaker in restrained (French) eaters, suggesting that dieting may be a potential explanation for the association between unhealthy and tasty (and thus forbidden) foods that seems more prominent in the American food culture (Werle et al., 2013).

Healthy food also is not necessarily associated with bad taste for people who consider "healthy" food as the obvious thing to do. This was shown in a study that demonstrated that people with high trait self-control who think of healthy food as part of their daily routine were not ambivalent at all about healthy foods and categorized them as straightforwardly positive (Gillebaart et al., 2015). The extent to which healthy food is associated with untasty (and unhealthy food with tasty) thus seems to depend on how people feel about healthy foods: when they consider healthy foods as the normal thing to do or simply like fruits and vegetables (which are healthy but not necessarily liked because they are healthy) they have no negative thoughts about these foods. In terms of promoting healthy food, it therefore may be worthwhile to avoid the label "healthy" because it communicates that this makes you give up on taste (as if it were a trade-off) and requires extra effort to invest in future benefits without immediate pleasure.

Summary

To sum up, whereas the biological function of eating implies that people derive pleasure from food, in rare cases it actually does nowadays. Instead, food has become a reason for concern. Many people are worrying about the diet–health link and ironically it seems that the more importance they attach to healthy eating the less they enjoy eating and the more they crave unhealthy food, which they consider tastier (while not actually eating less). This complicated association between food, health, and pleasure may also be one of the reasons why many people seem to turn to eating as a strategy to cope with negative emotions, which is one of the manifestations of emotional eating that we discuss in the next section.

NEGATIVE EMOTIONS LEAD TO OVEREATING, OR DON'T THEY?

For a long time negative emotions have been considered as important instigators of overeating (e.g., Bruch, 1964; Lehman & Rodin, 1989; Macht, 2008) and hence contributing to weight gain. The idea that negative emotions are responsible for overeating is rooted in psychosomatic theory (Bruch, 1964), stating that eating when experiencing negative emotions either results from the inability to distinguish hunger sensations from arousal due to other aversive internal states or results from having learned early on that eating is a means to alleviate negative emotional states. Emotional eating, generally defined as eating in response to negative emotions rather than hunger (e.g., Van Strien et al., 1986), has been the topic of extensive theoretical debate. Before we discuss empirical findings on emotional eating, we first elaborate on these theoretical notions. To put it bluntly, the exact process by which emotions affect eating behavior has largely remained unclear (Leith & Baumeister, 1996). Negative emotions bring about a bodily state similar to satiety, as increased autonomic emotional activity leads to the release of appetite-inhibiting hormones and to a variety of gastric changes similar to those that are involved in satiety (Blair, Wing, & Wald, 1991). The tendency to overeat in response to negative emotions, then, is surprising from a biological point of view. Also from a functional perspective, emotional eating seems maladaptive. Emotions prepare the organism for a set of diverse actions required to respond optimally to environmental demands and eating interferes with these demands. Accordingly, from a functional perspective on the role of emotions in behavior, a natural response to negative emotions would consist of *decreased* eating (Schachter, Goldman, & Gordon, 1968), with overeating while being emotional a response that is typical for individuals with eating pathology (such as, for example, binge eating disorder) rather than a normal reaction in healthy individuals (e.g., Herman & Polivy, 1988; Masheb & Grilo, 2006; Wiser & Telch, 1999).

Explaining the Role of Negative Emotions

In order to explain the seemingly irrational tendency to overeat in emotional situations in healthy individuals, several psychological explanations have been put forward. One group of theories has assumed that increased eating in response to negative emotions occurs in order to cope with these negative feelings. For example, it has been postulated that binging occurs as an attempt to escape from negative self-awareness (Heatherton & Baumeister, 1991). When individuals are confronted with ego-threatening information, they shift their attention to the immediate stimulus environment and away from higher cognition levels. This allows them to avoid having to deal with the implications of the threatening information. Such narrowing of attention results in reduced inhibitory actions, creating a situation where individuals are likely to engage in increased eating.

Another frequently posited assumption is that overeating increases the experience of positive emotions (note that this assumption is different from what we discussed in the previous section on eating rather than overeating creating a pleasurable experience). This perspective states that individuals derive pleasure from the consumption of food because of its hedonic qualities (Lehman & Rodin, 1989). Several studies have found that a binging episode does indeed temporarily improve one's mood (e.g., Deaver, Miltenberger, Smyth, Meidinger, & Crosby, 2003), but there are also accounts suggesting that overeating in fact only further increases negative mood (Macht & Dettmer, 2006; De Witt Huberts et al., 2013).

A third explanation for the role of negative emotions in overeating is the so-called masking theory, stating that overeating is an attempt to misattribute perceived stress to eating, so as to distract from the original source of distress (Herman & Polivy, 1988). These different accounts of negative emotions leading to overeating share the assumption that before overeating occurs, individuals experience negative feelings that they cannot regulate properly, prompting them to employ a strategy they do have access to, but that is highly maladaptive in the long run, that is, overeating (Evers, Stok, & de Ridder, 2010).

Emotional Eating and Dieting

Another group of theories has focused particularly on restrained eaters and posits that emotional eating in terms of overeating in response to negative emotions is only present in people who are trying to limit their food intake (Greeno & Wing, 1994). As we argued in the previous section, dietary restraint, defined as the intentional attempt to restrict caloric intake for the purpose of weight loss or weight maintenance (Herman & Mack, 1975), does not necessarily mean that actual caloric intake is restricted. Research has revealed that, in the long term, restrained eaters often fail in reaching their weight maintenance or weight loss goal (Stice, Presnell, Shaw, & Rohde, 2005; Stice et al., 2007). One of the reasons that many dieters are not able to lose weight is that they respond to (prolonged) restraint with disinhibited eating. Emotional distress is regarded as one of the typical triggers for disinhibition in restrained eaters, as the experience of distress imposes a more pressing concern than adhering to self-imposed dietary rules (Polivy, Herman, & McFarlane, 1994). Alternatively, it has also been theorized that the processing of emotionally distressing stimuli requires attention, which then is no longer available for cognitive control of one's diet because cognitive capacity is limited. This implies that restrained eaters are more prone to increase their food intake when negative emotions arise (Boon, Stroebe, Schut, & Jansen, 1998).

Negative Emotions and Eating: Empirical Findings

In contrast with the wide variety of theoretical accounts of *why* negative emotions would lead to overeating—either as a means to cope with negative emotions or otherwise—the actual empirical evidence that negative emotions lead to overeating is mixed, to say the least. In fact, a systematic review of experimental studies in "normal eaters"—that is, individuals with a normal weight and low scores on emotional and restrained eating—revealed that negative emotions can result in both decreased and increased eating (Macht, 2008). In this review of 25 studies, less than half of the studies (10) provided evidence of negative emotions leading to increased eating while one-third (7) suggested decreased eating and another one-third (8) articles pointed toward negative emotions not affecting eating behavior at all. Taken together, there is very limited evidence that negative emotions lead to overeating in normal eaters.

The same holds for restrained eaters. Studies that have examined the assumption that specifically restrained eaters are vulnerable to emotional eating have produced diverse findings. Greeno and Wing's (1994) classic systematic review supports the idea that restrained eating is the best predictor for increased eating in response to negative emotions. Their review reports that the eating patterns of unrestrained eaters and normal-weight individuals as well as obese individual, in contrast with those of restrained eaters, were unaffected by negative emotions. However, 20 years have passed since this review, and the role of restrained eating in emotional eating has been the topic of many additional studies since that time. Some studies have found support for the idea that typically restrained eaters overeat in response to negative emotions (e.g., Yeomans & Coughlan, 2009), but other studies did not replicate this finding (e.g., Oliver, Wardle, & Gibson, 2000). Consequently, it has been argued that restraint status is not a predictor of emotional eating (Spoor, Bekker, Van Strien, & Van Heck, 2007; Williams et al., 2002).

Emotion Regulation and Eating

As it is has proven difficult to predict when negative emotions result in emotional eating and in whom, it has been argued that it may not necessarily be the emotion itself that elicits overeating, but rather the manner in which the emotion is dealt with. That is, individuals who experience negative affect they cannot regulate properly, may be prone to turning to the maladaptive strategy of overeating. This line of reasoning has important implications, because it suggests that the problem is not necessarily related to the experience of negative emotions per se, but rather to the absence of adaptive emotion regulation strategies for dealing with negative affect. In our lab we have addressed this hypothesis in several studies and we specifically investigated how different emotion regulation strategies affect eating behavior.

In a series of experiments (Evers et al., 2010), participants were led to believe that they participated in two unrelated studies. In the so-called first study, negative emotions were induced, followed by a "second" study consisting of bogus taste test, actually meant to assess caloric intake. In the first experiment, focused on individual differences in reappraisal and suppression, sadness was induced by autobiographical recall contrasted against a control condition where participants had to recall an unemotional daily event. The taste test included comfort foods, pleasurable foods high in caloric content and palatability, such as chocolate and cookies. Results revealed that individuals regularly using suppression in their daily lives, indicating that they do not express their emotions, consumed more food when being emotional than individuals rarely using this strategy.

In two follow-up experiments, reappraisal and suppression were manipulated and contrasted against a spontaneous expression condition without any regulation instructions. Negative emotion was induced by a film excerpt and the so-called taste included both comfort and noncomfort foods, the latter being low in caloric value and palatability. Differences in food intake were especially expected for comfort foods, since these are the food types commonly expected to alleviate one's feelings (Lebel, Lu, & Dubé, 2008). Findings revealed that participants who were instructed to suppress their emotions ate more comfort foods compared to participants who were instructed to reappraise these emotions and compared to participants who were allowed to express their emotions spontaneously. The reappraisal and control condition did not differ in food consumption. Importantly, emotions per se did not affect food intake, which indicates that applying the maladaptive emotion regulation strategy of suppression was responsible for higher intake. These findings have been replicated in other studies with healthy, nonrestrained eaters (Taut, Renner, & Baban, 2012) and restrained eaters (Svaldi, Tuschen-Caffier, Lackner, Zimmermann, & Naumann, 2012).

In line with these findings, Taut and colleagues (2012) observed that reappraisal, an adaptive emotion regulation strategy that has been shown to decrease negative feelings, can also prevent emotional eating from occurring. Reappraisal refers to cognitively reframing the emotional situation so as to decrease its emotional impact. To assess eating behavior, Taut et al. used a nonforced free-eating setting, meaning that participants themselves could choose whether and how much they ate. This setting allowed for an analysis of whether or not eating was used to regulate emotions, in addition to an analysis of whether the amount of food that was consumed differed by emotion regulation strategies. Findings showed that about two-thirds of the participants in the control condition and the suppression condition turned to eating, while only one-third of the reappraisal group did. However, when participants in the reappraisal condition started to eat, they consumed as much as participants in the other conditions. These results suggest not only that maladaptive emotion regulation strategies can be responsible for emotional eating but also that adaptive emotion regulation strategies such as reappraisal decrease the likelihood of eating when being emotional. All in all, the findings on the role of emotion regulation strategies in overeating strongly support the notion that the way we deal with our emotions in daily life may be more relevant to explain emotional eating than the negative emotion itself.

Positive Emotions and Eating

The role of negative emotions in overeating has been the topic of much research, as can be inferred from the studies cited above. In contrast, the role of positive emotions as a potential cause of overeating has not been a topic of research until recently. A number of recent studies both in the lab and in the field make a strong case that positive emotions may be important triggers for increased eating (Bongers, Jansen, Havermans, Roefs & Nederkoorn, 2013; Evers, Adriaanse, De Ridder, & De Witt Huberts, 2013).

Although some studies could not find evidence for positive emotions being associated with overeating (e.g., Turner, Luszczynska, Warner, & Schwarzer, 2010; Yeomans & Coughlan, 2009), it makes theoretical sense that positive emotions, rather than negative emotions, are a trigger of increased eating. As suggested by the seminal work of Paul Rozin, in many cultures all over the world food plays an important role in celebrating important events such as weddings and birthdays that are generally accompanied by high levels of positive emotions (Rozin, 1999). As a result, positive emotions and eating may have become inherently interrelated, for example via an associative learning mechanism (Patel & Schlundt, 2001). Another reason why positive emotions may trigger increased eating is related to studies showing that people typically enjoy eating hedonic foods when in a positive mood (Macht, Roth, & Ellgring, 2002). The intention to eat is higher during joy than during sadness (Macht, 1999), and chocolate is considered most pleasant when experiencing positive emotions (Macht et al., 2002). Consequently, positive emotions may increase the pleasure of eating and result in increased consumption.

Currently, emotional eating is typically defined as increased eating in response to negative emotions (Arnow, Kenardy, & Agras, 1995; Van Strien et al., 1986), which is related to the origin of the emotional eating concept in psychosomatic theory (Bruch, 1964). The three most widely used emotional eater scales, measuring whether individuals perceive themselves as emotional eaters based on self-reports, are restricted to negative emotional states (EES by Arnow et al., 1995; TFEQ by Stunkard & Messick, 1985; DEBQ by Van Strien et al., 1986). More recently however, new initiatives for emotional eater scales have been developed with the inclusion of positive emotional states as well. For example, the Emotional Overeating Questionnaire (EOQ: Masheb & Grilo, 2006) was specifically developed for overweight patients with binge eating disorders and also includes a happiness subscale; the Emotional Appetite Questionnaire (EMAQ: Nolan, Halperin, & Geliebter, 2010) includes both positive and negative emotions; the EES has been modified into a version with several positive emotions such as happiness and enthusiasm (EES-II: Kenardy, Butler, Carter, & Moor, 2003). Although these newer emotional eater scales have not yet been validated, they provide at least a more complete reflection of the phenomenon of emotional eating.

Implicit Assessment of Emotional Eating

In the past years some controversy has risen about the validity of self-report questionnaires asking individuals to identify themselves as an emotional eater (Adriaanse et al., 2011; Evers, de Ridder & Adriaanse, 2009; Bongers, Jansen, Havermans, et al., 2013). Controversy not only relates to the inclusion of other affective states than negative emotions but also to the relevance of self-report as an adequate means to assess emotional eating. Evers et al. (2009) noted a potential triple bias in using self-reports for assessing emotional eating: people should be able to assess whether they were emotional at a specific occasion, whether and how much they ate at that moment, and whether there was an association between both—all these assessments are subject to severe bias of retrospective memory. As an alternative for self-report of emotional eating, Bongers, Jansen, Houben, and Roefs (2013) have proposed using a Single Target Implicit Association Test to measure the strength of associations between emotions and food concepts, based on the idea that emotional eaters show stronger associations between emotions and food concepts. In line with the idea that particularly positive emotions may be important triggers of overeating, the study revealed that participants with strong emotion-food associations consumed more during a positive emotion induction than during a negative emotion induction. Interestingly, only the IAT focused on associations between *positive* emotion and food had predictive value for eating under emotional load. Although speculative, this may indicate that it is easier to assess individual differences in positive emotional eaters rather than negative emotional eaters, as positive emotions may be more consistent in triggering *increased* eating than negative emotions.

Emotions as Justifications for Overeating

The suggestion of the studies presented earlier that particularly positive emotions may lead to eating more than one wants, is remarkable in view of the conventional idea that emotional distress is responsible for undesired behavior. Emotional distress is often portrayed as an impulsive force that undermines people's attempts at effective goal pursuit (such as eating healthily). However, a recent line of research suggests that long-term goals are sometimes deliberately violated when the context justifies doing so, a phenomenon labeled self-licensing (De Witt Huberts, Evers, & De Ridder, 2014; Kivetz & Zheng, 2006). Self-licensing is the act of making excuses for one's discrepant behavior before actual enactment, such that the forthcoming failure is made acceptable for oneself (De Witt Huberts et al., 2014). This novel perspective on self-regulation failure provides an additional but underresearched explanation for the self-defeating influence of emotions on (eating) behavior. Instead of emotions as impulsive forces, the self-licensing literature stipulates that emotions may be used as a justification for engaging in overeating. Typical justifications for overeating often relate to emotional states, such as "Because I am sad, I deserve chocolate," or "Because I am happy, I am allowed to take a cookie." Given the idea that particularly positive emotions may trigger increased eating, it may well be that positive emotional justifications are more often used as a license to eat than negative emotional justifications. Future research however, is needed to assess if such speculations have empirical merit.

Summary

The literature on emotional eating has examined to what extent affect influences eating behavior and has typically examined the role of negative emotions in overeating. In contrast with theoretical notions about emotional eating stating firmly that negative emotions should lead to increased consumption, empirical findings do not support that claim. In recent years it has become clear that the role of affect in eating behavior is more complex than previously assumed, with mixed evidence at best for the notion that negative emotions lead to increased eating and a more prominent role for positive emotions. In addition, the validity of self-report scales for assessing emotional eating has been questioned. Promising perspectives on the role of affect in eating behavior relate to the role of emotion regulation strategies and justifications as explanations for the observation that emotions and eating behavior seem so closely related. It should be noted that most studies on emotional eating so far have examined single emotional encounters without paying attention to the temporal dynamics of how affect and eating are interrelated. It has been suggested that emotional eaters may be better capable of balancing their eating behavior than hitherto assumed, and compensate for increased consumption during emotional distress by eating less in positive emotional encounters

(Sproesser, Schupp, & Renner, 2013). Future research should therefore consider emotional eating over time to account for the dynamics of consumption across situations.

OVERALL SUMMARY

In this chapter we have examined the role of affect in eating behavior from two perspectives: the dominant perspective that investigates how negative emotions may lead to overeating and as such is to blame for overweight, and a slightly less well known perspective examining how eating may lead to the experience of negative or positive affect. Taken together, both perspectives have more in common than one would expect. In the first part of this chapter it became clear that eating more often leads to negative affect than one would assume, especially insofar as people are preoccupied with the potential negative consequences of eating for their health and weight. The second part of this chapter shows that negative emotions do not necessarily result in overeating (different from what is generally assumed) unless people abuse emotions for overeating, either because they have poor emotion regulation strategies of because they use emotions as justifications for overeating—but primarily if they have a complicated relation with food in terms of dieting or otherwise trying to regulate their food intake. It thus seems that the once inherent pleasurable activity of eating has become quite complex in modern times where for many people eating is a cause of concern about health and overweight rather than simply enjoying good food. It remains to be seen whether a more positive view of eating as propagated by the new concept of Epicurean eating (Cornil & Chandon, 2016) can curb this trend.

REFERENCES

Adriaanse, M. A., De Ridder, D. T. D., & Evers, C. (2011). Emotional eating: Eating when emotional or emotional about eating? *Psychology and Health*, *26*, 23–39.

Andreyeva, T., Long, M. W., Henderson, K. E., & Grode, G. M. (2010). Trying to lose weight: Diet strategies among Americans with overweight or obesity in 1996 and 2003. *Journal of the American Dietetic Association*, *110*, 535–542.

Arnow, B., Kenardy, J., & Agras, W. S. (1995). The emotional eating scale: The development of a measure to assess coping with negative affect by eating. *International Journal of Eating Disorders*, *18*, 79–90.

Askegaard, S., Ordabayeva, N., Chandon, P., Cheung, T., Chytkova, Z., Cornil, Y., . . . &Werle, C. (2014). Moralities of food and health research. *Journal of Marketing Management*, *30*, 1800–1832.

Benton, E., & Donohoe, R. T. (1999). The effect of nutrients on mood. *Public Health Nutrition*, *2*, 403–409.

Berridge, K. C. (2000). Measuring hedonic impact in animals and infants: Microstructure of affective taste reactivity patterns. *Neuroscience and Biobehavioral Reviews*, *24*, 173–198.

Blair, E. H., Wing, R. R., & Wald, A. (1991). The effects of laboratory stressors on glycemic control and gastrointestinal transit time. *Psychosomatic Medicine*, *53*, 133–143.

Bongers, P., Jansen, A., Havermans, R., Roefs, A., & Nederkoorn, C. (2013). Happy eating: The underestimated role of overeating in a positive mood. *Appetite*, *67*, 74–80.

Bongers, P., Jansen, A., Houben, K., & Roefs, A. (2013). Happy eating: The single target implicit association test predicts overeating after positive emotions. *Eating Behaviors*, *14*, 348–355.

Boon, B., Stroebe, W., Schut, H., & Jansen, A. (1998). Food for thought: Cognitive regulation of food intake. *British Journal of Health Psychology*, *3*, 27–40.

Bruch, H. (1964). Psychological aspects in overeating and obesity. *Psychosomatics*, *5*, 269–274.

Cornil, Y., & Chandon, P. (2016). Pleasure as an ally of healthy eating? Contrasting visceral and Epicurean eating pleasure and their association with portion size preferences and wellbeing. *Appetite*, *104*, 52–59.

Deaver, C. M., Miltenberger, R. G., Smyth, J., Meidinger, A. M. Y., & Crosby, R. (2003). An evaluation of affect and binge eating. *Behavior Modification*, *27*, 578–599.

De Ridder, D. T. D., Adriaanse, M. A., Evers, C., & Verhoeven, A. (2014). Who diets? Most people and especially when they worry about food. *Appetite*, *80*, 103–108.

De Witt Huberts, J. C., Evers, C., & de Ridder, D. T. D. (2013). Double trouble: Restrained eaters do no teat less and feel worse. *Psychology and Health*, *28*, 686–700.

De Witt Huberts, J. C., Evers, C., & de Ridder, D. T. D. (2014). "Because I am worth it": A theoretical framework and empirical review of a justification-based account of self-regulation failure. *Personality and Social Psychology Review*, *18*, 119–138.

Evers, C., Adriaanse, M., de Ridder, D. T. D., & de Witt Huberts, J. C. (2013). Good mood food: Positive emotion as a neglected trigger for food intake. *Appetite*, *68*, 1–7.

Evers, C., de Ridder, D. T. D., & Adriaanse, M. A. (2009). Assessing yourself as an emotional eater: Mission impossible? *Health Psychology*, *28*, 717.

Evers, C., Stok, F. M., & de Ridder, D. T. D. (2010). Feeding your feelings: Emotion regulation strategies and emotional eating. *Personality and Social Psychology Bulletin*, *36*, 792–804.

Finkelstein, S. R., & Fishbach, A. (2010). When healthy food makes you hungry. *Journal of Consumer Research, 37,* 357–367.

Gillebaart, M., Schneider, I. K., & De Ridder, D. T. D. (2015). Effects of trait self-control on response conflict about healthy and unhealthy food. *Journal of Personality,* 1–10.

Greeno, C. G., & Wing, R. R. (1994). Stress-induced eating. *Psychological Bulletin, 115,* 444–464.

Heatherton, T. F., & Baumeister, R. F. (1991). Binge eating as escape from self-awareness. *Psychological Bulletin, 110,* 86–108.

Herman, C. P., & Mack, D. (1975). Restrained and unrestrained eating. *Journal of Personality, 43,* 647–660.

Herman, C. P., & Polivy, J. (1988). Excess and restraint in bulimia. In K. Pirke, W. Vandereycken, & E. Ploog (Eds.), *The psychobiology of bulimia* (pp. 33–41). New York, NY: Springer-Verlag.

Hofmann, W., Baumeister, R. F., Förster, G., & Vohs, K. D. (2012). Everyday temptations: An experience sampling study of desire, conflict, and self-control. *Journal of Personality and Social Psychology, 102,* 1318–1335.

Kenardy, J., Butler, A., Carter, C., & Moor, S. (2003). Eating, mood, and gender in a noneating disorder population. *Eating Behaviors, 4,* 149–158.

Kivetz, R., & Zheng, Y. (2006). Determinants of justification and self-control. *Journal of Experimental Psychology. General, 135,* 572–587.

Kroese, F. M., Evers, C., & De Ridder, D. T.D. (2013). If it's good it must be bad: The indirect effect of temptation strength on self-control through perceived unhealthiness. *Eating Behaviors, 14,* 522–524.

Lebel, J. L., Lu, J., & Dubé, L. (2008). Weakened biological signals: Highly-developed eating schemas amongst women are associated with maladaptive patterns of comfort food consumption. *Physiology and Behavior, 94,* 384–392.

Lehman, A. K., & Rodin, J. (1989). Styles of self-nurturance and disordered eating. *Journal of Consulting and Clinical Psychology, 57,* 117–122.

Leith, K. P., & Baumeister, R. F. (1996). Why do bad moods increase self-defeating behavior? *Journal of Personality and Social Psychology, 71,* 1250–1267.

Lindeman, M., & Stark, K. (2000). Loss of pleasure, ideological food choice reasons and eating pathology. *Appetite, 35,* 263–268.

Macht, M. (1999). Characteristics of eating in anger, fear, sadness and joy. *Appetite, 33,* 129–139.

Macht, M. (2008). How emotions affect eating: A five-way model. *Appetite, 50,* 1–11.

Macht, M., & Dettmer, D. (2006). Everyday mood and emotions after eating a chocolate bar or an apple. *Appetite, 46,* 332–336.

Macht, M., Gerer, J., & Ellgring, H. (2003). Emotions in overweight and normal-weight women immediately after eating foods differing in energy. *Physiology and Behavior, 80,* 367–374.

Macht, M., Roth, S., & Ellgring, H. (2002). Chocolate eating in healthy men during experimentally induced sadness and joy. *Appetite, 39,* 147–158.

Masheb, R. M., & Grilo, C. M. (2006). Emotional overeating and its associations with eating disorder psychopathology among overweight patients with binge eating disorder. *International Journal of Eating Disorders, 39,* 141–146.

Nederkoorn, C., Smulders, F. T. Y., & Jansen, A. (2000). Cephalic phase responses, craving and food intake in normal subjects. *Appetite, 35*, 45–55.

Nolan, L. J., Halperin, L. B., & Geliebter, A. (2010). Emotional Appetite Questionnaire. Construct validity and relationship with BMI. *Appetite, 54*, 314–319.

Oliver, G., Wardle, J., & Gibson, L. (2000). Stress and food choice: A laboratory study. *Psychosomatic Medicine, 62*, 853–865.

Papies, E. K., Barsalou, L. W., & Custers, R. (2012). Mindful attention prevents mindless impulses. *Social Psychological and Personality Science, 3*, 291–299.

Patel, K. A., & Schlundt, D. G. (2001). Impact of moods and social context on eating behavior. *Appetite, 36*, 111–118.

Pinel, J. P., Assanand, S., & Lehman, D. R. (2000). Hunger, eating, and ill health. *American Psychologist, 55*, 1105–1116.

Polivy, J., Herman, C. P., & McFarlane, T. (1994). Effects of anxiety on eating: Does palatability moderate distress-induced overeating in dieters? *Journal of Abnormal Psychology, 103*, 505–510.

Raghunathan, R., Naylor, R. W., & Hoyer, W. D. (2006). The unhealthy = tasty intuition and its effects on taste inferences, enjoyment, and choice of food products. *Journal of Marketing, 70*, 170–184.

Renaud, S., & de Lorgeril, M. (1992). Wine, alcohol, platelets, and the French paradox for coronary heart disease. *Lancet, 339*, 1523–1526.

Rozin, P. (1999). Food is fundamental, fun, frightening, and far-reaching. *Social Research, 66*, 9–30.

Rozin, P., Bauer, R., & Catanese, D. (2003). Food and life, pleasure and worry, among American college students: Gender differences and regional similarities. *Journal of Personality and Social Psychology, 85*, 132–141.

Rozin, P., Fischler, C., Imada, S., Sarubin, A., & Wrzesniewki, A. (1999). Attitudes to food and the role of food in life in the USA, Japan, Flemish Belgium and France: Possible implications for the diet-health debate. *Appetite, 33*, 163–180.

Rozin, P., Kabnick, K., Pete, E., Fischler, C., & Shields, C. (2003). The ecology of eating: Smaller portion sizes in France than in the United States help explain the French paradox. *Psychological Science, 14*, 450–455.

Schachter, S., Goldman, R., & Gordon, A. (1968). Effect of fear, food deprivation, and obesity on eating. *Journal of Personality and Social Psychology, 10*, 91–97.

Smith, A., Leekam, S., Ralph, A., & McNeill, G. (1988). The influence of meal composition on post-lunch changes in performance efficiency and mood. *Appetite, 10*, 195–203.

Spoor, S. T., Bekker, M. H., Van Strien T., & Van Heck, G. L. (2007). Relations between negative affect, coping, and emotional eating. *Appetite, 48*, 368–376.

Sproesser, G., Schupp, H. T., & Renner, B. (2013). The bright side of stress-induced eating: Eating more when stressed but less when pleased. *Psychological Science, 25*, 58–65.

Stice, E., Cooper, J. A., Schoeller, D. A., Tappe, K., & Lowe, M. R. (2007). Are dietary restraint scales valid measures of moderate to long-term dietary restriction? Objective biological and behavioral data suggest not. *Psychological Assessment, 19*, 339–458.

Stice, E., Presnell, K., Shaw, H., & Rohde, P. (2005). Psychological and behavioral risk factors for onset of obesity in adolescent girls: A prospective study. *Journal of Consulting and Clinical Psychology, 73*, 195–202.

Stunkard, A. J., & Messick, S. (1985). The three-factor eating questionnaire to measure dietary restraint, disinhibition, and hunger. *Journal of Psychosomatic Research, 29*, 71–83.

Svaldi, J., Tuschen-Caffier, B., Lackner, H. K., Zimmermann, S., & Naumann, E. (2012). The effects of emotion regulation on the desire to overeat in restrained eaters. *Appetite, 59*, 256–263.

Taut, D., Renner, B., & Baban, A. (2012). Reappraise the situation, but express your emotions: Impact of emotion regulation strategies on ad libitum food intake. *Frontiers in Psychology, 3*, 1–7.

Turner, S. A., Luszczynska, A., Warner, L., & Schwarzer, R. (2010). Emotional and uncontrolled eating styles and chocolate chip cookie consumption. A controlled trial of the effects of positive mood enhancement. *Appetite, 54*, 143–149.

Van Strien, T., Frijters, J. E. R., Bergers, G. P. A., & Defares, P. B. (1986). The Dutch Eating Behavior Questionnaire for assessment of restrained, emotional and external eating behavior. *International Journal of Eating Disorders, 5*, 295–315.

Werle, C. O. C., Trendel, O., & Ardito, G. (2013). Unhealthy food is not tastier for everybody: The "healthy = tasty" French intuition. *Food Quality and Preference, 28*, 116–121.

Williams, J. M. G., Healy, H., Eade, J., Windle, G., Cowen, P. J., Green, M. W., et al. (2002). Mood, eating behavior and attention. *Psychological Medicine, 32*, 469–481.

Wiser, S., & Telch, C.F. (1999). Dialectical behavior therapy for binge eating disorder. *Journal of Clinical Psychology, 55*, 755–768.

Yeomans, M., & Coughlan, E. (2009). Mood-induced eating: Interactive effects of restraint and tendency to overeat. *Appetite, 52*, 290–298.

13

Affective Determinants of Smoking

DANIELLE E. MCCARTHY, JESSICA W. COOK, TERESA M. LEYRO, HARUKA MINAMI, AND KRYSTEN W. BOLD

Tobacco use is the leading preventable cause of death in the United States (US Department of Health and Human Services [USDHHS], 2014) and a leading cause of mortality around the world (World Health Organization [WHO], 2011). Tobacco use prevalence in the United States continues to decline, but 15% of adults still smoke (Ward, Clarke, Nugent, & Schiller, 2016). The costs from tobacco use are staggering, with nearly $300 billion lost annually in productivity or healthcare expenses in the United States (USDHHS, 2014). Despite considerable progress made in tobacco control, this behavior remains a leading public health threat. Intractable relapse rates also suggest that this behavior is very difficult to change. Population data suggest that roughly half of all US cigarette smokers quit smoking for 24 hours in a given year, but only about 6% remain abstinent for 6 months or longer (Malarcher, Dube, Shaw, Babb, & Kaufmann, 2011). The direct pharmacological effects of nicotine and/or other constituents in tobacco help account for the low rates of successful cessation of tobacco use (e.g., Robinson & Berridge, 1993), but affective processes are also central to persistent motivation to use tobacco.

A commonly held expectancy among regular cigarette smokers is that smoking reduces tension or distress (Rash & Copeland, 2008). This may be because nicotine reliably ameliorates withdrawal-induced negative affect (e.g., Perkins, Karelitz, Conklin, Sayette, & Giedgowd, 2010), but not necessarily affect from other sources (Kassel, Stroud, & Paronis, 2003). Subtypes of smokers vary in the degree to which affect motivates smoking (Leventhal, 2010), but even intermittent (nondaily) smokers may be driven to smoke by internal distress (Shiffman et al., 2012). Data support affective dysregulation as both a risk factor for and a consequence of tobacco use (Breslau, Peterson, Schultz, Chilcoat, & Andreski, 1998; Pedersen & Von Soest, 2008), further demonstrating heterogeneity in affect-smoking relations.

Key questions regarding the nature of affective contributions to tobacco use and dependence remain unanswered. Namely, which affective dimensions predict use of tobacco, in which individuals, and under what circumstances? Research suggests that distinct dimensions of affective experience have independent relations with smoking. For example, mean levels, slopes, and volatility in daily withdrawal symptoms (characterized primarily by negative affect) over the first weeks of cessation attempts all contributed independent information about smoking cessation outcomes (Piasecki, Jorenby, Smith, Fiore, & Baker, 2002). Subsequent research showed that precessation negative affect was associated with smoking status 3 months post-quit (McCarthy, Piasecki, Fiore, & Baker, 2006) and that quit day levels of positive affect predicted smoking status 1 month post-quit (McCarthy et al., 2008). Heterogeneity in results across studies of the affective determinants of tobacco use highlights the need for greater attention to design, measurement, and analytical considerations in studies on this topic.

THEORETICAL MODELS

Theories of affective processing and drug motivation may be helpful in this regard. Although a comprehensive review of such theories is beyond the scope of this chapter, we highlight select relevant theories in this section.

Affect

For the sake of shared understanding, we define affect as an internal state (often accompanied by facial expressions or other measurable embodiments and related motivated behavior) induced by a stimulus (internal or external) and characterized in terms of both valence and arousal (Duncan & Feldman-Barratt, 2007). Positive affect is associated with approach motivation and positive mood states (e.g., joy, interest; Watson, Clark, & Tellegen, 1988). Negative affect (NA) is often defined as a general dimension of subjective distress or a broad range of aversive emotions (specific types of negative affect) including anger, anxiety, guilt, fear, and sadness (Watson et al., 1988). Negative affect and positive affect are empirically distinct psychological dimensions with unique biological and psychosocial correlates (Watson et al., 1988). We are particularly concerned with the tobacco motivational consequences of such states. We focus on the functional role of varied forms of affect on tobacco use posited by drug motivation models and supported by empirical findings.

Positive Reinforcement Models of Drug Use

Positive reinforcement models suggest that drug use is sustained primarily through positive reinforcement (introduction of a hedonically pleasant stimulus contingent on drug use that increases the probability of future drug use). Evidence in support of this model includes the psychomotor stimulant effects induced by nearly all drugs of abuse, including nicotine (Wise & Bozarth, 1987). Tobacco use induces positive feelings (Corrigall, 1999), particularly after a period of abstinence, but also induces unpleasant effects (e.g., dizziness, nausea), especially among those slow to metabolize nicotine (Tyndale & Sellers, 2001). Such countervalenced effects may reduce the effects of the mild positive consequences of tobacco on future use. The mildness of the positive effects of nicotine may sustain more frequent and chronic self-administration than would more intoxicating drugs, however (Hughes, 2001). Nicotine also potentiates responding to other appetitive stimuli (Caggiula et al., 2009). Thus, direct nicotine effects may be mild, but nicotine may also serve as an important modulator of responsivity to other rewards.

Rapid development of tolerance, an upward shift in hedonic set points, reduces the pleasurable effects of use (Ahmed & Koob, 1998). Rapid development of compensatory responses of opposite valence (i.e., opponent processes characterized by unpleasant effects) that grow more robust, emerge earlier, and last longer with more drug-use experience reduce net positive drug effects (Solomon, 1971). Both animal (Schulteis, Heyser, & Koob, 1997) and human research (Bickel, Stitzer, Liebson, & Bigelow, 1988) show that such compensatory or opponent processes can emerge very early, suggesting that avoidance or escape of withdrawal may become a potent motivator of drug use after a few experiences of drug use (Baker, Piper, McCarthy, Majeskie, & Fiore, 2004).

At the neural level, the role of positive reinforcement in drug motivation may decline over time, as drug use becomes less a process of rational stimulation-seeking mediated by prefrontal cortical processing and more a "habit" or compulsion mediated by striatal circuitry (Everitt & Robbins, 2005). This may help explain why heavy smokers dose themselves so frequently, even when the nicotinic acetylcholinergic receptors thought to be critical to nicotine dependence are already fully occupied from previous doses (Brody et al., 2006). Models of habit formation (in which behavior is thought to persist despite changes in reinforcement contingencies) have some support, but remain controversial (Root et al., 2009). In humans, even when persistent drug use carries extreme negative consequences, drug use behaviors may still produce favorable consequences such as ephemeral pleasure (i.e., positive reinforcement) or temporary relief from unpleasant states (i.e., negative reinforcement).

Negative Reinforcement Models of Drug Use

Tobacco withdrawal is characterized by affective distress (including both low-arousal states like depressed mood and high-arousal states such as anxiety and irritability), cognitive disturbances (e.g., difficulty concentrating), disturbed sleep, increased appetite, restlessness, and cravings or urges to use tobacco (Hughes & Hatsukami, 1986). Anhedonia (insensitivity to rewards) also appears to be a feature of tobacco withdrawal (Cook et al., 2015). Negative reinforcement models posit that avoidance of or escape from withdrawal symptoms is the central motive for continued drug use (Wikler, 1948). Refinements of this basic model suggest that withdrawal may be elicited (i.e., reinstated) by conditioned stimuli (O'Brien, Testa, O'Brien, Brady, & Wells, 1977). This refinement allows negative reinforcement models to better account for relapses that occur long after physiological withdrawal has resolved. Even so, it is difficult to square this model with several failures to detect relations between withdrawal and later smoking (Patten & Martin, 1996).

A refinement of the general negative reinforcement model suggests that apparent inconsistencies in the functional role of withdrawal may be resolved by a narrower focus on the central, motivationally potent components of withdrawal: negative affect and craving (Baker et al., 2004). This model stipulates that avoidance of or escape from negative affect is the central motive for continued drug use. The model further proposes that negative affect from diverse sources (not just falling blood drug levels) may elicit drug use responses through stimulus generalization or interoceptive conditioning processes (Baker et al., 2004). The model also specifies that affective distress may trigger awareness of drug motivation (i.e., craving) while undermining cognitive control processes (Baker et al., 2004). Taken together, these refinements mean that the reformulated affect-focused negative reinforcement model of drug motivation can account for drug use that occurs in the absence of withdrawal (but the presence of negative affect), while also positing conditions in which, and mechanisms by which, craving and affective distress may lead to drug use. Some of these hypotheses remain to be tested in smokers.

Other scholars have similarly proposed refinements of models to account for high rates of co-occurrence of smoking and other conditions, such as panic disorder (Zvolensky & Bernstein, 2005). These authors highlight the ways smoking and panic may influence one another, and posit that the tendency to monitor and react to bodily sensations that characterize panic may also heighten sensitivity to withdrawal (Zvolensky & Bernstein, 2005). Smokers may experience more unpleasant physical experiences (due to the direct effects of smoking but also to withdrawal) that they may be prone to monitor closely and interpret catastrophically if they also have a history of panic. In this way, smoking may feed panic and panic may feed smoking by making alleviation of withdrawal (through smoking) a particularly high priority (Zvolensky & Bernstein, 2005). Cognitive and affective processes may similarly account for the co-occurrence of smoking and other mood and anxiety disorders (Leventhal & Zvolensky, 2015).

Integrative Models

Other models similarly focus on individual vulnerabilities with implications for tobacco use. Gilbert's (1997) situation-by-trait adaptive response (STAR) model stipulates that interactions between individuals and situations are critical in determining the functional role of drug use. This affect-focused model posits that the adaptive value of drug use in terms of regulating emotion and motivation varies by person (e.g., personality, depression, personal goals), context (e.g., stress, drug availability), and their interaction. For example, drug motivation may be greater in the face of a social stressor for someone who values social standing highly than for someone who devalues social standing (Gilbert, 1997). This model suggests that drug use may be an instrumental effort to navigate changing situations and states.

Some models of drug motivation have incorporated both positive and negative reinforcement concepts and address the shifting relevance of these over the course of an individual's drug use career. The opponent-process model is a seminal model that posits that compensatory processes oppose affective or hedonic deflections from a set point in a "simple, dynamic affect control system" (Solomon, 1971, p. 82). This efficient model accounts for both the pleasurable effects of nicotine and the development of powerfully motivating withdrawal processes that set the stage for negative reinforcement of drug use (Solomon, 1971). The central tenet of this model is that repeated use of a drug trains opponent, compensatory processes that counter the effects of drug use. The opponent processes are slow to decay such that the withdrawal syndrome persists long after cessation of use (Solomon, 1971), which is particularly true in tobacco withdrawal (Hughes, 2001).

Others have augmented this opponent process model by highlighting tobacco effects on affect-relevant antireward processes. Koob and colleagues (Koob & LeMoal, 2008) have demonstrated that nicotine withdrawal elevates reward thresholds, such that greater stimulation is required to activate reward-related circuitry when individuals are experiencing withdrawal than when sated or drug-naïve. Withdrawal is therefore associated with not just craving for the drug of choice but also diminished positive affect and responding to nonnicotine rewards (e.g., D'Souza & Markou, 2010). Chronic drug use may trigger an antireward system that both suppresses reward responding and alters stress responding, both of which will have negative hedonic effects and will increase allostatic load for the user (Koob & LeMoal, 2008).

Incentive Sensitization and Habit Models

As the preceding review illustrates, many models of drug motivation, including tobacco motivation, are focused on affective processes. Other models focus less on hedonic tone and more on incentive salience. In the incentive sensitization theory of addiction, Robinson and Berridge (1993) assert that the direct pharmacological effects of drugs of abuse on mesotelencephalic dopaminergic circuits critical in processing incentive values (not hedonic rewards per se) cause drug-related cues to have outsized motivational consequences. This model posits that inflated incentive salience is a hallmark of drug abuse reflected by intense drug craving, which is distinct and separable from drug liking (and the hedonic value of drug effects). This account is not focused on affect per se, but Robinson and Berridge (1993) acknowledge that both positive and negative reinforcement processes may also contribute to drug motivation, and that withdrawal may inflate incentive salience (thus setting the stage for greater drug craving in withdrawal). As such, a full account of drug motivation likely will entail attention to affective processes.

EVIDENCE AND KNOWLEDGE GAPS

Answering the motivating question of this review, "Which affective dimensions predict use of tobacco, in which individuals, and under what circumstances?" may have important theoretical and clinical implications. Identifying the specific facets of affect that predict tobacco use may help us to better identify persons at risk or periods of risk within persons. This may enable tailoring of interventions to particular individuals and situations. The ready availability of personal tracking devices (e.g., mobile telephones and wearable technology) may facilitate real-time lapse vulnerability modeling within individuals trying to cease tobacco use. Indeed, some investigators are already tracking cigarette craving and linking this to real-time data about a smoker's proximity to tobacco retail outlets (Kirchner, Cantrell, Anesetti-Rothermel, & Abrams, 2013). This may soon facilitate just-in-time text or other messaging to remind people of their abstinence goals or to provide other interventions when they report spikes in craving or distress and/or proximity to a retail tobacco outlet. This is just one example of the implications of a more granular and context-specific understanding of the relations between affect and tobacco use.

The next portion of this chapter is dedicated to a review of what we currently know and what we still need to know regarding the roles of positive affect, anhedonia, negative affect, and negative-affect-related traits in tobacco use. Due to space limitations, these reviews are selective and illustrative rather than comprehensive. We focus on key concepts, seminal findings, and methodological issues, and will highlight critical knowledge gaps.

Anhedonia, Positive Affect, and Smoking

Anhedonia, the diminished experience of consummatory or anticipatory pleasure in rewards (Treadway & Zald, 2013), appears to play an important role in tobacco use. Nicotine enhancement of the appetitive effects of nondrug reinforcers (Caggiula et al., 2009) may be particularly salient for those who derive little pleasure from rewards. Positive affect, which may also influence smoking (McCarthy et al., 2008), is conceptually distinct from anhedonia in that it is not contingent on reward exposure. The moderate, inverse relation between positive affect and anhedonia (Cook, Spring, & McChargue, 2007) suggests that these constructs are distinct.

Several studies link anhedonia and positive affect with smoking initiation. Anhedonic adolescents are more likely to report smoking than their more hedonic peers (Audrain-McGovern et al., 2012). Conversely, elevated positive affect has been identified as a protective factor in longitudinal studies of adolescent smoking initiation (Wills Resko, Ainette, & Mendoza, 2004). Thus, adolescents who are relatively insensitive to environmental rewards may seek out compensatory behaviors, like smoking, that pharmacologically boost responsivity to rewards. Once smoking is initiated, nicotine enhancement of the appetitive effects of nondrug rewards may reinforce progression to more regular smoking. Tobacco dependence has also been linked with anhedonia both before (Leventhal, Piper, Japuntich, Baker, & Cook, 2014) and after a smoking cessation attempt (Cook et al., 2015). Although these data support the hypothesis that anhedonia leads to smoking progression and maintenance, other causal mechanisms (e.g., elevation of hedonic set points; Koob & LeMoal, 2008) cannot be ruled out.

Anhedonia might spur dependent patterns of tobacco use by enhancing the reward or incentive value of nicotine relative to nondrug rewards. For instance, anhedonia predicts an imbalance in choice of smoking over an alternative, monetary reward (Leventhal, Trujillo et al., 2014), illustrating anhedonic smokers' bias to pursue smoking over nonpharmacologic sources of reinforcement. Moreover, Cook et al. (2007) found that anhedonic smokers required nicotine to respond pleasurably to an appetitive nondrug stimulus; more hedonic smokers, on the other hand, responded to the appetitive stimulus regardless of nicotine exposure. Nicotine clearly inflates the value of nondrug rewards; conversely, nicotine deprivation leads to a deterioration in reward sensitivity and diminished positive affect (e.g., Cook et al., 2004). Such withdrawal-related decrements in reward functioning and positive affect could increase motivation to resume smoking following a quit attempt. Indeed, elevations in anhedonia before (Leventhal, Piper et al., 2014) and after quitting (Cook et al., 2015) are positively associated with cessation failure. Positive affect has also been linked with smoking abstinence (i.e., low post-quit positive affect predicts failure to quit; McCarthy et al., 2008). However, only anhedonia predicts smoking when included in a model with positive affect (Cook et al., 2015).

Negative Affect and Smoking

The role of negative affect across the different stages of smoking (initiation, maintenance, and cessation/relapse) has been extensively studied. Stressful life events and affective distress are relatively robust predictors of initial smoking and progression to regular smoking (Siqueira, Diab, Bodian, & Rolnitzky, 2000). Ecological momentary assessment (EMA) studies (Stone & Shiffman, 1994) that capture real-time (vs. recalled) relations among individual characteristics, contextual factors, fleeting affective states, and smoking behavior have demonstrated that teens with the greatest baseline negative mood variability at baseline show accelerated progression toward heavy smoking rather than time-limited experimentation with smoking (Weinstein, Mermelstein, Shiffman, & Flay, 2008).

Results of this study also suggest mood-stabilizing effects for those who escalate in smoking, indicating a potential process through which smoking is reinforced and maintained among youth.

Among dependent smokers, retrospective self-report studies identify negative-affect reduction as a primary reason for smoking (Rash & Copeland, 2008). Although this may be attributable to erroneous expectancies that smoking reduces negative affect from diverse sources (Shiffman, Paty, Gwaltney, & Dang, 2004), such expectancies may help maintain smoking (Kassel et al., 2003). Negative affect is also a barrier to smoking cessation; Smokers often report retrospectively that negative affect or stress preceded lapses during cessation (e.g., O'Connell & Martin, 1987). In addition, a prospective within-person EMA analysis showed that negative affect predicted a first lapse while other situational determinants (e.g., arousal, alcohol use) did not, and lapses preceded by negative affect were more likely to progress to relapse (Shiffman, Hickcox et al., 1996). Lapse events are also characterized by higher ratings of negative affect compared to temptation events (in which no smoking occurs), and temptation events are similarly characterized by greater negative affect compared to random, control reports (Shiffman, Paty, Gnys, Kassel, & Hickcox, 1996). A separate EMA study by Cooney et al. (2007) showed that negative affect predicted smoking lapses in a subsequent EMA report. These findings demonstrate that lapse events are driven by proximal (over a few hours) rather than distal (over days) affective influences (Shiffman & Waters, 2004). While these studies provide empirical support for the role of negative affect in smoking maintenance, several studies report no significant or very small relations between negative affect and subsequent smoking (e.g., Shiffman, Paty et al., 2004). The frequency and timing of assessments may critically influence observed relations and account for this heterogeneity in affect-smoking relations. Indeed, a recent experiment (McCarthy, Minami, Yeh, & Bold, 2015) found that frequent EMA monitoring (six daily prompts) suppressed several affect and withdrawal ratings (e.g., anxiety, anger) relative to low frequency monitoring (one daily report). More work is needed to identify the optimal frequency and duration of affect assessment during smoking cessation.

Extant evidence suggests that the effects of negative affect on smoking behavior are neither constant nor linear over time. Several studies indicate that the influence of negative affect on later smoking urges or smoking behavior is time-limited, lasting only a few hours, and these effects seem to decline in a nonlinear fashion (Minami, Yeh, Bold, Chapman, & McCarthy, 2014, Shiyko, Naab, Shiffman, & Li, 2014). These findings underscore the importance of examining the dynamic effects of affect on smoking behavior and suggest that time-varying effects may be missed if the assessment interval is nonoptimal. Furthermore, recent work suggests that distinct facets of negative affect operate differently in smokers during a quit attempt. A recent multilevel factor analysis supported a factor structure with two distinct facets of negative affect, agitation and distress (Bold, Witkiewitz, McCarthy, 2016), that differentiated smoking and temptation events in smokers during the first 3 weeks of a quit attempt. Greater momentary distress was uniquely related to smoking (compared to temptation events) while greater agitation was related to surviving a temptation without smoking (compared to smoking events; Bold et al., 2016). Thus, facets of negative affect may tap different smoking motivation processes that are obscured when examining global negative affect.

Depressive Symptoms

Depressive symptoms are among the most widely examined negative affective states in relation to smoking (e.g., Kenney, Holahan, North, & Holahan, 2006). While both cross-sectional and longitudinal studies suggest a link between depressive symptoms and smoking initiation (Brook, Cohen, & Brook, 1998), evidence of a prospective link is mixed (e.g., White, Pandina, & Chen, 2002). These data suggest that relations between depression and smoking initiation are complex and may differ across gender, cultural contexts, or assessment time frames. On the other hand, disproportionately high smoking rates are consistently found among depressed individuals (Morisano, Bacher, Audrain-McGovern, & George, 2009), and both major depressive disorder and elevated depressive symptoms are more prevalent in current smokers than in non- or former smokers (e.g., Goodwin et al., 2014). In addition, a history of major depression, especially recurrent major depression, predicts a greater likelihood of relapse (although findings are mixed; Hitsman et al., 2013). Precessation depressive symptoms are also associated with poor smoking cessation outcomes (e.g., Cooper, Borland, McKee, Yong, & Dugué, 2016). Different facets of depression (e.g., negative affect, somatic features, anhedonia) seem to have differential relations with smoking cessation success, which highlights the value of disaggregating depressive symptoms (Leventhal et al., 2008) to understand the role of affect in smoking cessation and relapse. Multiple mechanisms may link elevated depressive symptoms and difficulty quitting. Smokers with elevated depressive symptoms experience more severe negative affect, withdrawal, and craving post-quit (Pomerleau et al., 2005) and have lower cessation self-efficacy (Cinciripini et al., 2003), all of which are established predictors of lapses and relapses. Precessation depressive symptoms (and negative affectivity) seem to affect lapse and relapse risk, at least partly, through their influence on proximal antecedents of lapse (e.g., negative affect) during a quit attempt (e.g., Brodbeck, Bachmann, Brown, & Znoj, 2014).

Individual Difference Vulnerabilities

Individual differences related to negative affect may confer vulnerability for tobacco dependence and other forms of psychopathology. Cognitive-affective vulnerabilities that have received the most empirical support in smoking initiation, maintenance, and cessation include anxiety sensitivity, distress intolerance, and to a lesser extent, emotion dysregulation.

Anxiety sensitivity, the fear of anxiety and its potential negative social, physical, and cognitive consequences, is an established risk factor for anxiety and mood disorders (Naragon-Gainey, 2010). Individuals with this sensitivity tend to believe anxiety is dangerous and experience elevated distress and avoidance behaviors that promote the development of anxiety disorders and impede learning that anxiety may be tolerated.

Smokers high in anxiety sensitivity endorse smoking because it is habitual, addicting, and relieves negative affect (Leyro, Zvolensky, Vujanovic, & Bernstein, 2008) and they expect smoking to reduce affective distress (Leyro et al., 2008) more than do smokers lower in anxiety sensitivity. Smokers high in anxiety sensitivity also report lower confidence in quitting (Zvolensky et al., 2006) and perceive greater barriers to cessation (Gonzalez, Zvolensky, Vujanovic, Leyro, & Marshall, 2008) than do those lower in anxiety sensitivity. Prospective laboratory research has found that anxiety sensitivity predicts greater satisfaction, reward, pleasure, and positive-affect enhancement from smoking in the context of acute stress (Wong et al., 2013). Moreover, EMA studies have shown that elevations in negative affect among individuals high in anxiety sensitivity predict smoking lapse throughout a quit attempt (Langdon, Farris, Øverup, & Zvolensky, 2016). Although anxiety sensitivity is relatively stable, brief exposure-based cognitive-behavioral interventions significantly reduce this sensitivity (Smits, Berry, Tart, & Powers, 2008). A smoking-cessation intervention including interoceptive exercises led to reductions in anxiety sensitivity and panic symptoms (Schmidt et al., 2016). These findings suggest anxiety sensitivity is a malleable treatment target for smokers, although they have not yet demonstrated that anxiety sensitivity reductions mediated intervention effects on abstinence.

Distress tolerance is the perceived or measured ability to withstand perturbing emotional or physical experiences (Leyro, Zvolensky, & Bernstein, 2010). Like anxiety sensitivity, distress tolerance is empirically linked to a range of internalizing and externalizing symptoms and disorders, including tobacco dependence (Leyro et al., 2010). Low distress tolerance may heighten emotional reactivity and lead to avoidance of and escape from negative states (e.g., withdrawal; Leventhal & Zvolensky, 2015). Smokers lower in distress tolerance report greater perceived barriers to cessation (Kraemer, McLeish, Jeffries, Avallone, & Luberto, 2013) and are less likely to follow through with cessation treatment (MacPherson, Stipelman, Duplinsky, Brown, & Lejuez, 2008) than those with greater tolerance. A recent laboratory study found that nicotine-deprived smokers lower in distress tolerance smoked more puffs during a smoking choice task than those with greater tolerance (Bold, Yoon, Chapman, & McCarthy, 2013). Retrospective reports have found that low distress tolerance is associated with shorter times to lapse (Brown, Lejuez, Kahler, Strong, & Zvolensky, 2005) and total abstinence duration (Brown, Lejuez, Kahler, & Strong, 2002). Although some prospective studies have found that low distress tolerance is associated with difficulty initiating abstinence (Steinberg et al., 2012) and greater risk of lapse and relapse (Brown et al., 2009), others have not (e.g., Kalman, Hoskinson, Sambamoorthi, & Garvey, 2010). These inconsistencies may reflect differences in measurement or methods (e.g., self-report vs. behavioral indices of distress tolerance; Brown et al., 2009; Steinberg et al., 2012). More recently, an intervention designed to enhance tolerance of withdrawal (Brown et al., 2013) improved abstinence and lapse recovery while also reducing withdrawal distress, and a recent pilot study (Steinberg, Epstein, Stahl, Budsock, & Williams, 2015) of a task-persistence intervention yielded sizable (although not statistically significant) improvements in abstinence.

An additional transdiagnostic cognitive-affective vulnerability relevant to smoking is emotion regulation, broadly defined as the ability to adaptively respond to distressing emotional states with awareness, understanding, and acceptance (Aldao, Nolen-Hoeksema & Schweizer, 2010). Adaptive emotion regulation strategies include reappraisal and acceptance, whereas suppression and avoidance strategies are associated with psychopathological symptoms. Emerging research on the relation between emotion regulation and smoking suggests that emotion regulation may play a role in smoking maintenance and cessation. Cross-sectional work has found that self-reported use of nonjudging emotion regulation strategies is associated with greater odds of smoking cessation up to 6 weeks post-quit (Spears et al., 2015) and may promote quit resumption following early lapse (Heppner et al., 2016). In addition, mindfulness-based interventions may assist in both mood management and craving (Brewer et al., 2011). Daily smokers instructed to defuse (separate one's thoughts from the self) or reappraise craving, as opposed to suppress craving during a craving induction, were better able to resist smoking both immediately post-task and 1 week later (Beadman et al., 2015). In a recent low-contact intervention study, smokers randomized to digital device-guided mindfulness reported greater postpractice reduction in craving, less negative affect, and a greater reduction in smoking relative to those in a sham meditation control (Ruscio, Muench, Brede, & Waters, 2016). More intensive smoking cessation interventions that have sought to develop various emotion regulation strategies have also shown promise (de Souza et al., 2015). For example, acceptance and commitment therapy (ACT) designed to target smoking-specific experiential avoidance has been associated with improved long-term smoking cessation outcomes (Gifford et al., 2011).

Anxiety sensitivity, distress intolerance, and emotion dysregulation are conceptually and empirically related candidate cognitive-affective vulnerabilities linked to various forms of negative affect relevant to tobacco use. One study found that difficulties in emotion regulation mediate the relation between anxiety sensitivity and difficulty quitting smoking, stronger endorsement of negative reinforcement smoking motives, and positive smoking expectancies (Johnson, Farris, Schmidt, & Zvolensky, 2012). Also, emotion regulation training (e.g., reappraisal instruction) has also been shown to increase distress tolerance (Szasz, Szentagotai, & Hofmann, 2012). These findings support the notion that emotion regulation may be an explanatory mechanism linking anxiety sensitivity and distress tolerance to smoking processes. Clarifying these constructs and their roles in tobacco use and dependence is an important goal for future research. It is also important to advance our understanding of the methodological factors (e.g., deprivation state, affect induction, measurement models) that influence results and may contribute to inconsistency and failures to replicate in this literature. Nicotine deprivation seems to enhance relations between distress tolerance and smoking puff volume, whereas a social stressor (rather than nicotine deprivation) seems to enhance relations between anxiety sensitivity and negative affect relief from smoking (Perkins et al., 2010). Models that examine mediators of the relation between distress tolerance and smoking-relevant outcomes may help. A recent study found an indirect relation between distress tolerance and reduced nicotine withdrawal through lower stress-reactivity (Farris, Zvolensky, Otto, & Leyro, 2015). Understanding mediating processes in relations between cognitive-affective vulnerabilities and smoking outcomes may further elucidate the affective determinants of smoking.

CONCLUSIONS AND FUTURE DIRECTIONS

This review aimed to assess progress in answering the question "Which affective dimensions predict tobacco use, in which individuals, and under what circumstances?" The models and evidence reviewed in this chapter suggest that discrete dimensions of both positive affect and negative affect influence smoking. Whereas positive affect seems protective against tobacco use and dependence, evidence suggests that negative affect increases risk both tonically and phasically. Relations between affective variables and tobacco use also vary as a function of affective-processing individual difference variables, particularly anhedonia and negative reactions to arousal and distress. That is, there are identifiable individual differences, including gender and culture, that influence affective processing and appear to confer risk for chronic, problematic tobacco use. Data also suggest that affect–tobacco use relations vary as a function of time (e.g., since quit date), context (e.g., smoking opportunity, stressors; Sayette, Wertz, Martin, Perrott, & Hobel, 2003), and state (e.g., nicotine deprivation). Taken together, these data corroborate the importance of affective processing in tobacco use and dependence, but also suggest that a greater degree of specificity, granularity, and temporal resolution may be needed to fully unpack these relations.

Developing the right measures, scoring, and data analytic models to account for the time- and facet-varying effects of affect on smoking motivation is a work in progress. Enough signals have come through the noise to support the basic premise that affect modulates risk for smoking both short- and long-term. The volume of noise in the literature suggests, however, that these relations are stronger for some dimensions of affective experience, in some individuals, and in some contexts than others. Our models need to develop greater specificity and our methods greater precision in order to better distinguish signal from noise in this domain.

In addition, greater clarity regarding the distinctiveness and mediators of affective-processing vulnerabilities (i.e., anxiety sensitivity, distress intolerance, and emotion dysregulation) for tobacco use is needed. Although these individual differences help to identify those who are particularly reactive to negative affect, we need to understand better how these vulnerabilities interact and translate into smoking risk.

Empirical evidence demonstrating relations between affect and tobacco use does not necessarily speak to which drug motivational model is most accurate. Even incentive sensitization models that posit that nonassociative, nonaffective incentive salience inflation is the central process in drug motivation allow for affective modulation of incentive salience. As such, the empirical findings to date are consistent with several models of drug motivation, as these models generally lack sufficient specificity regarding affective processes to differentiate them with empirical findings.

To further elucidate the affective determinants of tobacco use, multiple methods and multiple measures will be needed. A combination of laboratory and clinical studies, supplemented by epidemiological research on transdiagnostic affective vulnerabilities and smoking will be needed to identify the circumstances and individuals in which specific dimensions predict tobacco use. Given that much of the motivational processing that leads to smoking and precipitates lapses may occur outside of awareness, and very low levels of affect may motivate tobacco use without entering conscious awareness as affective distress (Baker et al., 2004), it is important to move beyond self-report in the study of affect in smoking. Advances in mobile technology (e.g., wearable technology) provide new opportunities to track affect and smoking. Identifying optimal measurement frequency and timing will be critical for examining the role of affect in smoking and identifying cues for just-in-time interventions to prevent relapse.

The findings reviewed in this chapter have potential treatment implications. For example, treating anhedonia (behaviorally or pharmacologically) may prevent smoking initiation. Early evidence suggests that anxiety sensitivity and distress tolerance are malleable and that interventions targeting these vulnerabilities have promise as smoking cessation interventions (Brown et al., 2013; Steinberg et al., 2015). Diverse interventions that influence emotion regulation (self-monitoring, reframing or acceptance, mindfulness, and biofeedback), may be of use in preventing or treating smoking. Investigations of the efficacy of these interventions, likely as adjuncts to existing interventions, could advance our understanding of the role of affect in tobacco use and recovery. Careful mediation analyses could help identify the affective dimensions most closely related to success in quitting and affected by such interventions.

In sum, there is substantial evidence that both positive and negative affective processes play important roles in tobacco use trajectories, as acknowledged by prominent models of addiction. The specific facets of affective experiences and states that matter most to tobacco use are not yet entirely clear. Methodological considerations, including assessment and analytical choices, seem to influence results in investigations of affective influences on tobacco use. Refinement of these methods and mechanistic studies of emotion-focused interventions have the potential to further illuminate the affective determinants of tobacco use.

REFERENCES

Ahmed, S. H., & Koob, G. F. (1998). Transition from moderate to excessive drug intake: Change in hedonic setpoint. *Science, 282*, 298–300. doi:10.1126/science.282.5387.298

Aldao, A., Nolen-Hoeksema, S., & Schweizer, S. (2010). Emotion-regulation strategies across psychopathology: A meta-analytic review. *Clinical Psychology Review, 30*, 217–237. doi:10.1016/j.cpr.2009.11.004

Audrain-McGovern, J., Rodriguez, D., Leventhal, A. M., Cuevas, J., Rodgers, K., & Sass, J. (2012). Where is the pleasure in that? Low hedonic capacity predicts smoking onset and escalation. *Nicotine and Tobacco Research, 14*, 1187–1196. doi:10.1093/ntr/nts017

Baker, T. B., Piper, M. E., McCarthy, D. E., Majeskie, M. R., & Fiore, M. C. (2004). Addiction motivation reformulated: An affective processing model of negative reinforcement. *Psychological Review, 111*, 33–51. doi:10.1037/0033-295X.111.1.33

Beadman, M., Das, R. K., Freeman, T. P., Scragg, P., West, R., & Kamboj, S. K. (2015). A comparison of emotion regulation strategies in response to craving cognitions: Effects on smoking behaviour, craving and affect in dependent smokers. *Behaviour Research and Therapy, 69*, 29–39. doi:10.1016/j.brat.2015.03.013

Bickel, W. K., Stitzer, M. L., Liebson, I. A., & Bigelow, G. E. (1988). Acute physical dependence in man: Effects of naloxone after brief morphine exposure. *Journal of Pharmacology and Experimental Therapeutics, 244*, 126–132.

Bold, K. W., Yoon, H., Chapman, G. B., & McCarthy, D. E. (2013). Factors predicting smoking in a laboratory-based smoking-choice task. *Experimental and Clinical Psychopharmacology, 21*, 133–143. doi:10.1037/a0031559

Bold, K. W., Witkiewitz, K., & McCarthy, D. E. (2016). Multilevel factor analysis of smokers' real-time negative affect ratings while quitting. *Psychological Assessment, 28*, 1033–1042.

Breslau, N., Peterson, E. L., Schultz, L. R., Chilcoat, H. D., & Andreski, P. (1998). Major depression and stages of smoking: A longitudinal investigation. *Archives of General Psychiatry, 55*, 161–166. doi:10.1001/archpsych.55.2.161

Brewer, J. A., Mallik, S., Babuscio, T. A., Nich, C., Johnson, H. E., Deleone, C. M., . . . Carroll, K. M. (2011). Mindfulness training for smoking cessation: Results from a randomized controlled trial. *Drug and Alcohol Dependence, 119*, 72–80. doi:10.1016/j.drugalcdep.2011.05.027

Brodbeck, J., Bachmann, M. S., Brown, A., & Znoj, H. J. (2014). Effects of depressive symptoms on antecedents of lapses during a smoking cessation attempt: An ecological momentary assessment study. *Addiction, 109*, 1363–1370. doi:10.1111/add.12563

Brody, A. L., Mandelkern, M. A., London, E. D., Olmstead, R. E., Farahi, J., Scheibal, D., . . . Mukhin, A. G. (2006). Cigarette smoking saturates brain 4b nicotinic acetylecholine receptors. *Archives of General Psychiatry, 63*, 907–915. doi:10.1001/archpsyc.63.8.907

Brook, J. S., Cohen, P., & Brook, D. W. (1998). Longitudinal study of co-occurring psychiatric disorders and substance use. *Journal of the American Academy of Child and Adolescent Psychiatry, 37*, 322–330. doi:10.1097/00004583-199803000-00018

Brown, R. A., Lejuez, C. W., Kahler, C. W., & Strong, D. R. (2002). Distress tolerance and duration of past smoking cessation attempts. *Journal of Abnormal Psychology, 111*, 180–185. doi:10.1037/0021-843X.111.1.180

Brown, R. A., Lejuez, C. W., Kahler, C. W., Strong, D. R., & Zvolensky, M. J. (2005). Distress tolerance and early smoking lapse. *Clinical Psychology Review, 25*, 713–733. doi:10.1016/.cpr.2005.05.003

Brown, R. A., Lejuez, C. W., Strong, D. R., Kahler, C. W., Zvolensky, M. J., Carpenter, L. L., . . . Price, L. H. (2009). A prospective examination of distress tolerance and early smoking lapse in adult self-quitters. *Nicotine and Tobacco Research, 11*, 493–502. doi:10.1093/ntr/ntp041

Brown, R. A., Reed, K. M. P., Bloom, E. L., Minami, H., Strong, D. R., Lejuez, C. W., . . . Hayes, S. C. (2013). Development and preliminary randomized controlled trial of a distress tolerance treatment for smokers with a history of early lapse. *Nicotine and Tobacco Research, 15*, 2005–2015. doi:10.1093/ntr/ntt093.

Caggiula, A. R., Donny, E. C., Palmatier, M. I., Liu, X., Chaudhri, N., & Sved, A. F. (2009). The role of nicotine in smoking: A dual-reinforcement model. *Nebraska Symposium on Motivation, 55*, 91–109. doi:10.1007/978-0-387-78748-0_6

Cinciripini, P. M., Wetter, D. W., Fouladi, R. T., Blalock, J. A., Carter, B. L., Cinciripini, L. G., & Baile, W. F. (2003). The effects of depressed mood on smoking cessation: Mediation by postcessation self-efficacy. *Journal of Consulting and Clinical Psychology, 71*, 292–301. doi:10.1037/0022-006X.71.2.292

Cook, J. W., Piper, M. E., Leventhal, A. M., Schlam, T. R., Fiore, M. C., & Baker, T. B. (2015). Anhedonia as a component of the tobacco withdrawal syndrome. *Journal of Abnormal Psychology, 124*, 215–225. doi:10.1037/abn0000016

Cook, J. W., Spring, B., & McChargue, D. (2007). Influence of nicotine on positive affect in anhedonic smokers. *Psychopharmacology (Berl), 192*, 87–95. doi:10.1007/s00213-006-0688-5

Cook, J. W., Spring, B., McChargue, D. E., Borrelli, B., Hitsman, B., Niaura, R., . . . Kristeller, J. (2004). Influence of fluoxetine on positive and negative affect in a clinic-based smoking cessation trial. *Psychopharmacology, 173*, 153–159. doi:10.1007/s00213-003-1711-8

Cooney, N. L., Litt, M. D., Cooney, J. L., Pilkey, D. T., Steinberg, H. R., & Oncken, C. A. (2007). Alcohol and tobacco cessation in alcohol-dependent smokers: Analysis of real-time reports. *Psychology of Addictive Behaviors, 21*, 277–286. doi:10.1037/0893-164X.21.3.277

Cooper, J., Borland, R., McKee, S. A., Yong, H. H., & Dugué, P. A. (2016). Depression motivates quit attempts but predicts relapse: Differential findings for gender from the International Tobacco Control Study. *Addiction* [Published online February 17, 2015]. doi:10.1111/add.13290

Corrigall, W. A. (1999). Nicotine self-administration in animals as a dependence model. *Nicotine and Tobacco Research, 1*, 11–20. doi:10.1080/14622299050011121

de Souza, I. C. W., de Barros, V. V., Gomide, H. P., Miranda, T. C. M., de Paula Menezes, V., Kozasa, E. H., & Noto, A. R. (2015). Mindfulness-based interventions for the treatment of smoking: a systematic literature review. *Journal of Alternative and Complementary Medicine, 21*, 129–140. doi:10.1089/acm.2013.0471

D'Souza, M. S., & Markou, A. (2010). Neural substrates of psychostimulant withdrawal-induced anhedonia. *Current topics in Behavioral Neurosciences, 3*, 119–178. doi:10.1007/7854_2009_20

Duncan, S., & Feldman-Barratt, L. (2007). Affect is a form of cognition: A neurobiological analysis. *Cognition and Emotion, 21*, 1184–1211. doi: 10.1080/02699930701437931

Everitt, B. J., & Robbins, T. W. (2005). Neural systems of reinforcement for drug addiction; from actions to habit to compulsion. *Nature Neuroscience, 8*, 1481–1489. doi:10.1038/nn1579

Farris, S. G., Zvolensky, M. J., Otto, M. W., & Leyro, T. M. (2015). The role of distress intolerance for panic and nicotine withdrawal symptoms during a biological challenge. *Journal of Psychopharmacology, 29*, 783–791. doi: 10.1177/0269881115575536

Gifford, E. V., Kohlenberg, B. S., Hayes, S. C., Pierson, H. M., Piasecki, M. P., Antonuccio, D. O., & Palm, K. M. (2011). Does acceptance and relationship focused behavior therapy contribute to bupropion outcomes? A randomized controlled trial of functional analytic psychotherapy and acceptance and commitment therapy for smoking cessation. *Behavior Therapy, 42*, 700–715. doi: 10.1016/j.beth.2011.03.002

Gilbert, D. G. (1997). The situation x trait adaptive response (STAR) model of drug use, drug effects, and craving. *Human Psychopharmacology, 12,* S89–S102. doi: 10.1002/(SICI)1099-1077(199706)12:2+<S89::AID-HUP906>3.0.CO;2-P

Gonzalez, A., Zvolensky, M. J., Vujanovic, A. A., Leyro, T. M., & Marshall, E. C. (2008). An evaluation of anxiety sensitivity, emotional dysregulation, and negative affectivity among daily cigarette smokers: Relation to smoking motives and barriers to quitting. *Journal of Psychiatric Research, 43,* 138–147. doi: 10.1016/j.jpsychires.2008.03.002

Goodwin, R. D., Wall, M. M., Choo, T., Galea, S., Horowitz, J., Nomura, Y., . . . Hasin, D.S. (2014). Changes in the prevalence of mood and anxiety disorders among male and female current smokers in the United States: 1990-2001. *Annals of Epidemiology, 24,* 493–497. doi: 10.1016/j.annepidem.2014.01.014

Heppner, W. L., Spears, C. A., Correa-Fernández, V., Castro, Y., Li, Y., Guo, B., . . . Cinciripini, P. M. (2016). Dispositional mindfulness predicts enhanced smoking cessation and smoking lapse recovery. *Annals of Behavioral Medicine, 50,* 337–347. doi: 10.1007/s12160-015-9759-3

Hitsman, B., Papandonatos, G. D., McChargue, D. E., DeMott, A., Herrera, M. J., Spring, B., Borrelli, B., & Niaura, R. (2013). Past major depression and smoking cessation outcome: A systematic review and meta-analysis update *Addiction, 108,* 294–306. doi: 10.1111/add.12009

Hughes, J. R. (2001). Why does smoking so often produce dependence? A somewhat different view. *Tobacco Control, 10,* 62–64. doi: 10.1136/tc.10.1.62

Hughes, J. R., & Hatsukami, D. K. (1986). Signs and symptoms of tobacco withdrawal. *Archives of General Psychiatry, 43,* 289–294. doi:10.1001/archpsyc.1986.01800030107013

Johnson, K. A., Farris, S. G., Schmidt, N. B., & Zvolensky, M. J. (2012). Anxiety sensitivity and cognitive-based smoking processes: Testing the mediating role of emotion dysregulation among treatment-seeking daily smokers. *Journal of Addictive Diseases, 31,* 143–157. doi: 10.1080/10550887.2012.665695

Kalman, D., Hoskinson, R., Sambamoorthi, U., & Garvey, A. J. (2010). A prospective study of persistence in the prediction of smoking cessation outcome: Results from a randomized clinical trial. *Addictive Behaviors, 35,* 179–182. doi:10.1016/j.addbeh.2009.09.017

Kassel, J. D., Stroud, L. R., & Paronis, C. A. (2003). Smoking, stress, and negative affect: Correlation, causation, and context across stages of smoking. *Psychological Bulletin, 129,* 270–304. doi: 10.1037/0033-2909.129.2.270

Kenney, B. A., Holahan, C. J., North, R. J., & Holahan, C. K. (2006). Depressive symptoms and cigarette smoking in American workers. *American Journal of Health Promotion, 20,* 179–182. doi: 10.4278/0890-1171-20.3.179

Kirchner, T. R., Cantrell, J., Anesetti-Rothermel, A., & Abrams, D. B. (2013). Geospatial exposure to point-of-sale tobacco: Real-time craving and smoking-cessation outcomes. *American Journal of Preventive Medicine, 45,* 379–385. doi: 10.1016/j.amepre.2013.05.016

Koob, G. F., & LeMoal, M. (2008). Addiction and the brain antireward system. *Annual Review of Psychology, 59,* 29–53. doi: 10.1146/annurev.psych.59.103006.093548

Kraemer, K. M., McLeish, A. C., Jeffries, E. R., Avallone, K. M., & Luberto, C. M. (2013). Distress tolerance and perceived barriers to smoking cessation. *Substance Abuse, 34*, 277–282. doi: 10.1080/08897077.2013.771597

Langdon, K. J., Farris, S. G., Øverup, C. S., & Zvolensky, M. J. (2016). Associations between anxiety sensitivity, negative affect, and smoking during a self-guided smoking cessation attempt. *Nicotine and Tobacco Research, 18*, 1188–1195. doi: 10.1093/ntr/ntv253

Leventhal, A. M. (2010). Do individual differences in reinforcement smoking moderate the relationship between affect and urge to smoke? *Behavioral Medicine, 36*, 1–6. doi: 10.1080/08964280903521347

Leventhal, A. M., Piper, M. E., Japuntich, S. J., Baker, T. B., & Cook, J. W. (2014). Anhedonia, depressed mood, and smoking cessation outcome. *Journal of Consulting and Clinical Psychology, 82*, 122–129. doi:10.1037/a0035046

Leventhal, A. M., Ramsey, S. E., Brown, R. A., LaChance, H. R., & Kahler, C. W. (2008). Dimensions of depressive symptoms and smoking cessation. *Nicotine & Tobacco Research, 10*, 507–517. doi:10.1080/14622200801901971

Leventhal, A. M., Trujillo, M., Ameringer, K. J., Tidey, J. W., Sussman, S., & Kahler, C. W. (2014). Anhedonia and the relative reward value of drug and nondrug reinforcers in cigarette smokers. *Journal of Abnormal Psychology, 123*, 375–386. doi:10.1037/a0036384

Leventhal, A. M., & Zvolensky, M. J. (2015). Anxiety, depression, and cigarette smoking: A transdiagnostic vulnerability framework to understanding emotion-smoking comorbidity. *Psychological Bulletin, 141*, 176–212. doi:10.1037/bul0000003

Leyro, T. M., Zvolensky, M. J., & Bernstein, A. (2010). Distress tolerance and psychopathological symptoms and disorders: A review of the empirical literature among adults. *Psychological Bulletin, 136*, 576–600. doi: http://dx.doi.org/10.1037/a0019712.

Leyro, T. M., Zvolensky, M. J., Vujanovic, A. A., & Bernstein, A. (2008). Anxiety sensitivity and smoking motives and outcome expectancies among adult daily smokers: Replication and extension. *Nicotine and Tobacco Research, 10*, 985–994. doi: 10.1080/14622200802097555

MacPherson, L., Stipelman, B. A., Duplinsky, M., Brown, R. A., & Lejuez, C. W. (2008). Distress tolerance and pre-smoking treatment attrition: Examination of moderating relationships. *Addictive Behaviors, 33*, 1385–1393. doi: 10.1016/j.addbeh.2008.07.001

Malarcher, A., Dube, S., Shaw, L., Babb, S., & Kaufmann, R. (2011). Quitting smoking among adults—United States, 2001–2010. *Morbidity and Mortality Weekly Report, 60*, 1513–1519.

McCarthy, D. E., Piasecki, T. M., Fiore, M. C., & Baker, T. B. (2006). Life before and after quitting smoking: An electronic diary study. *Journal of Abnormal Psychology, 115*, 454–466. doi: 10.1037/0021-843X.115.3.454

McCarthy, D. E., Piasecki, T. M., Lawrence, D. L., Jorenby, D. E., Shiffman, S., & Baker, T. B. (2008). Psychological mediators of bupropion sustained-release treatment for smoking cessation. *Addiction, 103*, 1521–1533. doi:10.1111/j.1360-0443.2008.02275.x

McCarthy, D. E., Minami, H., Yeh, V. M., & Bold, K. W. (2015). An experimental investigation of reactivity to ecological momentary assessment frequency among adults trying to quit smoking. *Addiction, 110*, 1549–1560. doi: 0.1111/add.12996

Minami, H., Yeh, V. M., Bold, K. W., Chapman, G. B., & McCarthy, D. E. (2014). Relations among affect, abstinence motivation and confidence, and daily smoking lapse risk. *Psychology of Addictive Behaviors, 28*, 376–388. doi: 10.1037/a0034445

Morisano, D., Bacher, I., Audrain-McGovern, J., & George, T. P. (2009). Mechanisms underlying the comorbidity of tobacco use in mental health and addictive disorders. *Canadian Journal of Psychiatry, 54*, 356–367. doi: 10.1177/070674370905400603

Naragon-Gainey, K. (2010). Meta-analysis of the relations of anxiety sensitivity to the depressive and anxiety disorders. *Psychological Bulletin, 136*, 128–150. doi: 10.1037/a0018055

O'Brien, C. P., Testa, T., O'Brien, T. J., Brady, J. P., & Wells, B. (1977). Conditioned narcotic withdrawal in humans. *Science, 195*, 1000–1002.

O'Connell, K. A., & Martin, E. J. (1987). Highly tempting situations associated with abstinence, temporary lapse, and relapse among participants in smoking cessation programs. *Journal of Consulting and Clinical Psychology, 55*, 367–371.

Patten, C. A., & Martin, J. E. (1996). Does nicotine withdrawal affect smoking cessation? Clinical and theoretical issues. *Annals of Behavioral Medicine, 183*, 190–200.

Pedersen, W., & Von Soest, T. (2008). Smoking, nicotine dependence and mental health among young adults: A 13-year population-based longitudinal study. *Addiction, 104*, 129–137. doi: 10.1111/j.1360-0443.2008.02395.x

Perkins, K. A., Karelitz, J. L., Giedgowd, G. E., Conklin, C. A., & Sayette, M. A. (2010). Differences in negative mood-induced smoking reinforcement due to distress tolerance, anxiety sensitivity, and depression history. *Psychopharmacology, 210*, 25–34. doi: 10.1007/s00213-010-1811-1

Piasecki, T. M., Jorenby, D. E., Smith, S. S., Fiore, M. C., & Baker, T. B. (2002). Smoking withdrawal dynamics: II. Improved tests of withdrawal-relapse relations. *Journal of Abnormal Psychology, 112*, 14–27. doi: 10.1037/0021-843X.112.1.14

Pomerleau, O. F., Pomerleau, C. S., Mehringer, A. M., Snedecor, S. M., Ninowski, R., & Sen, A. (2005). Nicotine dependence, depression, and gender: Characterizing phenotypes based on withdrawal discomfort, response to smoking, and ability to abstain. *Nicotine and Tobacco Research, 7*, 91–102.

Rash, C. J., & Copeland, A. (2008). The Brief Smoking Consequences Questionnaire—Adult (BSCQ-A): Development of a short form of the SCQ-A. *Nicotine and Tobacco Research, 10*, 1633–1643. doi: 10.1080/14622200802409990

Robinson T. E., & Berridge, K. C. (1993). The neural basis of drug craving: An incentive sensitization theory of addiction. *Brain Research Reviews, 18*, 247–291. doi: 10.1016/0165-0173(93)90013-P

Root, D. H., Fabbricatore, A. T., Barker, D. J., Ma, S., Pawlak, A. P., & West, M. O. (2009). Evidence for habitual and goal-directed behavior following devaluation of cocaine: a multifaceted interpretation of relapse. *PLoS ONE, 4*, e7170. doi:10.1371/journal.pone.0007170

Ruscio, A. C., Muench, C., Brede, E., & Waters, A. J. (2016). Effect of brief mindfulness practice on self-reported affect, craving, and smoking: A pilot randomized controlled trial using ecological momentary assessment. *Nicotine and Tobacco Research, 18*, 64–73. doi: 10.1093/ntr/ntv074

Sayette, M. A., Wertz, J. M., Martin, C. S., Perrott, M. A., & Hobel, J. (2003). Effects of smoking opportunity on cue-elicited urge: A facial coding analysis. *Experimental and Clinical Psychopharmacology, 11*, 218–227. doi: 10.1093/acprof:oso/9780195179644.003.0029

Schmidt, N. B., Raines, A. M., Allan, N. P., & Zvolensky, M. J. (2016). Anxiety sensitivity risk reduction in smokers: A randomized control trial examining effects on panic. *Behaviour Research and Therapy, 77*, 138–146. doi: 10.1016/j.brat.2015.12.011

Schulteis, G., Heyser, C. J., & Koob, G. F. (1997). Opiate withdrawal signs precipitated by naloxone following a single exposure to morphine: Potentiation with a second morphine exposure. *Psychopharmacology, 129*, 59–65. doi: 10.1007/s002130050162

Shiffman, S., Hickcox, M., Paty, J. A., Gnys, M., Kassel, J. D., & Richards, T. J. (1996). Progression from a smoking lapse to relapse: Prediction from abstinence violation effects, nicotine dependence, and lapse characteristics. *Journal of Consulting and Clinical Psychology, 64*, 993–1002. doi: 10.1037/0022-006X.64.5.993

Shiffman S., Paty, J. A., Gnys, M., Kassel, J. D., Hickcox, M. (1996). First lapses to smoking: Within-subjects analysis of real-time reports. *Journal of Consulting and Clinical Psychology, 64*, 366–379. doi: 10.1037/0022-006X.64.2.366

Shiffman, S., Paty, J. A., Gwaltney, C. J., & Dang, Q. (2004). Immediate antecedents of cigarette smoking: An analysis of unrestricted smoking patterns. *Journal of Abnormal Psychology, 113*, 166–171. doi: 0.1037/1064-1297.13.3.219

Shiffman, S., Tindle, H., Li, X., Scholl, S., Dunbar, M., & Mitchell-Miland, C. (2012). Characteristics and smoking patterns of intermittent smokers. *Experimental and Clinical Psychopharmacology, 20*, 264–277. doi: 10.1037/a0027546

Shiffman, S., & Waters, A. J. (2004). Negative affect and smoking lapses: A prospective analysis. *Journal of Consulting and Clinical Psychology, 72*, 192–201. doi: 10.1037/0022-006X.72.2.192

Shiyko, M., Naab, P., Shiffman, S., & Li, R. (2014). Modeling complexity of EMA data: Time-varying lagged effects of negative affect on smoking urges for subgroups of nicotine addiction. *Nicotine and Tobacco Research,16*, S144–S150. doi: 10.1093/ntr/ntt109

Siqueira, L., Diab, M., Bodian, C., & Rolnitzky, L. (2000). Adolescents becoming smokers: The roles of stress and coping methods. *Journal of Adolescent Health, 27*, 399–408. doi: 10.1016/S1054-139X(00)00167-1

Smits, J. A., Berry, A. C., Tart, C. D., & Powers, M. B. (2008). The efficacy of cognitive-behavioral interventions for reducing anxiety sensitivity: A meta-analytic review. *Behaviour Research and Therapy, 46*, 1047–1054. doi: 10.1016/j.brat.2008.06.010

Solomon, R. L. (1971). An opponent-process theory of acquired motivation: The affective dynamics of addiction. In J. E. Maser & M. E. P. Seligman (Eds.), *Psychopathology: Experimental models* (pp. 66–103). San Francisco: Freeman.

Spears, C. A., Houchins, S. C., Stewart, D. W., Chen, M., Correa-Fernández, V., Cano, M. Á., . . . Wetter, D. W. (2015). Nonjudging facet of mindfulness predicts enhanced smoking cessation in Hispanics. *Psychology of Addictive Behaviors, 29*, 918–923. doi: 10.1037/adb0000087

Steinberg, M. L., Epstein, E. E., Stahl, N. F., Budsock, T. D., & Williams, J. M. (2015). Task persistence as a target for tobacco dependence treatment. *Drug and Alcohol Dependence, 146*, e108. doi: 10.1016/j.drugalcdep.2014.09.661

Steinberg, M. L., Williams, J. M., Gandhi, K. K., Foulds, J., Epstein, E. E., & Brandon, T. H. (2012). Task persistence predicts smoking cessation in smokers with and without schizophrenia. *Psychology of Addictive Behaviors, 26*, 850–858. doi:10.1037/a0028375

Stone, A. A., & Shiffman, S. (1994). Ecological momentary assessment in behavioral medicine. *Annals of Behavioral Medicine, 16*, 199–202.

Szasz, P. L., Szentagotai, A., & Hofmann, S. G. (2012). Effects of emotion regulation strategies on smoking craving, attentional bias, and task persistence. *Behaviour Research and Therapy, 50*, 333–340. doi:10.1016/j.brat.2012.02.010

Treadway, M. T., & Zald, D. H. (2013). Parsing anhedonia: Translational models of reward-processing deficits in psychopathology. *Current Directions in Psychological Science, 22*, 244–249. doi:10.1177/0963721412474460

Tyndale, R. F., & Sellers, E. M. (2001). Variable CYP2A6-mediated nicotine metabolism alters smoking behavior and risk. *Drug Metabolism and Disposition, 29*, 548–552. doi: 0090-9556/01/2904-548–552

US Department of Health and Human Services. (2014). *The health consequences of smoking: 50 years of progress. A report of the surgeon general.* Atlanta, GA: US Department of Health and Human Services, Centers for Disease Control and Prevention, National Center for Chronic Disease Prevention and Health Promotion, Office on Smoking and Health, 2014. Printed with corrections, January 2014.

Ward, B. W., Clarke, T. C., Nugent, C. N., & Schiller, J. S. (2016). *Early release of selected estimates based on data from the 2015 National Health Interview Survey.* National Center for Health Statistics. Retrieved May 24, 2016, from: http://www.cdc.gov/nchs/nhis.htm.

Watson, D., Clark, L. A., & Tellegen, A. (1988). Development and validation of brief measures of positive and negative affect: The PANAS scales. *Journal of Personality and Social Psychology, 54*, 1063–1070. doi:10.1037/0022-3514.54.6.1063

Weinstein, S.M., Mermelstein, R., Shiffman, S., & Flay, B. (2008). Mood variability and cigarette smoking escalation among adolescents. *Psychology of Addictive Behaviors, 22*, 504–513. doi: 10.1037%2F0893-164X.22.4.504

White, H. R., Pandina, R. J., & Chen, P. H. (2002). Developmental trajectories of cigarette use from early adolescence into young adulthood. *Drug and Alcohol Dependence, 65*, 167–178. doi: 10.1016/S0376-8716(01)00159-4

Wikler, A. (1948). Recent progress in research on the neurophysiological basis of morphine addiction. *American Journal of Psychiatry, 105*, 329–338.

Wills, T. A., Resko, J. A., Ainette, M. G., & Mendoza, D. (2004). Smoking onset in adolescence: A person-centered analysis with time-varying predictors. *Health Psychology, 23*, 158–167. doi:10.1037/0278-6133.23.2.158

Wise, R. A., & Bozarth, M. A. (1987). A psychomotor stimulant theory of addiction. *Psychological Review, 94*, 469–492.

Wong, M., Krajisnik, A., Truong, L., Lisha, N. E., Trujillo, M., Greenberg, J. B., . . . Leventhal, A. M. (2013). Anxiety sensitivity as a predictor of acute subjective effects of smoking. *Nicotine and Tobacco Research, 15*, 1084–1090. doi: 10.1093/ntr/nts208

World Health Organization. (2011). WHO report on the global tobacco epidemic, 2011. Geneva: World Health Organization, 2011 [accessed May 24, 2016].

Zvolensky, M. J., & Bernstein, A. (2005). Cigarette smoking and panic psychopathology. *Current Directions in Psychological Science*, *14*, 301–305. doi: 10.1111/j.0963-7214.2005.00386.x

Zvolensky, M. J., Bonn-Miller, M. O., Feldner, M. T., Leen-Feldner, E., McLeish, A. C., & Gregor, K. (2006). Anxiety sensitivity: Concurrent associations with negative affect smoking motives and abstinence self-confidence among young adult smokers. *Addictive Behaviors*, *31*, 429–439. doi:10.1016/j.addbeh.2005.05.027

14

The Role of Negative Affect in the Course of Substance Use Disorders

ELIZABETH D. REESE, JENNIFER Y. YI, RYAN P. BELL, AND STACEY B. DAUGHTERS

INTRODUCTION

Beginning stages of substance use (i.e., initiation, development of consistent self-administration) are characterized by a positive reinforcement process (Wise & Koob, 2014), such that initially, substance use is accompanied by increased positive affect (PA; e.g., euphoria and pleasure), which occurs through the substance's influence on reward-related brain regions. However as recreational substance use transitions into chronic use, the motive for drug self-administration transitions into a negative reinforcement process, wherein substances are used to alleviate various aversive physical and psychological experiences associated with withdrawal symptoms (Baker, Piper, McCarthy, Majeskie, & Fiore, 2004; Wise & Koob, 2014). Psychological distress, namely negative affect (NA), factors into the perpetuation of chronic substance use and contributes to the increased risk of relapse. Thus in this chapter, we review the processes by which NA contributes to the course of substance use disorders, and overview treatment approaches that directly target affective components of substance use.

Theoretical perspectives on the dimensionality of PA and NA are important to consider when evaluating the contribution of literature discussed in this chapter to substance use disorders. One widely used theory of affect conceptualizes PA and NA as bipolar opposites existing along a continuous valence dimension (Russell & Carroll, 1999). This conceptualization allows for the interpretation of increases in NA to reflect simultaneous decreases in PA. Another prominent conceptualization of affect identifies PA and NA as two separable dimensions that adequately subsume the range of human emotional experiences (Watson & Tellegen, 1999). In this chapter, we discuss NA as an independent construct, which should be interpreted as separable from PA. This follows accepted conceptualizations of the development of substance use as influenced first by PA in early stages of use and later by NA as substance use transitions from recreational to chronic intake (Wise & Koob, 2014). We acknowledge the importance of both PA and NA in the onset and maintenance of substance use, however as this chapter focuses on affect in relation to disordered substance use, we intentionally emphasize the role of NA within processes related to chronic use, which are central to this chapter.

OVERVIEW OF SUBSTANCE USE AND SUBSTANCE USE DISORDERS

According to a 2012 international report of substance use, approximately 1 in 20 adults (~230 million) have used an illicit substance since 2010. Of those, 12% are estimated to be problem substance users (UNODC, 2012). Problem substance use contributes to the global burden of diseases, evidenced by increased rates of substance use disorder diagnoses and substance-related health outcomes. As estimated in 2010, one in every three new HIV infections reported is attributed to injection drug use, while the estimated number of injection drug users living with Hepatitis B or C is 2.3 million (14.5%) and 7.4 million (46.7%), respectively (UNODC, 2012). Through this increase in disease burden worldwide, research suggests that 1 in every 100 adult deaths can be attributed to substance use (UNODC, 2012).

Consistent with the criteria set forth by the *Diagnostic and Statistical Manual of Mental Disorders, Fifth Edition* (DSM-5; American Psychiatric Association, 2013), a substance use disorder (SUD) is a chronic, relapsing disorder diagnosed when the repeated intake of a substance (alcohol or drug) results in clinical and functional impairment, including significant health-related problems or failure to meet job-related and/or familial obligations. Such disorders are diagnosed based on evidence of impaired control, risky use, social impairment, and pharmacological criteria and can range in severity from mild to moderate to severe depending on the quantity of symptoms present. The SUD diagnostic criteria in the DSM-5 combine criteria used to diagnose substance abuse and dependence in the *Diagnostic and Statistical Manual of Mental Disorders, Fourth Edition* (DSM-IV; American Psychiatric Association, 1994). While a key component of substance abuse in the DSM-IV included legal issues, this criterion has been discarded due to poor fit with other criteria and relatively low prevalence rates among adults (Hasin et al., 2013). Additionally, craving has been added as a criterion in the DSM-5 in part because of evidence that craving is a central component of SUDs, as well as to increase consistency between the DSM-5 and other prominent mental health classification systems (Hasin et al., 2013) such as the International Classification of Diseases (World Health Organization, 1992).

THEORETICAL MODELS OF ADDICTION

Opponent Process Theory and Allostatic Model of Addiction

An influential early theory of addiction, the opponent process theory, posits that during initial substance use and early acute drug administration, individuals experience intense hedonic and rewarding effects such as pleasure and euphoria, resulting in the reinforcement of substance use (Solomon, 1980; Solomon & Corbit, 1974) and highlighting the importance of positive reinforcement in the early stages of substance use (Wise & Koob, 2014). We now know that the rewarding effects of substance use result because both drugs and alcohol act on reward-related regions of the brain (Koob & Volkow, 2010). However, according to the opponent process theory, this powerful hedonic reaction to substance use is opposed or counteracted by a stress response system, the hypothalamic-pituitary-adrenal (HPA) axis, which governs levels of stress-related hormones in the body. The increase in HPA axis activity is a biological reaction to the body's response to intense pleasure and reward and serves to bring our bodies back to a neutral, or homeostatic state. Koob and LeMoal's allostatic model of addiction (Koob & Le Moal, 1997, 2001, 2008) furthers this theory by suggesting that with repeated drug administrations, there is an overstimulation of the brain's reward system. In response to this overstimulation across time, our body's stress response intensifies, masking the hedonic effects of substance use and resulting in a perpetual state of withdrawal/NA. Thus, as addiction develops, the overactivation of the stress response results in an allostatic, or dysregulated mood state. Negative reinforcement becomes the primary motivation for substance use, such that substances are consumed in order to alleviate the NA state that persists after the effects of a substance begin to subside.

Negative Reinforcement Theory

Extending Koob and LeMoal's allostatic model of addiction, Baker and colleagues' (2004) negative reinforcement theory posits that once individuals begin experiencing withdrawal symptoms, they develop a learned association between substance use and NA relief. Thus, individuals begin chronic drug self-administration in order to alleviate withdrawal-related NA, which is hypothesized to occur both with and without cognitive awareness. At low levels of affective response, drug administration is largely an automatized process where individuals are unaware of NA, which is detected primarily through interoceptive cues. Alternatively, at high levels of NA, when NA states are most salient to the individual (perhaps when a substance is unavailable for immediate consumption), the user's substance valuation increases, resulting in compulsive drug-seeking behavior. This model hypothesizes that cognitive control resources, (e.g., choosing an alternative response during affective distress rather than substance use), are readily accessible at moderate levels of NA. Only in such cases will the substance user have the ability to respond adaptively when faced with situations that may elicit substance use as a response. The negative reinforcement theory further proposes that because substance users learn to respond to NA resulting from substance withdrawal, they extend this learned behavioral response pattern to other non-substance-related affective states (e.g., environmental stress). Through this generalization from withdrawal states to NA states arising from environmental stressors, addicted individuals will begin to self-administer drugs in response to NA experiences across substance-related and non-substance-related situations, increasing relapse risk even when withdrawal symptoms are no longer present.

Taken together, several theories of addiction focus on NA as a central component in the progression of SUD development. Specifically, both NA within addiction-related processes (e.g., withdrawal from substance use) as well as generalized NA in response to environmental factors are theorized to impact the course of addiction, perpetuating substance use behavior and leading to negative health outcomes. To validate such theoretical models, it is imperative to closely examine the evidence linking NA to substance use behavior throughout the course of the addiction cycle. This includes close inspection of NA within SUD development, maintenance, and relapse.

SUBSTANCE USE RISK

Past year prevalence rates for co-occurring substance use and mood disorders are roughly 19%, and co-occurring substance use and anxiety disorders are approximately 17% (Grant, Hasin, Chou, Stinson, & Dawson, 2004). Lifetime rates of comorbid SUD and major depression are estimated at 40.3% for alcohol use disorder and 17.2% for illicit drug use disorders (Pettinati, O'Brien, & Dundon, 2013). Though comorbidity estimates between mood-related disorders and SUDs do not provide information about temporal order of onset, evidence suggests that individuals with a prior diagnosis of an affect-related disorder may be at higher risk for subsequent SUD development. Results of the Epidemiological Catchment Area study suggest that individuals diagnosed with an anxiety disorder have a 50% increase in odds of a lifetime alcohol use disorder diagnosis (Regier et al., 1990). This relationship is further supported by the results from a 7-year longitudinal study showing that the odds of developing a new alcohol dependence diagnosis at year 7 increases from 3.5 to 5.0 for individuals diagnosed with an anxiety disorder at years 1 and 4 (Kushner, Sher, & Erickson, 1999). In addition to affect-related psychopathology, negatively valenced life experiences have also been linked to the development of SUDs. For example, Keyes, Hatzenbuehler, and Hasin (2011) found that specific stressful life events including divorce and job loss increases the risk of developing disordered alcohol use, while childhood maltreatment predicts early-onset drinking in adolescents and adults diagnosed with alcohol use disorders. Moreover, the inability to tolerate NA (i.e., low distress tolerance) is associated with increased frequency of alcohol use and heavy episodic drinking among adolescents (Daughters et al., 2009; Winward, Bekman, Hanson, Lejuez, & Brown, 2014). Taken together, this work provides evidence of an increased risk for substance use among individuals with a comorbid mood or anxiety disorder and/or an inability to tolerate NA states.

SUBSTANCE USE MAINTENANCE AND RELAPSE

Substantial evidence exists linking NA to substance use maintenance and relapse. In much of the literature, NA is examined as a separate construct from two core components of the addiction cycle, namely *withdrawal* and *craving*, both of which are known to induce and perpetuate NA states.

As such, it is often difficult to definitively disentangle the experience of withdrawal and craving from much of the literature examining NA and substance use. With that caveat in mind, in the following section we provide a review of the link between NA and substance use maintenance and relapse among studies examining NA states more generally as well as from those in the context of withdrawal and craving.

Negative Affect

Substance use appears to be a common response to experiences of NA, which contributes to the maintenance of both NA and substance use. For example, men often turn to substance use in response to depression and stress, which exacerbates state NA (Whittle et al., 2015). This aligns with previous research demonstrating heavy drinking in response to chronic stress (e.g., unfavorable marital status, unfavorable employment status) and acute stress (e.g., victim of a crime, financial problems, divorce) for women and men, respectively (San Jose, Van Oers, Van De Mheen, Garretsen, & Mackenbach, 2000), and increased drinking behavior directly following a stress task across multiple studies (de Wit, Söderpalm, Nikolayev, & Young, 2003; McGrath, Jones, & Field, 2016). In an ecological momentary assessment study investigating combat veterans with co-occurring SUD and post-traumatic stress disorder, the exacerbation of post-traumatic stress disorder symptoms is associated with an increase in alcohol consumption within the same time period (Possemato et al., 2015). Additionally, college students and household-residing women who have experienced sexual revictimization are more likely to report monthly binge drinking, marijuana use, and other illicit drug use as compared to nonvictims (Walsh et al., 2014). Moreover, Furnari et al. (2015) show a significant increase in stress severity in the days preceding cocaine use in a sample of polysubstance users, while Keyes and colleagues (2011) found higher rates of drinking to cope with traumatic events among those with a history of alcohol use disorder.

Negative affect also predicts relapse vulnerability (Kenford et al., 2002; Piasecki et al., 2000), as relapse has the tendency of occurring in the context of NA (Baker et al., 2004; Kassel, Stroud, & Paronis, 2003). In a study of depressed male veterans, Curran, Flynn, Kirchner, and Booth (2000) found that compared to nondepressed men, men with mild to moderate depressive symptoms are three times more likely to relapse to alcohol while those with severe depression are five times more likely to be at risk of alcohol relapse over a 3-month follow-up period. These results are supported by another study linking depressive symptomology to relapse risk and shortened time to first drink (Greenfield et al., 1998), as well as increased odds of smoking relapse at a 10-year follow-up (Zvolensky, Bakhshaie, Sheffer, Perez, & Goodwin, 2015). In addition, research suggests stress-related experiences are specifically linked to relapse in substance users. In a study of male and female smokers, perceived stress predicts risk of smoking relapse specifically for men (Nakajima & al'Absi, 2012), while another study demonstrates that stress induction is specifically predictive of shorter time to relapse among alcohol-dependent patients (Sinha et al., 2011).

Furthermore, distress tolerance, defined as an individual's ability to persist in goal-directed behavior while experiencing physical or psychological distress, is linked to substance use outcomes across drug classes. This behavioral proxy for negative reinforcement behavior allows researchers to induce distress in a controlled setting and evaluate one's ability to persist with a task despite psychological discomfort, modeling a recovering substance user's attempt to remain abstinent while simultaneously experiencing intense NA and psychological withdrawal symptoms. Indeed, among smokers and illicit drug users, low distress tolerance is associated with an increased likelihood of treatment dropout (Daughters et al., 2005; Tull, Gratz, Coffey, Weiss, & McDermott, 2013), shorter abstinence durations (Daughters et al., 2005), and relapse (Brandon et al., 2003; Cameron, Reed & Ninnemann, 2013; Strong et al., 2012).

Withdrawal

In line with negative reinforcement theories discussed previously in this chapter, numerous studies suggest that alleviation of NA experienced specifically during addiction-related processes such as substance use withdrawal characterize the primary motivation for continued substance use. Although the withdrawal experience is heterogeneous across substance types, NA is understood as a universal and central component of withdrawal (Baker et al., 2004) and can manifest as a variety of emotions including anxiety, sadness, anger, depression, dysphoria, and irritability (Gold, Washton, & Dackis, 1985; Hall, Muñoz, Reus, & Sees, 1993; Kosman & Unna, 1967; Mansky, 1978). For instance, substances such as cocaine, nicotine, and buprenorphine that have fewer or milder somatic and physical withdrawal symptoms are strongly associated with NA during withdrawal (Coffey, Dansky, Carrigan, & Brady, 2000; Fudala, Jaffe, Dax, & Johnson, 1990; Jorenby et al., 1996; Lago & Kosten, 1994). In addition, Rigg and Ibañez (2010) show that the alleviation of withdrawal symptoms, anxiety, and stress are among the most commonly reported motives for non-prescription-drug use among current and recovering illicit drug users.

This more progressive understanding of the withdrawal syndrome has been developed and accompanied by advancements in the ability to detect and measure affective changes during withdrawal experiences, such as with neuroimaging, neurochemical and neuromolecular examinations, and refined animal models that inform the course of substance use (Heilig, Egli, Crabbe, & Becker, 2010). During acute withdrawal, animals demonstrate central nervous system hyperexcitability as well as increased sensory reactivity, which is hypothesized to reflect altered affective processing in humans (Heilig et al., 2010). Additional animal models propose the involvement of the central nervous system during acute withdrawal as demonstrated by motivational signs of withdrawal such as increased anxiety-like responses (Doremus, Brunell, Varlinskaya, & Spear, 2003; Gehlert et al., 2007; Prediger, da Silva, Batista, Bittencourt, & Takahashi, 2006) and withdrawal-induced drug self-administration which correspond to human responses during acute withdrawal, such as self-medication through substance use (Koob & Mason, 2016). Together, both human and animal research support the experience of NA during withdrawal.

Additional evidence builds on the role of NA during withdrawal, suggesting that substance use during withdrawal may be motivated by the alleviation of NA. In conjunction with previously mentioned findings, Kenford and colleagues (2002) demonstrate that NA, specifically post-quit affect, is a potent predictor of relapse to smoking in a large sample of smokers more so than physiological symptomology. Compared to nonaffective withdrawal symptoms, such as somatic and physical symptoms, NA is more commonly reported as a precipitant for substance use and relapse (Brandon, Tiffany, Obremski, & Baker, 1990; Marlatt & Gordon, 1980). In particular, the severity of NA during withdrawal is predictive of relapse vulnerability, such that there exists a roughly linear relationship between the magnitude of affective disturbance and duration of abstinence during the withdrawal period (Fendt & Mucha, 2001; Jarvik et al., 2000). Additionally, habitual smokers that relapse within the first 24-hour abstinence period of a quit attempt report a greater reduction in PA (i.e., cheerfulness, content, calmness, controllability, and interest) than those who maintain abstinence (al'Absi, Hatsukami, Davis, & Wittmers, 2004). Similarly, rapid increases in NA predict relapse among smokers experiencing withdrawal during quit attempts (Shiffman & Waters, 2004). Together, such findings suggest that NA sensitively indexes substance use outcomes during the experience of withdrawal.

Craving

Craving is understood as the subjective experience of *wanting to use a substance*, and is associated with a compulsion to seek and take a substance (Tiffany & Wray, 2012). Negative affect is positively correlated with craving for nicotine (McCarthy, Piasecki, Fiore, & Baker, 2006; Shiyko, Burkhalter, Li, & Park, 2014; Van Zundert, Engels, & Kuntsche, 2011), cannabis (Buckner, Crosby, Wonderlich, & Schmidt, 2012), cocaine (Epstein et al., 2009; Kennedy et al., 2013), and heroin (Epstein et al., 2009). More specifically, ecological momentary assessment results demonstrate that craving for cocaine, heroin, and tobacco occurs when users experience

NA states consisting of feeling "worried, anxious, or tense," "angry or frustrated" (either "with myself or because things were not going my way" or "because of my relationship with someone else"), or that "others were being critical of me" (Preston & Epstein, 2011).

In order to study the effects of craving on substance use behavior, researchers often induce NA (e.g., stress) using behavioral stress imagery to manipulate craving states (Sinha, Catapano, & O'Malley, 1999). This is important as studies show a positive correlation between craving and nicotine (Tiffany & Drobes, 1991), cocaine (Tiffany, Singleton, Haertzen, & Henningfield, 1993), alcohol (Singleton et al., 1994), and heroin (Tiffany, Fields, Singleton, Haertzen, & Henningfield, 1996) use. Neuroimaging investigations show that in response to stress, higher activation in neural regions associated with inhibitory control, interoception, and habitual behavior is associated with increased cocaine craving (Sinha et al., 2005), and higher activation of the ventral striatum and ventromedial prefrontal cortex is associated with increased stress-induced alcohol craving (Seo et al., 2013).

Furthermore, NA-related substance craving is associated with increased risk for relapse. Biological and neuroimaging research shows that alcohol-related brain changes (e.g., brain volume, brain function, biological stress responses) are associated with higher craving and increased alcohol relapse risk (Sinha, 2012). Specifically, NA-related alcohol craving predicts time to alcohol relapse after treatment (Breese et al., 2005; Cooney, Litt, Morse, Bauer, & Gaupp, 1997), and stress-induced cocaine craving is predictive of time to cocaine relapse (Sinha, Garcia, Paliwal, Kreek, & Rounsaville, 2006). However, the relationship between craving and relapse among opiate users is not well supported. While one study shows increased craving associated with opiate use at a 1-week follow-up (McHugh, Park, & Weiss, 2014), another reports no association between relapse and cue-induced craving among opiate users engaged in methadone/buprenorphine maintenance treatment (Fatseas et al., 2011).

Taken together, there is sufficient evidence to suggest that NA, experienced in daily life as a function of affect-related psychopathology or within addiction-specific processes such as withdrawal and craving, contributes significantly to the course of addiction. As such, addiction treatment and intervention approaches targeting NA may be particularly useful for individuals navigating NA experiences during recovery attempts.

SUBSTANCE USE TREATMENT

Multiple treatment approaches have been developed to address NA associated with substance use behavior and comorbid psychopathology. Acceptance-based behavioral treatments (e.g., acceptance and commitment therapy; Hayes, Strosahl, & Wilson, 1999); dialectical behavior therapy; Linehan, 1993), which focus on increasing emotional acceptance, may be useful in treating substance use by targeting NA experiences. For example, several studies find significantly less substance use at follow-up for individuals who receive acceptance and commitment therapy (Hayes, 2004), and higher rates of post-treatment abstinence for those who receive dialectical behavior therapy (Linehan et al., 2002). What is more, several new treatment approaches have been developed with the goal of increasing an individual's ability to cope with NA experiences. Initial results from a randomized controlled trial of a distress tolerance treatment show that those receiving distress tolerance treatment evidence greater improvements on distress tolerance behavioral measures as well as clinically significant change in depressive symptoms compared to individuals in a supportive counseling condition and those in a treatment as usual condition (Bornovalova, Gratz, Daughters, Hunt, & Lejuez, 2012). Mindfulness-based relapse prevention is another treatment aimed at developing awareness and acceptance of negative thoughts and feelings as a more effective coping strategy in the face of high-risk situations for substance users (Witkiewitz, Marlatt, & Walker, 2005). Individuals receiving mindfulness-based relapse prevention evidence significant improvements in substance use outcomes as compared to treatment as usual and basic relapse prevention, including significantly fewer days of substance use and decreased heavy drinking at a 1-year follow-up (Bowen et al., 2014). One additionally important therapeutic approach, behavioral activation treatment for depression, aims to decrease depressive symptoms by increasing positive reinforcement within the patient's daily experience. Behavioral activation treatment has been adapted for use with addicted individuals and is linked to decreased depression and anxiety symptom severity in illicit drug users with elevated depressive symptoms (Daughters et al., 2008) and increased treatment retention rates in a study comparing behavioral activation for substance use to a supportive counseling condition (Magidson et al., 2011).

In addition to empirically validated behavioral treatments aimed at increasing an individual's ability to tolerate NA states, pharmacological and neurobiological treatments that target stress-induced substance craving and normalization of the HPA axis during distress states may also be of benefit. In particular, corticotropin-releasing factor antagonists and 2-adrenergic agonists have been found to decrease stress-induced reinstatement of cocaine seeking, and glucocorticoid antagonists have been found to decrease cocaine reinforcement in drug-experienced laboratory animals (Erb et al., 2000; Goeders, 2002). Moreover, an exciting new treatment, noninvasive brain stimulation, shows promising results in preliminary studies. Repetitive transcranial magnetic stimulation is an approved treatment method of refractory major depression, a disorder characterized by increases in NA (O'Reardon et al., 2007). In addition, transcranial electrical stimulation applied to prefrontal regions associated with stress imagery-induced substance craving has been shown to decrease cortisol, a physiological measure of stress (Antal et al., 2014; Brunoni et al., 2013). When using both techniques, reduced substance craving is evident across multiple substances including nicotine, alcohol, and cocaine (Hone-Blanchet, Ciraulo, Pascual-Leone, & Fecteau, 2015), highlighting the utility of noninvasive brain stimulation as a candidate treatment for targeting NA associated with substance use.

SUMMARY

In sum, numerous theories emphasize the central role of NA in SUDs. Negative affect relief is highlighted as a primary motivation for continued substance use as recreational use transitions into disordered or problematic use. Support for NA models of addiction comes from empirical evidence supporting the connection between NA and risk for SUD development, maintenance, and relapse, in addition to the central role of NA in addiction-specific processes including withdrawal and craving. As a result, treatment approaches have been developed to address NA experiences integrated within SUDs and have demonstrated promising results.

REFERENCES

al'Absi, M., Hatsukami, D., Davis, G. L., & Wittmers, L. E. (2004). Prospective examination of effects of smoking abstinence on cortisol and withdrawal symptoms as predictors of early smoking relapse. *Drug and Alcohol Dependence, 73*, 267–278. doi: 10.1016/j.drugalcdep.2003.10.014

American Psychiatric Association. (2013). *Diagnostic and statistical manual of mental disorders, fifth edition (DSM-5®)*. Arlington, VA: American Psychiatric Association.

Antal, A., Fischer, T., Saiote, C., Miller, R., Chaieb, L., Wang, D. J., . . . Kirschbaum, C. (2014). Transcranial electrical stimulation modifies the neuronal response to psychosocial stress exposure. *Human Brain Mapping, 35*, 3750–3759. doi: 10.1002/hbm.22434

Baker, T. B., Piper, M. E., McCarthy, D. E., Majeskie, M. R., & Fiore, M. C. (2004). Addiction motivation reformulated: An affective processing model of negative reinforcement. *Psychological Review, 111*, 33–51. doi: 10.1037/0033-295X.111.1.33

Bornovalova, M. A., Gratz, K. L., Daughters, S. B., Hunt, E. D., & Lejuez, C. W. (2012). Initial RCT of a distress tolerance treatment for individuals with substance use disorders. *Drug and Alcohol Dependence, 122*(1–2), 70–76. doi: 10.1016/j.drugalcdep.2011.09.012

Bowen, S., Witkiewitz, K., Clifasefi, S. L., Grow, J., Chawla, N., Hsu, S. H., . . . Lustyk, M. K. (2014). Relative efficacy of mindfulness-based relapse prevention, standard relapse prevention, and treatment as usual for substance use disorders: A randomized clinical trial. *JAMA Psychiatry, 71*, 547–556.

Brandon, T. H., Herzog, T. A., Juliano, L. M., Irvin, J. E., Lazev, A. B., & Simmons, V. N. (2003). Pretreatment task persistence predicts smoking cessation outcome. *Journal of Abnormal Psychology, 112*, 448–456.

Brandon, T. H., Tiffany, S. T., Obremski, K. M., & Baker, T. B. (1990). Postcessation cigarette use: The process of relapse. *Addictive Behaviors, 15*, 105–114.

Breese, G. R., Chu, K., Dayas, C. V., Funk, D., Knapp, D. J., Koob, G. F., . . . Weiss, F. (2005). Stress enhancement of craving during sobriety: A risk for relapse. *Alcoholism, Clinical and Experimental Research, 29*, 185–195.

Brunoni, A. R., Vanderhasselt, M. A., Boggio, P. S., Fregni, F., Dantas, E. M., Mill, J. G., . . . Bensenor, I. M. (2013). Polarity- and valence-dependent effects of prefrontal transcranial direct current stimulation on heart rate variability and salivary cortisol. *Psychoneuroendocrinology, 38*, 58–66. doi: 10.1016/j.psyneuen.2012.04.020

Buckner, J. D., Crosby, R. D., Wonderlich, S. A., & Schmidt, N. B. (2012). Social anxiety and cannabis use: An analysis from ecological momentary assessment. *Journal of Anxiety Disorders, 26*, 297–304. doi: 10.1016/j.janxdis.2011.12.006

Cameron, A., Reed, K. P., & Ninnemann, A. (2013). Reactivity to negative affect in smokers: The role of implicit associations and distress tolerance in smoking cessation. *Addictive Behaviors, 38*, 2905–2912.

Coffey, S. F., Dansky, B. S., Carrigan, M. H., & Brady, K. T. (2000). Acute and protracted cocaine abstinence in an outpatient population: A prospective study of mood, sleep and withdrawal symptoms. *Drug and Alcohol Dependence, 59*, 277–286.

Cooney, N. L., Litt, M. D., Morse, P. A., Bauer, L. O., & Gaupp, L. (1997). Alcohol cue reactivity, negative-mood reactivity, and relapse in treated alcoholic men. *Journal of Abnormal Psychology, 106*, 243–250.

Curran, G. M., Flynn, H. A., Kirchner, J., & Booth, B. M. (2000). Depression after alcohol treatment as a risk factor for relapse among male veterans. *Journal of Substance Abuse Treatment, 19*, 259–265.

Daughters, S. B., Braun, A. R., Sargeant, M. N., Reynolds, E. K., Hopko, D. R., Blanco, C., & Lejuez, C. (2008). Effectiveness of a brief behavioral treatment for inner-city illicit drug users with elevated depressive symptoms: The life enhancement treatment for substance use (LETS Act!). *Journal of Clinical Psychiatry, 69*, 122.

Daughters, S. B., Lejuez, C., Kahler, C. W., Strong, D. R., & Brown, R. A. (2005). Psychological distress tolerance and duration of most recent abstinence attempt among residential treatment-seeking substance abusers. *Psychology of Addictive Behaviors, 19*, 208.

Daughters, S. B., Lejuez, C. W., Bornovalova, M. A., Kahler, C. W., Strong, D. R., & Brown, R. A. (2005). Distress tolerance as a predictor of early treatment dropout in a residential substance abuse treatment facility. *Journal of Abnormal Psychology, 114*, 729–734.

Daughters, S. B., Reynolds, E. K., MacPherson, L., Kahler, C. W., Danielson, C. K., Zvolensky, M., & Lejuez, C. W. (2009). Distress tolerance and early adolescent externalizing and internalizing symptoms: The moderating role of gender and ethnicity. *Behaviour Research and Therapy, 47*, 198–205.

de Wit, H., Söderpalm, A. H., Nikolayev, L., & Young, E. (2003). Effects of acute social stress on alcohol consumption in healthy subjects. *Alcoholism: Clinical and Experimental Research, 27*, 1270–1277.

Doremus, T. L., Brunell, S. C., Varlinskaya, E. I., & Spear, L. P. (2003). Anxiogenic effects during withdrawal from acute ethanol in adolescent and adult rats. *Pharmacology Biochemistry and Behavior, 75*, 411–418.

Epstein, D. H., Willner-Reid, J., Vahabzadeh, M., Mezghanni, M., Lin, J. L., & Preston, K. L. (2009). Real-time electronic diary reports of cue exposure and mood in the hours before cocaine and heroin craving and use. *Archives of General Psychiatry, 66,* 88–94. doi: 10.1001/archgenpsychiatry.2008.509

Erb, S., Hitchcott, P. K., Rajabi, H., Mueller, D., Shaham, Y., & Stewart, J. (2000). Alpha-2 adrenergic receptor agonists block stress-induced reinstatement of cocaine seeking. *Neuropsychopharmacology, 23,* 138–150.

Fatseas, M., Denis, C., Massida, Z., Verger, M., Franques-Rénéric, P., & Auriacombe, M. (2011). Cue-induced reactivity, cortisol response and substance use outcome in treated heroin dependent individuals. *Biological Psychiatry, 70,* 720–727.

Fendt, M., & Mucha, R. F. (2001). Anxiogenic-like effects of opiate withdrawal seen in the fear-potentiated startle test, an interdisciplinary probe for drug-related motivational states. *Psychopharmacology, 155,* 242–250.

American Psychiatric Association. (1994). *Diagnostic and statistical manual of mental disorder, Fourth Edition (DSM-4).* Washington, D.C.: American Psychiatric Association.

Fudala, P. J., Jaffe, J. H., Dax, E. M., & Johnson, R. E. (1990). Use of buprenorphine in the treatment of opioid addiction: II. Physiologic and behavioral effects of daily and alternate-day administration and abrupt withdrawal. *Clinical Pharmacology and Therapeutics, 47,* 525–534.

Furnari, M., Epstein, D. H., Phillips, K. A., Jobes, M. L., Kowalczyk, W. J., Vahabzadeh, M., . . . Preston, K. L. (2015). Some of the people, some of the time: Field evidence for associations and dissociations between stress and drug use. *Psychopharmacology, 232,* 3529–3537.

Gehlert, D. R., Cippitelli, A., Thorsell, A., Lê, A. D., Hipskind, P. A., Hamdouchi, C., . . . Song, M. (2007). 3-(4-Chloro-2-morpholin-4-yl-thiazol-5-yl)-8-(1-ethylpropyl)-2, 6-dimethyl-imidazo [1, 2-b] pyridazine: A novel brain-penetrant, orally available corticotropin-releasing factor receptor 1 antagonist with efficacy in animal models of alcoholism. *Journal of Neuroscience, 27,* 2718–2726.

Goeders, N. E. (2002). Stress and cocaine addiction. *Journal of Pharmacology and Experimental Therapeutics, 301,* 785–789.

Gold, M. S., Washton, A. M., & Dackis, C. A. (1985). Cocaine abuse: Neurochemistry, phenomenology, and treatment. *Cocaine use in America: Epidemiologic and clinical perspectives. National Institute on Drug Abuse Research Monograph, 61,* 130–150.

Grant, B. F., Hasin, D. S., Chou, S. P., Stinson, F. S., & Dawson, D. A. (2004). Nicotine dependence and psychiatric disorders in the United States: Results from the national epidemiologic survey on alcohol and related conditions. *Archives of General Psychiatry, 61,* 1107–1115.

Greenfield, S. F., Weiss, R. D., Muenz, L. R., Vagge, L. M., Kelly, J. F., Bello, L. R., & Michael, J. (1998). The effect of depression on return to drinking: A prospective study. *Archives of General Psychiatry, 55,* 259–265.

Hall, S. M., Muñoz, R. F., Reus, V. I., & Sees, K. L. (1993). Nicotine, negative affect, and depression. *Journal of Consulting and Clinical Psychology, 61,* 761.

Hasin, D. S., O'Brien, C. P., Auriacombe, M., Borges, G., Bucholz, K., Budney, A., . . . Petry, N. M. (2013). DSM-5 criteria for substance use disorders: Recommendations and rationale. *American Journal of Psychiatry, 170,* 834–851.

Hayes, S. C. (2004). Acceptance and commitment therapy, relational frame theory, and the third wave of behavioral and cognitive therapies. *Behavior Therapy, 35*, 639–665.

Hayes, S. C., Strosahl, K. D., & Wilson, K. G. (1999). *Acceptance and commitment therapy*: New York, NY: Guilford Press.

Heilig, M., Egli, M., Crabbe, J. C., & Becker, H. C. (2010). Review: Acute withdrawal, protracted abstinence and negative affect in alcoholism: Are they linked? *Addiction Biology, 15*, 169–184.

Hone-Blanchet, A., Ciraulo, D. A., Pascual-Leone, A., & Fecteau, S. (2015). Noninvasive brain stimulation to suppress craving in substance use disorders: Review of human evidence and methodological considerations for future work. *Neuroscience and Biobehavioral Reviews, 59*, 184–200. doi: 10.1016/j.neubiorev.2015.10.001

Jarvik, M. E., Madsen, D. C., Olmstead, R. E., Iwamoto-Schaap, P. N., Elins, J. L., & Benowitz, N. L. (2000). Nicotine blood levels and subjective craving for cigarettes. *Pharmacology Biochemistry and Behavior, 66*, 553–558.

Jorenby, D. E., Hatsukami, D. K., Smith, S. S., Fiore, M. C., Allen, S., Jensen, J., & Baker, T. B. (1996). Characterization of tobacco withdrawal symptoms: Transdermal nicotine reduces hunger and weight gain. *Psychopharmacology, 128*, 130–138.

Kassel, J. D., Stroud, L. R., & Paronis, C. A. (2003). Smoking, stress, and negative affect: Correlation, causation, and context across stages of smoking. *Psychological Bulletin, 129*, 270.

Kenford, S. L., Smith, S. S., Wetter, D. W., Jorenby, D. E., Fiore, M. C., & Baker, T. B. (2002). Predicting relapse back to smoking: Contrasting affective and physical models of dependence. *Journal of Consulting and Clinical Psychology, 70*, 216.

Kennedy, A. P., Epstein, D. H., Phillips, K. A., & Preston, K. L., (2013). Sex differences in cocaine/heroin users: Drug-use triggers and craving in daily life. *Drug and Alcohol Dependence, 132*, 29–37.

Keyes, K. M., Hatzenbuehler, M. L., & Hasin, D. S. (2011). Stressful life experiences, alcohol consumption, and alcohol use disorders: The epidemiologic evidence for four main types of stressors. *Psychopharmacology, 218*, 1–17.

Koob, G. F., & Le Moal, M. (1997). Drug abuse: Hedonic homeostatic dysregulation. *Science, 278*(5335), 52–58.

Koob, G. F., & Le Moal, M. (2001). Drug addiction, dysregulation of reward, and allostasis. *Neuropsychopharmacology, 24*, 97–129.

Koob, G. F., & Le Moal, M. (2008). Neurobiological mechanisms for opponent motivational processes in addiction. *Philosophical Transactions of the Royal Society of London B: Biological Sciences, 363*, 3113–3123.

Koob, G. F., & Mason, B. J. (2016). Existing and future drugs for the treatment of the dark side of addiction. *Annual Review of Pharmacology and Toxicology, 56*, 299–322. doi: 10.1146/annurev-pharmtox-010715-103143

Koob, G. F., & Volkow, N. D. (2010). Neurocircuitry of addiction. *Neuropsychopharmacology, 35*, 217–238.

Kosman, M. E., & Unna, D. (1967). Effects of chronic administration of the amphetamines and other stimulants on behavior. *Clinical Pharmacology and Therapeutics, 9*, 240–254.

Kushner, M. G., Sher, K. J., & Erickson, D. J. (1999). Prospective analysis of the relation between DSM-III anxiety disorders and alcohol use disorders. *American Journal of Psychiatry, 156*, 723–732.

Lago, J. A., & Kosten, T. R. (1994). Stimulant withdrawal. *Addiction, 89*, 1477–1481.

Linehan, M. (1993). *Cognitive-behavioral treatment of borderline personality disorder*. New York, NY: Guilford Press.

Linehan, M. M., Dimeff, L. A., Reynolds, S. K., Comtois, K. A., Welch, S. S., Heagerty, P., & Kivlahan, D. R. (2002). Dialectical behavior therapy versus comprehensive validation therapy plus 12-step for the treatment of opioid dependent women meeting criteria for borderline personality disorder. *Drug and Alcohol Dependence, 67*, 13–26.

Magidson, J. F., Gorka, S. M., MacPherson, L., Hopko, D. R., Blanco, C., Lejuez, C., & Daughters, S. B. (2011). Examining the effect of the Life Enhancement Treatment for Substance Use (LETS ACT) on residential substance abuse treatment retention. *Addictive Behaviors, 36*, 615–623.

Mansky, P. A. (1978). Opiates: Human psychopharmacology. In L. L. Iversen (Ed.), *Handbook of Psychopharmacology: Drugs of abuse* (pp. 95–185). New York, NY: Springer US.

Marlatt, G. A., & Gordon, J. R. (1980). Determinants of relapse: Implications for the maintenance of behavioral change. In P. O. Davison & S. M. Davidson (Eds.), *Behavioral medicine: Changing health lifestyles* (pp. 410–452). New York, NY: Brunner/Mazel.

McCarthy, D. E., Piasecki, T. M., Fiore, M. C., & Baker, T. B. (2006). Life before and after quitting smoking: An electronic diary study. *Journal of Abnormal Psychology, 115*, 454–466. doi: 10.1037/0021-843X.115.3.454

McGrath, E., Jones, A., & Field, M. (2016). Acute stress increases ad-libitum alcohol consumption in heavy drinkers, but not through impaired inhibitory control. *Psychopharmacology, 233*, 1227–1234.

McHugh, R. K., Park, S., & Weiss, R. D. (2014). Cue-induced craving in dependence upon prescription opioids and heroin. *American Journal on Addictions, 23*, 453–458.

Nakajima, M., & al'Absi, M. (2012). Predictors of risk for smoking relapse in men and women: A prospective examination. *Psychology of Addictive Behaviors, 26*, 633.

O'Reardon, J. P., Solvason, H. B., Janicak, P. G., Sampson, S., Isenberg, K. E., Nahas, Z., . . . Sackeim, H. A. (2007). Efficacy and safety of transcranial magnetic stimulation in the acute treatment of major depression: A multisite randomized controlled trial. *Biological Psychiatry, 62*, 1208–1216. doi: 10.1016/j.biopsych.2007.01.018

Pettinati, H. M., O'Brien, C. P., & Dundon, W. D. (2013). Current status of co-occurring mood and substance use disorders: A new therapeutic target. *American Journal of Psychiatry, 170*, 23–30.

Piasecki, T. M., Niaura, R., Shadel, W. G., Abrams, D., Goldstein, M., Fiore, M. C., & Baker, T. B. (2000). Smoking withdrawal dynamics in unaided quitters. *Journal of Abnormal Psychology, 109*, 74.

Possemato, K., Maisto, S. A., Wade, M., Barrie, K., McKenzie, S., Lantinga, L. J., & Ouimette, P. (2015). Ecological momentary assessment of PTSD symptoms and alcohol use in combat veterans. *Psychology of Addictive Behaviors, 29*, 894.

Prediger, R. D., da Silva, G. E., Batista, L. C., Bittencourt, A. L., & Takahashi, R. N. (2006). Activation of adenosine A1 receptors reduces anxiety-like behavior during acute ethanol withdrawal (hangover) in mice. *Neuropsychopharmacology, 31*, 2210–2220.

Preston, K. L., & Epstein, D. H. (2011). Stress in the daily lives of cocaine and heroin users: Relationship to mood, craving, relapse triggers, and cocaine use. *Psychopharmacology, 218*, 29–37. doi: 10.1007/s00213-011-2183-x

Regier, D. A., Farmer, M. E., Rae, D. S., Locke, B. Z., Keith, S. J., Judd, L. L., & Goodwin, F. K. (1990). Comorbidity of mental disorders with alcohol and other drug abuse: Results from the Epidemiologic Catchment Area (ECA) Study. *Journal of the American Medical Association, 264*, 2511–2518.

Rigg, K. K., & Ibañez, G. E. (2010). Motivations for non-medical prescription drug use: A mixed methods analysis. *Journal of Substance Abuse Treatment, 39*, 236–247.

Russell, J. A., & Carroll, J. M. (1999). On the bipolarity of positive and negative affect. *Psychological Bulletin, 125*, 3–30.

San Jose, B., Van Oers, H. A., Van De Mheen, H. D., Garretsen, H. F., & Mackenbach, J. P. (2000). Stressors and alcohol consumption. *Alcohol and Alcoholism, 35*, 307–312.

Seo, D., Lacadie, C. M., Tuit, K., Hong, K. I., Constable, R. T., & Sinha, R. (2013). Disrupted ventromedial prefrontal function, alcohol craving, and subsequent relapse risk. *JAMA Psychiatry, 70*, 727–739. doi: 10.1001/jamapsychiatry.2013.762

Shiffman, S., & Waters, A. J. (2004). Negative affect and smoking lapses: A prospective analysis. *Journal of Consulting and Clinical Psychology, 72*, 192–201. doi: 10.1037/0022-006X.72.2.192

Shiyko, M. P., Burkhalter, J., Li, R., & Park, B. J. (2014). Modeling nonlinear time-dependent treatment effects: An application of the generalized time-varying effect model (TVEM). *Journal of Consulting and Clinical Psychology, 82*, 760–772. doi: 10.1037/a0035267

Singleton, E. G., Tiffany, S. T., & Henningfield, J. E. (1994). *The multidimensional aspects of craving for alcohol.* Intramural Research Program Report. Baltimore, MD: National Institute on Drug Abuse, National Institutes of Health.

Sinha, R. (2012). How does stress lead to risk of alcohol relapse? *Alcohol Research: Current Reviews, 34*, 432.

Sinha, R., Catapano, D., & O'Malley, S. (1999). Stress-induced craving and stress response in cocaine dependent individuals. *Psychopharmacology, 142*, 343–351.

Sinha, R., Fox, H. C., Hong, K.-I. A., Hansen, J., Tuit, K., & Kreek, M. J. (2011). Effects of adrenal sensitivity, stress-and cue-induced craving, and anxiety on subsequent alcohol relapse and treatment outcomes. *Archives of General Psychiatry, 68*, 942–952.

Sinha, R., Garcia, M., Paliwal, P., Kreek, M. J., & Rounsaville, B. J. (2006). Stress-induced cocaine craving and hypothalamic-pituitary adrenal responses are predictive of cocaine relapse outcomes. *Archives of General Psychiatry, 63*, 324–331.

Sinha, R., Lacadie, C., Skudlarski, P., Fulbright, R. K., Rounsaville, B. J., Kosten, T. R., & Wexler, B. E. (2005). Neural activity associated with stress-induced cocaine craving: a functional magnetic resonance imaging study. *Psychopharmacology, 183*, 171–180. doi: 10.1007/s00213-005-0147-8

Solomon, R. L. (1980). The opponent-process theory of acquired motivation: The costs of pleasure and the benefits of pain. *American Psychologist, 35*, 691.

Solomon, R. L., & Corbit, J. D. (1974). An opponent-process theory of motivation: I. Temporal dynamics of affect. *Psychological Review, 81*, 119.

Strong, D. R., Brown, R. A., Sims, M., Herman, D. S., Anderson, B. J., & Stein, M. D. (2012). Persistence on a stress-challenge task before initiating buprenorphine treatment was associated with successful transition from opioid use to early abstinence. *Journal of Addiction Medicine, 6*, 219–225. doi: 10.1097/ADM.0b013e31825d927f

Tiffany, S. T., & Drobes, D. J. (1991). The development and initial validation of a questionnaire on smoking urges. *British Journal of Addiction, 86*, 1467–1476.

Tiffany, S. T., Fields, L., Singleton, E., Haertzen, C., & Henningfield, J. E. (1996). The development of a heroin craving questionnaire. *Unpublished raw data* (1995).

Tiffany, S. T., Singleton, E., Haertzen, C. A., & Henningfield, J. E. (1993). The development of a cocaine craving questionnaire. *Drug and Alcohol Dependence, 34*, 19–28.

Tiffany, S. T., & Wray, J. M. (2012). The clinical significance of drug craving. *Annals of the New York Academy of Sciences, 1248*, 1–17. doi: 10.1111/j.1749-6632.2011.06298.x

Tull, M. T., Gratz, K. L., Coffey, S. F., Weiss, N. H., & McDermott, M. J. (2013). Examining the interactive effect of posttraumatic stress disorder, distress tolerance, and gender on residential substance use disorder treatment retention. *Psychology of Addictive Behaviors, 27*, 763–773. doi: 10.1037/a0029911

UNODC. (2012). *World drug report 2012* (Vol. E.12.XI.1): United Nations Publications.

Van Zundert, R. M., Engels, R. C., & Kuntsche, E. (2011). Contextual correlates of adolescents' self-efficacy after smoking cessation. *Psychology of Addictive Behaviors, 25*, 301–311. doi: 10.1037/a0023629

Walsh, K., Resnick, H. S., Danielson, C. K., McCauley, J. L., Saunders, B. E., & Kilpatrick, D. G. (2014). Patterns of drug and alcohol use associated with lifetime sexual revictimization and current posttraumatic stress disorder among three national samples of adolescent, college, and household-residing women. *Addictive Behaviors, 39*, 684–689.

Watson, D., & Tellegen, A. (1999). Issues in the dimensional structure of affect—Effects of descriptors, measurement error, and response formats: Comment on Russell and Carroll. *Psychological Bulletin, 125*, 601–610.

Whittle, E. L., Fogarty, A. S., Tugendrajch, S., Player, M. J., Christensen, H., Wilhelm, K., . . . Proudfoot, J. (2015). Men, depression, and coping: Are we on the right path? *Psychology of Men and Masculinity, 16*, 426.

Winward, J. L., Bekman, N. M., Hanson, K. L., Lejuez, C. W., & Brown, S. A. (2014). Changes in emotional reactivity and distress tolerance among heavy drinking adolescents during sustained abstinence. *Alcoholism: Clinical and Experimental Research, 38*, 1761–1769. doi: 10.1111/acer.12415

Wise, R. A., & Koob, G. F. (2014). The development and maintenance of drug addiction. *Neuropsychopharmacology, 39*, 254–262.

Witkiewitz, K., Marlatt, G. A., & Walker, D. (2005). Mindfulness-based relapse prevention for alcohol and substance use disorders. *Journal of Cognitive Psychotherapy, 19*, 211–228.

World Health Organization. (1992). *The ICD-10 classification of mental and behavioural disorders: Clinical descriptions and diagnostic guidelines*: Geneva: World Health Organization.

Zvolensky, M. J., Bakhshaie, J., Sheffer, C., Perez, A., & Goodwin, R. D. (2015). Major depressive disorder and smoking relapse among adults in the United States: A 10-year, prospective investigation. *Psychiatry Research, 226*, 73–77.

15

Feeling Hot Hot Hot

Affective Determinants of Sexual Behavior

NATASHA S. HANSEN, ARIELLE S. GILLMAN,
SARAH W. FELDSTEIN EWING, AND ANGELA D. BRYAN

Sex in its many forms is an almost universal human practice. According to data from the Centers for Disease Control (CDC), 97% of men and 98% of women aged 15–44 in the United States report having had penile-vaginal intercourse; 90% of men and 88% of women report having had oral sex with an opposite sex partner; 40% of men and 35% of women report have had anal sex with an opposite sex partner; 6.5% of men report having had oral or anal sex with another man; and 11% of women report having had a sexual experience with another woman (Mosher, Chandra, & Jones, 2005). Further, in a global survey of over 26,000 adults spanning 26 countries, two-thirds (67%) reported having had sex at least once in the past week, with rates ranging from 38% in Japan, and 57% in the United States, to 89% in Greece (Wylie, 2009). Sex is also an important health behavior, one that has been shown to have significant impacts spanning physiological, psychological, and interpersonal domains.

Given its ubiquity and its potential for widespread health impacts, understanding the determinants of sexual behaviors has become a topic of considerable scientific investigation. There are numerous cognitive, hormonal, cultural, and situational factors that may influence the likelihood that an individual will engage in a particular sexual behavior, and it would take volumes to detail all that is known about each of these determinants. Instead, this chapter begins by briefly describing the evidence for why sex should be considered an important health behavior, including the health benefits associated with certain sexual behaviors and risks associated with others, and then outlines the research on affective determinants of sexual behavior. The scientific literature on this topic is complex and still growing, but it is our hope to provide an overview of the intricate ways in which our emotions may help shape our sexual experiences.

A brief note on terminology: the distinguished affective scientist James Gross notes that there has been considerable debate in the scientific community about the best way to define the closely-related terms "affect," "mood," and "emotion," largely because these terms are derived from the vernacular and are commonly used interchangeably to refer to a wide array of internal states ranging from mild to intense, and momentary to prolonged (see Gross, 2010). Gross defines "affect" as an umbrella term referring to internal states ranging from positive to negative in valance, and this definition is consistent with other widely used definitions of affect that describe the "global affective space" of pleasure/displeasure (Ekkekakis, 2009). According to Gross's perspective, there are three types of affective states: *moods, emotions*, and *attitudes. Attitude* refers to a person's relatively stable valenced judgments about the goodness or badness of a person or thing that influence how that person will feel, think, or behave toward that person or thing. *Mood* is a more diffuse and undirected global state, lasting longer than an emotion but not as long as an attitude. *Emotion*, the most transient of the affective states, is an immediate internal response to a stimulus event, often leading to physiological, behavioral, and experiential changes. Despite the apparent utility of such precise definitions, much of the literature on affect and sexual behavior does not align directly with these subtle distinctions, and many authors still use the terms interchangeably. Thus, for this chapter, we use the original descriptions, and note when we are referring to the construct of affect more broadly, or emotion, mood, or attitudes more specifically.

SEX AS AN IMPORTANT HEALTH BEHAVIOR: PHYSIOLOGICAL AND PSYCHOLOGICAL BENEFITS

In terms of physiological health benefits, greater frequency of sexual intercourse has been shown to predict increased cardiovascular health in both men and women (Brody, Veit, & Rau, 2000), as well as healthier blood pressure (Brody, 2006), and improved resting heart rate variability, a measure associated with lower mortality rates, greater self-regulation, and improved stress resilience (Brody et al., 2000). Vaginal intercourse has been shown to help improve and maintain women's vaginal health and pelvic function (Levin, 2003), and vaginal self-stimulation appears to have pain-relieving properties above and beyond the effects of distraction (Whipple & Komisaruk, 1988). Other studies have similarly found that women with more lifetime sex partners had lower rates of breast cancer (Rossing, Stanford, Weiss, & Daling, 1996), and that exposure to semen through unprotected penile-vaginal intercourse is associated with decreased risk of breast cancer (Lê, Bacheloti, & Hill, 1989). There is also evidence of a negative correlation between intercourse frequency and incidence of prostate cancer (Bosland, 1988).

Consensual sexual activity has also been linked to numerous psychological and interpersonal health benefits. More frequent sexual intercourse has been associated with increased mental health satisfaction, and relationship satisfaction in both genders (Brody, 2007; Brody & Costa, 2009). There is even some suggestion that people with a more active sex life live longer. One longitudinal study that followed 918 men for 10 years found that those with the greatest frequency of orgasms were 50% less likely to die, even after controlling for age, social class, blood pressure, smoking, and coronary heart disease at baseline (Smith, Frankel, & Yarnell, 1997). Another longitudinal study, tracking both men and women (total

N = 252) for 25 years, found that more frequent sex predicted a lower annual death rate among men (Palmore, 1982). Interestingly, for women in this same study it was the *quality* rather than quantity of intercourse that predicted mortality—in other words, enjoyment of intercourse rather than frequency predicted lowered likelihood of premature death for women (Palmore, 1982).

SEX AS AN IMPORTANT HEALTH BEHAVIOR: PHYSIOLOGICAL AND PSYCHOLOGICAL RISKS

There are also significant physiological and psychological health risks associated with certain sexual behaviors.[1] More than any other sexual behavior, penetrative sex without a condom puts people at risk of sexually transmitted infections (STIs) and unplanned pregnancy (CDC, 2016). Unplanned pregnancies, especially among teenagers, often have costly health consequences for both mother and child, including putting the mother at increased risk for depression, substance abuse, intimate partner violence, low educational attainment, and poverty, and her child at risk for abuse, neglect, mental illness, addiction, inferior cognitive and language skills, low educational attainment, poverty, prison, and becoming a teen parent (Ruedinger & Cox, 2012). Sexually transmitted infections can pose equally serious health threats. According to data from the World Health Organization, more than 1 million STIs are acquired daily worldwide (World Health Organization, 2016). While the majority of STIs have only mild symptoms and can be treated easily, several of the diseases spread through unprotected sex can have devastating health consequences and some, such as HIV/AIDS, are still incurable and if left untreated can be fatal (WHO, 2016). In November 2016, the United Nations AIDS Organization reported that there were 36.7 million people living with HIV/AIDS globally, with 2.1 million new infections occurring in 2015 alone (UN AIDS Organization, 2016). Although AIDS-related deaths have been on the decline since 2005, at least 46% of people living with the virus worldwide still do not have access to treatment, and there were an estimated 1.1 million deaths attributable to the effects of HIV/AIDs in 2015 alone (UN AIDS Organization, 2016). The spread of HIV/AIDS and other STIs is by no means limited to developing nations. In 2015, 29,747 people in the European Union and Economic Area, and 39,513 people in the United States were diagnosed with HIV (ECDC, 2016; CDC, 2016). Although HIV/AIDS can be transmitted through other means, such as contaminated drug injection equipment, the vast majority of infections are attributable to unprotected sex, both penile-vaginal and penile-anal (ECDC, 2016; CDC, 2016).

AFFECTIVE DETERMINANTS OF SEXUAL BEHAVIORS: SEXUAL INTERCOURSE FREQUENCY

Given that sex is often a highly emotionally charged experience, it is unsurprising that certain affective states have been closely tied to sexual behaviors. Numerous studies have examined the connection between affect and the frequency of sexual intercourse. These studies have consistently demonstrated a strong positive association between self-reported happiness, as well as overall mental health and emotional well-being, and greater sexual intercourse frequency (e.g., Blanchflower & Oswald, 2004; Brody & Costa, 2009; Cheng & Smyth, 2015). Due to the correlational nature of the vast majority of this research, it is challenging to establish the nature of the causal relationship between affective states and intercourse frequency. Nevertheless, it is certainly reasonable to posit that happy people engage in more frequent sex, and the association between happiness and sex has been shown in research conducted around the world and in several sizable samples. For example, happiness was shown to predict higher intercourse frequency in a nationally representative US sample of 16,000 men and women of all ages (Blanchflower & Oswald, 2004), and the same positive correlation was observed in a sample of 3,800 Chinese adults (Cheng & Smyth, 2015). Furthermore, happier people have been shown to have better quality sex, and more emotional and physical satisfaction with their sex partners (Cheng & Smyth, 2015), and positive mood has been shown to predict increased sexual activity the subsequent day (Burleson, Trevathan, & Todd, 2007). There is also evidence that elevated mood states can cause increased sexual desire and higher intercourse frequency. At the extreme high end of the positive affect spectrum, hypomania and mania are states characterized by expansive mood, euphoria (and/or irritability), and elevated energy levels. Heightened sex drive is a hallmark of hypomania/mania and is included as a core symptom on common clinical diagnostic scales for the condition (e.g., Young, Biggs, Ziegler, & Meyer, 1978). During such elevated mood states, adolescents with symptoms of mania have been shown to seek out more and riskier sexual behaviors than age-matched controls (Brown et al., 2010).

The effects of *low* positive affect and of negative mood on intercourse frequency and sexual interest have been less consistent. At the extreme low end of the positive affect spectrum, depression is a state characterized by hopelessness, lethargy, and lack of interest or pleasure in formerly enjoyed activities. Diminished interest in sex is one of the symptoms on commonly used depression evaluation scales (Beck, Steer, & Carbin, 1988; Reynolds & Kobak, 1995), and individuals with elevated symptoms of depression tend to report low libido (e.g., Casper et al., 1985) as well as significantly less sexual arousal and fewer orgasms than those experiencing higher levels of positive affect (Frohlich & Meston, 2002). However, in a study of 663 undergraduate women, although negative mood states such as depression and anxiety predicted diminished interest in sex in most participants, 40% of the women reported no relationship between negative mood and sex, and a small minority (9.5%) reported an *increase* in sexual interest while feeling anxious or depressed (Lykins, Janssen, & Graham, 2006).

AFFECT AND SEX IN THE CONTEXT OF ROMANTIC RELATIONSHIPS

A large body of research in the affect and sex domain has focused on sex in the context of a relationship. Overall, the literature has shown a strong association between relationship satisfaction and sexual satisfaction within that relationship, which in turn is often positively correlated with intercourse frequency (e.g., Brody & Costa, 2009; Byers, 2005; Hurlbert & Apt, 1994; Laumann et al., 2006). This association between emotional satisfaction and sexual satisfaction appears to be cross-cultural. For example, a large cross-national study that surveyed 27,500 men and women, aged 40–80 years, spanning 29 countries found a strong association between emotional satisfaction within a relationship and the couple's frequency of sexual intercourse, as well as the amount of time spent in foreplay (Laumann et al., 2006).

There is some suggestion that relationship satisfaction may be associated with certain sexual behaviors more than others. In a study of heterosexual American couples, marital satisfaction was shown to be significantly related to the frequency of penile-vaginal intercourse (PVI) but not oral sex (Hurlbert & Apt, 1994). Similar results were reported for a small sample of Portuguese women: those who reported the highest levels of love, trust, intimacy, passion, and emotional satisfaction with their partners also reported the highest frequency of orgasms during PVI (Costa & Brody, 2007). A large study of Swedish couples (n = 2,810) similarly found a positive correlation between relationship satisfaction and PVI specifically (Brody & Costa, 2009). More research is needed to examine the affective predictors of specific sexual behaviors within gay, lesbian, and transgender couples.

Though these correlational studies cannot provide evidence for the presence or direction of a causal relationship, several longitudinal studies suggest a temporal association between affective states and sex between romantic couples. A longitudinal study of 87 long-term couples tracked over 18 months showed that each partner's affective evaluation of the relationship and their sexual satisfaction varied concurrently (Byers, 2005). Another longitudinal study of mood and sexual activity tracked middle-aged women for 9 months and showed that positive mood one day predicted increased physical affection and sexual activity with the partner the following day, though interestingly negative mood was shown to be unrelated to sexual activity (Burleson et al., 2007). Together, these studies suggest a relationship between mood, emotional intimacy with the partner, and sexual activity whereby couples experiencing more positive mood states and greater feelings of emotional satisfaction within a relationship are more likely to engage in more sexual activity, and satisfying sexual interactions with the romantic partner may in turn lift mood and promote further emotional intimacy.

AFFECTIVE DETERMINANTS OF SEXUAL AROUSAL

Another aspect of sexual behavior that has received considerable scientific attention is the relationship between affect and sexual arousal. Mood has been shown to significantly impact the likelihood that an individual will become aroused in a sexual context. Such studies either measure naturally occurring affective states, or induce desired states, and then assess subjective and/or physiological arousal in response to an erotic stimulus. For example, in an empirical study of sexually functional males (n = 24), a within-subjects design was used to test whether inducing positive versus negative mood would influence subjective arousal and/or erectile response during an erotic film (Mitchell, Dibartolo, Brown, & Barlow, 1998). Mood was assessed with the Positive and Negative Affect Schedule (PANAS; Watson, Clark, & Tellegen, 1988), a widely used 20-item scale specifically designed to measure levels of both positive activated affective states (e.g., inspired, interested, enthusiastic, proud) and negative activated affective states (e.g., distressed, ashamed, hostile, scared). Mood manipulation was achieved by means of selected musical pieces, shown in previous studies to reliably alter mood in the desired manner. Participants showed significantly increased subjective and objective sexual arousal following the positive mood induction. Other studies of sexually functional males have similarly found that positive affect was subsequently associated with higher subjective and physiological sexual arousal (Nobre et al., 2004). Results for negative mood in men have been less consistent. The previously described empirical mood induction study (Mitchell et al., 1998) found that negative mood induction resulted in significantly diminished objective sexual arousal, but not subjective arousal, relative to baseline and a neutral condition. Another study found that negative mood induction produced diminished and delayed subjective but not physiological sexual arousal in men (Meisler & Carey, 1991), and a further investigation found that state negative affect was unrelated to subsequent arousal, and that trait negative affect was associated with lower subjective sexual arousal but marginally heightened erectile response (Nobre et al., 2004).

Fewer studies have examined the relationship between affect and sexual arousal in women, but there is some evidence to suggest the pattern may differ slightly between the genders. In a study similar to those described previously, positive affect was shown to have a strong positive correlation with both physiological and self-reported sexual arousal in response to a variety of erotic film clips in both men and women, but negative affect had only limited predictive power overall (Peterson & Janssen, 2007). Interestingly, in the same study ambivalence (co-occurring high levels of positive and negative affect) was shown to be a strong positive predictor of sexual arousal in both genders, and indifference (co-occurring low positive and low negative affect) predicted the lowest levels of genital response, particularly among women. A subsequent study showed that inducing happiness in heterosexual women significantly increased subjective sexual arousal and perceived genital sensations in response to an erotic film (Ter Kuile, Both, & Van Uden, 2010). In contrast, after a sad mood induction, women reported experiencing marginally less sexual arousal and fewer genital sensations, although no difference in objective arousal was detected.

Taken together, the results of these studies suggest positive affect may be a stronger predictor of sexual arousal than negative affect, particularly among women, and that lack of sexual arousal may be more attributable to low levels of positive activated affect than high levels of negative activated affect (Ter Kuile et al., 2010). Further research will be needed to parse out more fine-grained distinctions between the effects of specific emotions under the broader umbrellas of positive versus negative affect. For example, it seems plausible that *inspiration* may have a different effect on sexual arousal than *pride*, although both are classified as positive affective states, and similarly that *shame* and *hostility* may have distinct effects on sexual arousal, although both are broadly classified as negative affective states (Watson et al., 1988).

AFFECTIVE DETERMINANTS OF RISKY SEX

Affect appears to play an important role in determining the likelihood that an individual will choose to have unprotected sex, thereby putting themselves and/or their partner at risk for contracting an STI, or of experiencing an unplanned pregnancy. One of the first studies to investigate the affective determinants of sexual risk behavior involved in-depth interviews with self-identified gay men in San Francisco about the emotional contexts in which they were most likely to engage in unprotected sex (Díaz, 1999). The men reported that they felt driven to these encounters to fulfill emotional needs beyond simple sexual satisfaction. They said episodes of unprotected sex in particular were most likely to occur in contexts where they were experiencing extreme loneliness or despair, and felt an intense emotional need for interpersonal connection and social acceptance. Abuse of alcohol and other drugs was reported to increase the likelihood of anal sex without a condom by facilitating or justifying sexual encounters that would otherwise have been perceived as frightening or distasteful (Díaz, 1999). Interestingly, negative affect, especially negative emotions such as guilt and regret, after past unprotected sex was reported to increase the likelihood of future unprotected sexual encounters (Díaz, 1999).

Other studies have investigated the role of emotion dysregulation as a mechanism behind risky sexual behavior. Emotion dysregulation may include difficulty managing emotional states, particularly when experiencing emotional distress (Gratz & Roemer, 2004). Emotion dysregulation has been posited to be a component of other health risk behaviors, including substance use (Dvorak et al., 2014), self-harm (Gratz & Tull, 2010), and suicidal ideation (Anestis, Bagge, Tull, & Joiner, 2011). Some have suggested that risky sex, including intercourse without a condom and sex under the influence of substances, may also represent a strategy that individuals employ in an effort to increase positive affect and/or diminish negative affect and distress (e.g., Orcutt, Cooper, & Garcia, 2005). Others have theorized that individuals seek out risky sex because they hope that it will mitigate powerful negative affective states such as shame, anger, or sadness (Crepaz & Marks, 2001). A study of 752 college-aged women showed that higher emotion dysregulation predicted disuse of condoms or other form of contraception, along with higher lifetime number of sexual partners, and greater likelihood of sexual intercourse under the influence of alcohol or other drugs (Messman-Moore, Walsh, & DiLillo, 2010). Of note, emotion dysregulation significantly predicted condomless sex with a stranger, but not with a long-term dating partner. Emotion dysregulation has also been linked to other sexual risk behaviors, including sex for money or drugs, sex while intoxicated, and sex without a condom among individuals with a substance use disorder (Tull, Weiss, Adams, & Gratz, 2012). These relationships remained robust even after controlling for other known contributors to risky sex, including depression, trauma exposure, sensation seeking, substance use, and demographic factors (e.g., age, gender, marital status).

Although research in this area has focused primarily on *negative* mood states, at least one study has suggested that *positive* emotional urgency, defined as "the tendency to engage in rash action in response to extreme positive affect" (Cyders & Smith, 2008, p. 807), also predicted increased risky sexual behaviors among young adults ($n = 407$), including sex without a condom, sex without birth control, and sex in the context of substance use (Zapolski, Cyders, & Smith, 2009). Negative emotional urgency, defined as "the tendency to engage in rash action in response to extreme negative affect" (Cyders & Smith, 2008; p. 807), was also predictive of risky sex, even after controlling for gender and personality dispositions toward impulsivity. Although positive emotional urgency and negative emotional urgency were significantly correlated with one another, both constructs independently predicted risky sex.

It is noteworthy that most of the research on affective determinants of sexual risk behavior has included the role of substance use in this equation, either as a predictor of unprotected sex, or as one type of risky sexual behavior (e.g., sex while under the influence). One hypothesis is that intoxicants, such as alcohol, may interfere with emotion regulation and self-control resources, thereby increasing the likelihood of engaging in risky sex (Orcutt et al., 2005; Tull et al., 2012). Another possibility is that drugs such as alcohol may heighten states of positive or negative emotional urgency (Zapolski et al., 2009), and/or may hamper the experience of negative affective states (e.g., fear, reluctance, distaste) that might otherwise protect individuals from engaging in dangerous sexual situations (Díaz, 1999). Future research that clarifies the interplay between affect and emotion dysregulation, substance use, and risky sex could help inform interventions aimed at decreasing unwanted pregnancies and the transmission of HIV/AIDS and other STIs.

AFFECTIVE ATTITUDES AND RISKY SEX

Affect and risky sexual behavior have also been studied in the context of explicitly endorsed affective attitudes about factors contributing to safer or unsafe sex (e.g., attitudes toward condom use or having casual partners). Much of this research draws on the social cognitive tradition, in which theories assume behavior to be intentional, planned, and deliberate. A popular theory that often frames this work is the theory of planned behavior (TPB; Ajzen & Madden, 1986), which states that attitudes (along with social norms and perceived behavioral control) influence behavior consciously through their impact on explicit intentions to engage in the behavior. That is, if a person feels positively about condom use (e.g., believes they will feel safer if they use condoms), they will plan to use condoms during their sexual encounters (e.g., making explicit plans, buying condoms), and these intentions should translate to behavior engagement (i.e., actually using a condom during sex). The TPB model has been used extensively to study the influence of attitudes in the context of risky sexual behavior, and condom use in particular; a 2001 meta-analysis of the TPB in the context of condom use found that attitudes about condoms were correlated with intentions to use condoms at .58, more strongly than perceived behavioral control and norms (correlated at .45 and .39, respectively) (Albarracín, Johnson, Fishbein, & Muellerleile, 2001).

While social-cognitive models of behavior (i.e., TPB) traditionally assume that attitudes strictly influence behavior through intentions, recently, others have argued that health behavior is often engaged in automatically or impulsively, without conscious awareness, and is informed by "gut" reactions (Sheeran, Gollwitzer, & Bargh, 2013). In support of this idea, the authors of the 2001 meta-analysis tested a model of the alternative hypothesis that attitudes may directly predict behavior, rather than solely working through more elaborate intentions. This model also fit the data well, and the strength of the relationship between attitudes and behavior (.21) was similar to that of intentions and behavior (.26) (Albarracín et al., 2001). These findings suggest that there may be some situations under which attitudes influence behavior more directly rather than through intentions.

To refine this theory further, some have argued that the measurement of attitudes in the TPB framework should be more nuanced; attitudes are typically measured as responses to semantic differential scales representing an individual's explicit beliefs regarding condoms across several global evaluative dimensions ("I think using condoms every time I have sex would be: beneficial/harmful, good/bad, healthy/unhealthy, pleasant/unpleasant, enjoyable/unenjoyable) (Ajzen & Madden, 1986; Conner, Graham, & Moore, 1999; Montanaro & Bryan, 2014). Other studies have separated the measurement of attitudes into *cognitive/instrumental attitudes*, or those representing an individual's beliefs about the utility or benefit of using condoms for one's health, and *affective/experiential attitudes*, or those representing an individual's valenced/emotionally laden evaluation of condom use (e.g., "Condoms take away the pleasure of sex."). Studies that have measured affective attitudes separately have found these types of attitudes to explain variance in condom use intentions over and above cognitive factors (Bryan, Aiken, & West, 1996, 1997) and to also correlate with condom use even when controlling for intentions (Bryan, Aiken, & West, 2004; Bryan, Rocheleau, Robbins, & Hutchison, 2005), providing support for the idea that affective attitudes in particular may influence behavior without working through conscious awareness.

Studies that have measured or manipulated affective attitudes implicitly (rather than through a self-report questionnaire) further support their potential influence on automatic routes to risky sexual behavior engagement. For example, a study by Czopp, Monteith, Zimmerman, and Lynam (2004) used an implicit associations task (IAT) to measure implicit positive versus negative associations with condom use and also measured self-reported explicit attitudes. They found that while *explicit* attitudes toward condoms significantly predicted intentions to use condoms in a situation with strong explicit cues for safer sexual behavior (thus theoretically calling for a more "controlled" process of decision-making), *implicit* attitudes predicted intentions to use condoms in a situation with fewer cues for safer sex (theoretically leading to a more "automatic" route to decision-making) (Czopp et al., 2004).[2] Another study by Ellis et al. manipulated affective associations with condoms using an evaluative conditioning procedure, in which images of condoms were either paired with positive words or neutral words. Participants in the condom-positive condition were more likely to take free condoms when leaving the laboratory than those in the neutral condition (Ellis, Homish, Parks, Collins, & Kiviniemi, 2015). Finally, Tybur and colleagues implicitly manipulated the emotion of disgust by exposing one group of participants to a noxious smell while completing study procedures, in order to examine whether olfactory pathogen cues might lead to disease avoidance behavior (operationalized as intentions to use condoms). Participants in this condition reported stronger intentions to use condoms after experiencing the emotion of disgust as compared to those in the control condition (Tybur, Bryan, Magnan, & Hooper, 2011).

ANTICIPATED AFFECTIVE RESPONSES AND RISKY SEX

A substantial body of literature also supports *anticipated* affect as a way that affect and emotion influence decisions to engage in risky sexual behavior, over and above TPB variables and affective attitudes. Anticipated affect differs from affective attitudes in that they do not describe an individual's evaluation (implicit or explicit) of a particular behavior, but rather involve that person's expected emotional state if a behavior were (or were not) to be engaged in. Together, both affective attitudes and anticipated affect have been shown to predict health behavior intentions across a wide range of behaviors over and above TPB variables (Conner, McEachan, Taylor, O'Hara, & Lawton, 2015). Most commonly, research on anticipated affective responses center around expectations regarding the emotion of regret. Regret has been identified by affective scientists as a specific negative emotional state that induces individuals to change or desire to change their behavior after a negative course of action caused by the self (Roseman, Wiest, & Swartz, 1994; Zeelenberg, van Dijk, Manstead, & der Pligt, 1998). In general, people seek to avoid regret (Gilovich & Medvec, 1995), and thus, will modify their behavior if they anticipate that they might feel regretful in the future. Interestingly, the largest area of the literature on anticipated regret in health behavior is in the context of safer/unsafe sexual practices (Koch, 2014). Anticipated regret significantly predicts intentions to use condoms over and above TPB variables (Abraham, Henderson, & Der, 2004; Conner et al., 1999; Hynie, MacDonald, & Marques, 2006). Supporting the idea that regret is focused toward a negative outcome caused by the self, a study by Barker, Buunk, and Manstead (1997) found that participants were more likely to report using condoms if they anticipated negative feelings if they were not to use a condom (and positive feelings having used them). This association was moderated by self-efficacy, such that this relationship was particularly strong if participants felt that condom use was under their control (Barker et al., 1997). Expanding beyond condom use, Conner and Flesch (2001) found that more positive anticipated affective reactions toward a hypothetical casual sex scenario were associated with stronger intentions to engage in casual sex. Notably, gender may be an important consideration when examining the influence of anticipated regret on sexual behavior; one study found that women are generally more likely to regret sexual actions compared to men, who are more likely to regret sexual *in*action (Galperin et al., 2013).

SUMMARY AND CONCLUSION

Consensual sex is an almost universal human experience that is associated with stress resilience, improved cardiovascular health, lower rates of prostate and breast cancer, and increased life expectancy. At the same time, sexual activity can pose the risk of significant negative health impacts such as unplanned pregnancy or STIs. Affect has been shown to be a potentially significant determinant of both healthy and risky sexual behaviors. Happy people tend to have a higher frequency of sexual intercourse, and for those in relationships, higher affective relationship satisfaction predicts both the frequency and quality of sexual activity. Mood influences the likelihood that a person will become sexually aroused, and positive affect may be a stronger predictor of sexual arousal than negative affect, particularly among women. Risky sex may serve as a maladaptive emotion regulation strategy, especially in combination with intoxicants. Both implicit and explicit affective attitudes have also been shown to play a role in determining the likelihood that an individual will engage in risky sex, predicting both the intention to use condoms and condom use behavior directly.

Because sex is such an important and ubiquitous health behavior, one that influences multiple domains of physical and psychological health, it is essential that the role of affect, mood, and emotion in sexual behavior be acknowledged, particularly in the context of intervention efforts to improve positive sexual outcomes and reduce sexual risk behavior. Indeed some criticisms of traditional social cognitive perspectives focus on the lack of emphasis on the influence of affect and emotion on health behavior (Conner, Godin, Sheeran, & Germain, 2013; Sniehotta, Presseau, & Araújo-Soares, 2014), and perhaps nowhere is that criticism more appropriate than when examining or trying to change such an emotionally laden health behavior as sexual activity. Our review suggests that important areas for future research involve better methods of establishing the causal effects of affect on sexual behavior, as in many cases the relationships are surely complex and bidirectional, and cross-sectional survey studies simply cannot provide evidence of temporal precedence, much less casual direction. Thus we hope to see more longitudinal and experimental studies, so that the causal role of affect on sexual behavior can be better understood and more effectively used in health behavior interventions.

NOTES

1. We recognize that sexual violence represents a huge risk to both physical and mental health (e.g., Brener, McMahon, Warren, & Douglas, 1999; Faravelli, Giugni, Salvatori, & Ricca, 2004; Fergusson, McLeod, & Horwood, 2013). As such this topic deserves its own treatment and is therefore beyond the scope of this chapter.
2. Interestingly, in this study, implicit attitudes toward condoms were positive at the mean level, that is, people generally had positive automatic associations with condoms.

REFERENCES

Abraham, C., Henderson, M., & Der, G. (2004). Cognitive impact of a research-based school sex education programme. *Psychology and Health, 19*, 689–703. http://doi.org/10.1080/08870440410001722921

Ajzen, I., & Madden, T. J. (1986). Prediction of goal-directed behavior: Attitudes, intentions, and perceived behavioral control. *Journal of Experimental Social Psychology, 22*(5), 453–474. http://doi.org/10.1016/0022-1031(86)90045-4

Albarracín, D., Johnson, B. T., Fishbein, M., & Muellerleile, P. A. (2001). Theories of reasoned action and planned behavior as models of condom use: A meta-analysis. *Psychological Bulletin, 127*, 142–161. http://doi.org/10.1037/0033-2909.127.1.142

Anestis, M. D., Bagge, C. L., Tull, M. T., & Joiner, T. E. (2011). Clarifying the role of emotion dysregulation in the interpersonal-psychological theory of suicidal behavior in an undergraduate sample. *Journal of Psychiatric Research, 45*, 603–611. http://doi.org/10.1016/j.jpsychires.2010.10.013

Barker, A. B., Buunk, B. P., & Manstead, A. S. R. (1997). The moderating role of self-efficacy beliefs in the relationship between anticipated feelings of regret and condom use. *Journal of Applied Social Psychology, 27*, 2001–2014. http://doi.org/10.1111/j.1559-1816.1997.tb01637.x

Beck, A. T., Steer, R. A., & Carbin, M. G. (1988). Psychometric properties of the Beck Depression Inventory: Twenty-five years of evaluation. *Clinical Psychology Review, 8*, 77–100. http://doi.org/10.1016/0272-735890050-5

Blanchflower, D. G., & Oswald, A. J. (2004). Money, sex and happiness: An empirical study. *Scandinavian Journal of Economics, 106*, 393–415. http://doi.org/10.1111/j.0347-0520.2004.00369.x

Bosland, M. C. (1988). The etiopathogenesis of prostatic cancer with special reference to environmental factors. *Advances in Cancer Research, 51*, 1–106. Retrieved from http://www.ncbi.nlm.nih.gov/pubmed/3066144

Brener, N. D., McMahon, P. M., Warren, C. W., & Douglas, K. A. (1999). Forced sexual intercourse and associated health-risk behaviors among female college students in the United States. *Journal of Consulting and Clinical Psychology, 67*, 252–259. Retrieved from http://www.ncbi.nlm.nih.gov/pubmed/10224736

Brody, S. (2006). Blood pressure reactivity to stress is better for people who recently had penile-vaginal intercourse than for people who had other or no sexual activity. *Biological Psychology, 71*, 214–222. http://doi.org/10.1016/j.biopsycho.2005.03.005

Brody, S. (2007). Vaginal orgasm is associated with better psychological function. *Sexual and Relationship Therapy, 22*, 173–191. http://doi.org/10.1080/14681990601059669

Brody, S., & Costa, R. M. (2009). Satisfaction (sexual, life, relationship, and mental health) is associated directly with penile-vaginal intercourse, but inversely with other sexual behavior frequencies. *Journal of Sexual Medicine, 6*, 1947–1954. http://doi.org/10.1111/j.1743-6109.2009.01303.x

Brody, S., Veit, R., & Rau, H. (2000). A preliminary report relating frequency of vaginal intercourse to heart rate variability, Valsalva ratio, blood pressure, and cohabitation status. *Biological Psychology, 52*, 251–257. Retrieved from http://www.ncbi.nlm.nih.gov/pubmed/10725567

Brown, L. K., Hadley, W., Stewart, A., Lescano, C., Whiteley, L., Donenberg, G., . . . Project STYLE Study Group. (2010). Psychiatric disorders and sexual risk among adolescents in mental health treatment. *Journal of Consulting and Clinical Psychology, 78*, 590–597. http://doi.org/10.1037/a0019632

Bryan, A. D., Aiken, L. S., & West, S. G. (1996). Increasing condom use: Evaluation of a theory-based intervention to prevent sexually transmitted diseases in young women. *Health Psychology, 15*, 371–382. http://doi.org/10.1037/0278-6133.15.5.371

Bryan, A. D., Aiken, L. S., & West, S. G. (1997). Young women's condom use: The influence of acceptance of sexuality, control over the sexual encounter, and perceived susceptibility to common STDs. *Health Psychology, 16*, 468–479. http://doi.org/10.1037/0278-6133.16.5.468

Bryan, A., Aiken, L. S., & West, S. G. (2004). HIV/STD risk among incarcerated adolescents: Optimism about the future and self-esteem as predictors of condom use self-efficacy. *Journal of Applied Social Psychology, 34*, 912–936. http://doi.org/10.1111/j.1559-1816.2004.tb02577.x

Bryan, A., Rocheleau, C. A., Robbins, R. N., & Hutchison, K. E. (2005). Condom use among high-risk adolescents: Testing the influence of alcohol use on the relationship of cognitive correlates of behavior. *Health Psychology, 24*, 133–142. http://doi.org/10.1037/0278-6133.24.2.133

Burleson, M. H., Trevathan, W. R., & Todd, M. (2007). In the mood for love or vice versa? Exploring the relations among sexual activity, physical affection, affect, and stress in the daily lives of mid-aged women. *Archives of Sexual Behavior, 36*, 357–368. http://doi.org/10.1007/s10508-006-9071-1

Byers, E. S. (2005). Relationship satisfaction and sexual satisfaction: A longitudinal study of individuals in long-term relationships. *Journal of Sex Research*, *42*, 113–118. http://doi.org/10.1080/00224490509552264

Casper, R. C., Redmond, D. E., Katz, M. M., Schaffer, C. B., Davis, J. M., & Koslow, S. H. (1985). Somatic symptoms in primary affective disorder: Presence and relationship to the classification of depression. *Archives of General Psychiatry*, *42*, 1098–104. Retrieved from http://www.ncbi.nlm.nih.gov/pubmed/3863548

Centers for Disease Control and Prevention. (2016). *HIV in the United States: At a glance*. Retrieved January 8, 2017, from https://www.cdc.gov/hiv/statistics/overview/ataglance.html

Cheng, Z., & Smyth, R. (2015). Sex and happiness. *Journal of Economic Behavior and Organization*, *112*, 26–32. http://doi.org/10.1016/j.jebo.2014.12.030

Conner, M., & Flesch, D. (2001). Having Casual Sex: Additive and Interactive Effects of Alcohol and Condom Availability on the Determinants of Intentions. *Journal of Applied Social Psychology*, *31*(1), 89–112. http://doi.org/10.1111/j.1559-1816.2001.tb02484.x

Conner, M., Godin, G., Sheeran, P., & Germain, M. (2013). Some feelings are more important: Cognitive attitudes, affective attitudes, anticipated affect, and blood donation. *Health Psychology*, *32*, 264–272. http://doi.org/10.1037/a0028500

Conner, M., Graham, S., & Moore, B. (1999). Alcohol and intentions to use condoms: Applying the theory of planned behaviour. *Psychology and Health*, *14*, 795–812. http://doi.org/10.1080/08870449908407348

Conner, M., McEachan, R., Taylor, N., O'Hara, J., & Lawton, R. (2015). Role of affective attitudes and anticipated affective reactions in predicting health behaviors. *Health Psychology*, *34*, 642–652. http://doi.org/10.1037/hea0000143

Costa, R. M., & Brody, S. (2007). Women's relationship quality is associated with specifically penile-vaginal intercourse orgasm and frequency. *Journal of Sex and Marital Therapy*, *33*, 319–327. http://doi.org/10.1080/00926230701385548

Crepaz, N., & Marks, G. (2001). Are negative affective states associated with HIV sexual risk behaviors? A meta-analytic review. *Health Psychology*, *20*, 291–299. http://doi.org/10.1037/0278-6133.20.4.291

Cyders, M. A., & Smith, G. T. (2008). Emotion-based dispositions to rash action: Positive and negative urgency. *Psychological Bulletin*, *134*, 807–828. http://doi.org/10.1037/a0013341

Czopp, A. M., Monteith, M. J., Zimmerman, R. S., & Lynam, D. R. (2004). Implicit attitudes as potential protection from risky sex: Predicting condom use with the IAT. *Basic and Applied Social Psychology*, *26*, 227–236. http://doi.org/10.1080/01973533.2004.9646407

Díaz, R. M. (1999). Trips to Fantasy Island: Contexts of risky sex for San Francisco gay men. *Sexualities*, *2*, 89–112.

Dvorak, R. D., Sargent, E. M., Kilwein, T. M., Stevenson, B. L., Kuvaas, N. J., & Williams, T. J. (2014). Alcohol use and alcohol-related consequences: Associations with emotion regulation difficulties. *American Journal of Drug and Alcohol Abuse*, *40*, 125–130. http://doi.org/10.3109/00952990.2013.877920

Ekkekakis, P. (2009). The dual-mode theory of affective responses to exercise in metatheoretical context: I. Initial impetus, basic postulates, and philosophical framework. *International Review of Sport and Exercise Psychology, 2*, 73–94. http://doi.org/10.1080/17509840802705920

Ellis, E. M., Homish, G. G., Parks, K. A., Collins, R. L., & Kiviniemi, M. T. (2015). Increasing condom use by changing people's feelings about them: An experimental study. *Health Psychology, 34*, 941–950. http://doi.org/10.1037/hea0000205

European Centre for Disease Prevention and Control, & WHO Regional Office for Europe. (2016). *HIV/AIDS surveillance in Europe 2015*. Retrieved from http://ecdc.europa.eu/en/publications/Publications/HIV-AIDS-surveillance-Europe-2015.pdf

Faravelli, C., Giugni, A., Salvatori, S., & Ricca, V. (2004). Psychopathology after rape. *American Journal of Psychiatry, 161*, 1483–1485. http://doi.org/10.1176/appi.ajp.161.8.1483

Fergusson, D. M., McLeod, G. F. H., & Horwood, L. J. (2013). Childhood sexual abuse and adult developmental outcomes: Findings from a 30-year longitudinal study in New Zealand. *Child Abuse and Neglect, 37*, 664–674. http://doi.org/10.1016/j.chiabu.2013.03.013

Frohlich, P., & Meston, C. (2002). Sexual functioning and self-reported depressive symptoms among college women. *Journal of Sex Research, 39*, 321–325. http://doi.org/10.1080/00224490209552156

Galperin, A., Haselton, M. G., Frederick, D. A., Poore, J., von Hippel, W., Buss, D. M., & Gonzaga, G. C. (2013). Sexual regret: Evidence for evolved sex differences. *Archives of Sexual Behavior, 42*, 1145–1161. http://doi.org/10.1007/s10508-012-0019-3

Gilovich, T., & Medvec, V. H. (1995). The experience of regret: What, when, and why. *Psychological Review, 102*, 379–395. http://doi.org/10.1037/0033-295X.102.2.379

Gratz, K. L., & Roemer, L. (2004). Multidimensional assessment of emotion regulation and dysregulation: Development, factor structure, and initial validation of the difficulties in emotion regulation scale. *Journal of Psychopathology and Behavioral Assessment, 26*, 41–54. http://doi.org/10.1023/B:JOBA.0000007455.08539.94

Gratz, K. L., & Tull, M. T. (2010). The relationship between emotion dysregulation and deliberate self-harm among inpatients with substance use disorders. *Cognitive Therapy and Research, 34*, 544–553. http://doi.org/10.1007/s10608-009-9268-4

Gross, J. J. (2010). The future's so bright, I gotta wear shades. *Emotion Review, 2*, 212–216. http://doi.org/10.1177/1754073910361982

Hurlbert, D. F., & Apt, C. (1994). Female sexual desire, response, and behavior. *Behavior Modification, 18*, 488–504. Retrieved from http://www.ncbi.nlm.nih.gov/pubmed/7980375

Hynie, M., MacDonald, T. K., & Marques, S. (2006). Self-conscious emotions and self-regulation in the promotion of condom use. *Personality and Social Psychology Bulletin, 32*, 1072–1084. http://doi.org/10.1177/0146167206288060

Koch, E. J. (2014). How does anticipated regret influence health and safety decisions? A literature review. *Basic and Applied Social Psychology, 36*, 397–412. http://doi.org/10.1080/01973533.2014.935379

Laumann, E. O., Paik, A., Glasser, D. B., Kang, J.-H., Wang, T., Levinson, B., . . . Gingell, C. (2006). A cross-national study of subjective sexual well-being among older women and men: Findings from the global study of sexual attitudes and behaviors. *Archives of Sexual Behavior, 35*, 143–159. http://doi.org/10.1007/s10508-005-9005-3

Lê, M. G., Bacheloti, A., & Hill, C. (1989). Characteristics of reproductive life and risk of breast cancer in a case-control study of young nulliparous women. *Journal of Clinical Epidemiology, 42*, 1227–1233. http://doi.org/10.1016/0895-435690121-2

Levin, R. J. (2003). Do women gain anything from coitus apart from pregnancy? Changes in the human female genital tract activated by coitus pain disorders: Responses to a web-based survey. *Journal of Sex and Marital Therapy, 29*(suppl 1), 59–69. http://doi.org/10.1080/713847134

Lykins, A. D., Janssen, E., & Graham, C. A. (2006). The relationship between negative mood and sexuality in heterosexual college women and men. *Journal of Sex Research, 43*, 136–143. http://doi.org/10.1080/00224490609552308

Meisler, A. W., & Carey, M. P. (1991). Depressed affect and male sexual arousal. *Archives of Sexual Behavior, 20*, 541–554. Retrieved from http://www.ncbi.nlm.nih.gov/pubmed/1768221

Messman-Moore, T. L., Walsh, K. L., & DiLillo, D. (2010). Emotion dysregulation and risky sexual behavior in revictimization. *Child Abuse and Neglect, 34*, 967–976. http://doi.org/10.1016/j.chiabu.2010.06.004

Mitchell, W. B., Dibartolo, P. M., Brown, T. A., & Barlow, D. H. (1998). Effects of positive and negative mood on sexual arousal in sexually functional males. *Archives of Sexual Behavior, 27*, 197–207. http://doi.org/10.1023/A:1018686631428

Montanaro, E. A., & Bryan, A. D. (2014). Comparing theory-based condom interventions: Health belief model versus theory of planned behavior. *Health Psychology, 33*, 1251–1260. http://doi.org/10.1037/a0033969

Mosher, W. D., Chandra, A., & Jones, J. (2005). Sexual behavior and selected health measures: Men and women 15–44 years of age, United States, 2002. *Advance Data, 362*, 1–55. Retrieved from http://www.ncbi.nlm.nih.gov/pubmed/16250464

Nobre, P. J., Wiegel, M., Bach, A. K., Weisberg, R. B., Brown, T. A., Wincze, J. P., & Barlow, D. H. (2004). Determinants of sexual arousal and the accuracy of its self-estimation in sexually functional males. *Source: The Journal of Sex Research, 41*, 363–371. Retrieved from http://www.jstor.org/stable/3813544

Orcutt, H. K., Cooper, M. L., & Garcia, M. (2005). Use of sexual intercourse to reduce negative affect as a prospective mediator of sexual revictimization. *Journal of Traumatic Stress, 18*, 729–739. http://doi.org/10.1002/jts.20081

Palmore, E. B. (1982). Predictors of the longevity difference: A 25-year follow-up. *The Gerontologist, 22*, 513–518. http://doi.org/10.1093/GERONT/22.6.513

Peterson, Z. D., & Janssen, E. (2007). Ambivalent affect and sexual response: The impact of co-occurring positive and negative emotions on subjective and physiological sexual responses to erotic stimuli. *Archives of Sexual Behavior, 36*, 793–807. http://doi.org/10.1007/s10508-006-9145-0

Reynolds, W. M., & Kobak, K. A. (1995). Reliability and validity of the Hamilton Depression Inventory: A paper-and-pencil version of the Hamilton Depression

Rating Scale Clinical Interview. *Psychological Assessment*, *7*, 472–483. http://doi.org/10.1037/1040-3590.7.4.472

Roseman, I. J., Wiest, C., & Swartz, T. S. (1994). Phenomenology, behaviors, and goals differentiate discrete emotions. *Journal of Personality and Social Psychology*, *67*, 206–221. http://doi.org/10.1037/0022-3514.67.2.206

Rossing, M. A., Stanford, J. L., Weiss, N. S., & Daling, J. R. (1996). Indices of exposure to fetal and sperm antigens in relation to the occurrence of breast cancer. *Epidemiology (Cambridge, Mass.)*, *7*, 309–311. Retrieved from http://www.ncbi.nlm.nih.gov/pubmed/8728448

Ruedinger, E., & Cox, J. E. (2012). Adolescent childbearing. *Current Opinion in Pediatrics*, *24*, 446–452. http://doi.org/10.1097/MOP.0b013e3283557b89

Sheeran, P., Gollwitzer, P. M., & Bargh, J. A. (2013). Nonconscious processes and health. *Health Psychology*, *32*, 460–473. http://doi.org/10.1037/a0029203

Smith, G. D., Frankel, S., & Yarnell, J. (1997). Sex and death: Are they related? Findings from the Caerphilly cohort study. *BMJ*, *315*, 1641–1644.

Sniehotta, F. F., Presseau, J., & Araújo-Soares, V. (2014). Time to retire the theory of planned behaviour. *Health Psychology Review*, *8*, 1–7. http://doi.org/10.1080/17437199.2013.869710

Ter Kuile, M. M., Both, S., & Van Uden, J. (2010). The effects of experimentally-induced sad and happy mood on sexual arousal in sexually healthy women. *Journal of Sexual Medicine*, *7*, 1177–1184. http://doi.org/10.1111/j.1743-6109.2009.01632.x

Tull, M. T., Weiss, N. H., Adams, C. E., & Gratz, K. L. (2012). The contribution of emotion regulation difficulties to risky sexual behavior within a sample of patients in residential substance abuse treatment. *Addictive Behaviors*, *37*, 1084–1092. http://doi.org/10.1016/j.addbeh.2012.05.001

Tybur, J. M., Bryan, A. D., Magnan, R. E., & Hooper, A. E. C. (2011). Smells like safe sex. *Psychological Science*, *22*, 478–480. http://doi.org/10.1177/0956797611400096

United Nations AIDS Organization. (2016). *UNAIDS Fact sheet 2016: Global HIV Statistics*. Retrieved January 7, 2017, from http://www.unaids.org/en/resources/fact-sheet

Watson, D., Clark, L. A., & Tellegen, A. (1988). Development and validation of brief measures of positive and negative affect: The PANAS scales. *Journal of Personality and Social Psychology*, *54*, 1063–1070. Retrieved from http://www.ncbi.nlm.nih.gov/pubmed/3397865

Whipple, B., & Komisaruk, B. R. (1988). Analgesia produced in women by genital self-stimulation. *Journal of Sex Research*, *24*, 130–140. http://doi.org/10.1080/00224498809551403

World Health Organization. (2016). *Sexually transmitted infections (STIs)*. Retrieved January 7, 2017, from http://www.who.int/mediacentre/factsheets/fs110/en/

Wylie, K. (2009). A global survey of sexual behaviours. *Journal of Family and Reproductive Health*, *3*, 39–49.

Young, R. C., Biggs, J. T., Ziegler, V. E., & Meyer, D. A. (1978). A rating scale for mania: reliability, validity and sensitivity. *The British Journal of Psychiatry : The Journal of Mental Science*, *133*, 429–35. Retrieved from http://www.ncbi.nlm.nih.gov/pubmed/728692

Zapolski, T. C. B., Cyders, M. A., & Smith, G. T. (2009). Positive urgency predicts illegal drug use and risky sexual behavior. *Psychology of Addictive Behaviors, 23*, 348–354. http://doi.org/10.1037/a0014684

Zeelenberg, M., van Dijk, W. W., Manstead, A. S. R., & der Pligt, J. (1998). The experience of regret and disappointment. *Cognition and Emotion, 12*, 221–230. http://doi.org/10.1080/026999398379727

16

Affect and Tanning Behaviors

ASHLEY K. DAY AND ELLIOT J. COUPS

TANNING BEHAVIORS: A BRIEF HISTORY

The belief that tanned skin is attractive and desirable can be traced to the industrial revolution. The advent of industrial machinery moved laborers from fields to factories, and a darkened complexion was no longer a sign of being a member of the working class. A tanned appearance became fashionable, and a sign that one could afford to spend leisure time outdoors. As the beauty industry began to capitalize on this shift in societal beauty ideals, the medical industry began to espouse numerous—and in hindsight, mostly false—health benefits of ultraviolet (UV) radiation exposure, including treatment for skin conditions, fatigue, and tuberculosis. By the 1920s, psychiatric facilities were treating patients with UV light, and in 1929 "the need for ultra-violet ray apparatus in every medical hospital [was] urged both for treatment of mental and physical conditions" (Cormac, 1929, p. 455). Further, in 1926 a scientific journal dedicated to "sunlight therapy" was first published, and artificial UV lamps were being marketed as both medical apparatus to be used by trained health professionals and as devices to purchase for home use (Carter, 2007). Coco Chanel summarized the mood of the time, stating in *Vogue* magazine, "the 1929 girl must be tanned" (Vogue Magazine, 1929, p. 99, cited in Randle, 1997).

At the same time as the desire for a tanned appearance began to emerge, understanding of the health risks associated with excessive UV exposure also advanced. By the 1930s, UV radiation was considered a carcinogen by many in the medical industry. Today it is known that both sunburns and lifetime levels of UV radiation exposure increase the risk of melanoma—the most lethal form of skin cancer—as well as the risk of nonmelanoma skin cancers, including basal and squamous cell carcinomas. In 2014, 88 years after it was first discovered that exposure to UV radiation causes skin cancer in mice (Findlay, 1979), the US Surgeon General released a Call to Action to Prevent Skin Cancer (US Department of Health and Human Services, 2014), acknowledging the disease as a major public health problem. Worldwide, there were an estimated 232,000 new cases of melanoma and 55,000 melanoma-related deaths in 2012 (Ferlay et al., 2015). There is a lack of reliable data regarding the worldwide incidence of nonmelanoma skin cancers, but an estimated 3.3 million people in the United States are treated for more than 5.4 million cases of nonmelanoma skin cancer annually (Rogers, Weinstock, Feldman, & Coldiron, 2015). The incidence rates of melanoma and nonmelanoma skin cancers have increased considerably over the last 40 years (Chen, Geller, & Tsao, 2013; Lomas, Leonardi-Bee, & Bath-Hextall, 2012), which stands in contrast to the decreasing or stable rates for most other types of cancer. The World Health Organization estimates that, globally, excessive UV exposure causes over 1.5 million days of lost activity annually (McMichael et al., 2006). However, despite the risks, a large number of individuals continue to engage in tanning behaviors, particularly young white women.

Importantly, the term "tanning" can refer to one of three behaviors: sunbathing outdoors, indoor tanning, or artificial tanning. Sunbathing refers to the traditional behavior of exposing oneself to the sun's UV rays for the purposes of getting a tan. Indoor tanning refers to the use of tanning beds or booths that provide concentrated UV radiation exposure. Indoor tanning beds minimize levels of UV-B radiation, which can allow individuals to tan without burning the skin, sometimes giving indoor tanners the false sense of security that they are not damaging their skin (Lessin, Perlis, & Zook, 2012; Miyamura et al., 2011). In Western countries, 19.3% of adolescents (≤19 years old), 55.0% of university students, and 35.7% of all adults report having indoor tanned one or more times (Wehner et al., 2014). Past year indoor tanning rates for these groups are 18.3%, 43.1%, and 14.0%, respectively. Artificial tanning refers to the use of cosmetic products to temporarily give the skin a tanned appearance without exposure to UV radiation. This chapter focuses on sunbathing and indoor tanning, as these tanning behaviors are associated adverse health risks, including skin cancer.

AFFECTIVE DETERMINANTS OF TANNING BEHAVIORS: AN OVERVIEW

Since the late 1980s, researchers have been investigating why people engage in tanning behaviors and how we might be able to influence this behavior. Although the majority of research has involved health behavior theories that emphasize social cognitive factors, a number of studies have explored the role of affective factors, including feelings of relaxation, improved mood, and endorphin release in response to UV exposure. In this chapter, we outline relevant research on affective determinants of tanning behaviors. Early research measured affective constructs without any clear theoretical basis, but rather because they were "commonly thought to promote or limit dependent behavior" (Zeller, Lazovich, Forster, & Widome, 2006, p. 590). As the literature grew, evidence for the role of affective attitudes in tanning behaviors became established. Other research has examined affective responses to tanning behaviors, and we provide examples of literature that shows changes in affect as a result of tanning behavior as well as research exploring the role of anticipated mood changes in predicting tanning behaviors.

Affective Attitudes to Tanning

Conceptualization and understanding of the role of affective factors as determinants of tanning behaviors has evolved over time. Initial studies focused primarily on perceived affective reasons for tanning. One of the first studies that explored reasons for tanning was published in 1987 (Keesling & Friedman, 1987). Although a single theoretical model did not guide the predictors selected, some constructs from the health belief model (Janz & Becker, 1984) were included, as well as cultural and social learning variables. The authors hypothesized that "regarding mood . . . sunbathers would report less depression, less anxiety, and more relaxation than those who do not sunbathe . . . based on anecdotal accounts that indicate that sunbathing is extremely relaxing and on recent research that demonstrates the positive effect of exposure to sunlight on mental health" (p. 482). However, time spent sunbathing and time spent outdoors in general were not significantly associated with participants' reported current levels of depression, anxiety, or relaxation. Another early tanning research study surveyed a sample of 476 people aged over 15 years who were recruited at either a shopping mall, a social function, or on a vacation cruise ship. Of the indoor tanning users in the sample, 58% reported that indoor tanning made them feel relaxed and 14% reported that it made them feel happy (Mawn & Fleischer, 1993).

Subsequent studies moved away from examining potential affective attitudes to tanning and instead focused primarily on the role of social cognitive factors. When they were considered, affective factors (such as feelings of relaxation or improved mood) were typically nested into broader attitudinal measures that also included nonaffective variables (e.g., beliefs that indoor tanning is safe and that a tan represents a healthy appearance) (e.g., Knight, Kirincich, Farmer, & Hood, 2002; Rhainds, De Guire, & Claveau, 1999). One social cognitive framework that has been regularly used in the tanning literature is the theory of planned behavior (Ajzen, 1991). The theory of planned behavior hypothesizes that behavioral intentions are the best predictor of behavior, and that behavioral intentions are influenced by attitudes toward the behavior, subjective norms concerning the behavior, and perceived behavioral control. Hillhouse, Adler, Drinnon, and Turrisi (1997) were the first to apply the full model to tanning behavior. Affective variables were included in a broader measure, which considered attitudes toward tanning and included participants' level of agreement that indoor tanning or sunbathing were relaxing versus not relaxing, stimulating versus boring, and pleasant versus unpleasant. Overall, more favorable attitudes were significantly associated with lower intentions to use sunscreen and greater intentions to sunbathe and indoor tan.

More recently, researchers have returned to isolating affective determinants of tanning behaviors from broader attitudinal scales and report results from single-item measures of affective constructs. Such studies have also examined associations between affective factors and tanning beliefs and behaviors. For example, in a study of 163 Midwestern American college students, 72.2% of sunbathers and 35% of indoor tanning users reported tanning because "[they] think it is relaxing" (Dennis, Lowe, & Snetselaar, 2009). Students who indicated that they feel better with a tan perceived greater importance of tanning. In a telephone interview study of 1,275 adolescents in Massachusetts and Minnesota, agreement that indoor tanning "lifts my spirits" was significantly associated with greater self-reported difficulty to quit indoor tanning, after controlling for other variables (Zeller et al., 2006).

Acute Affective Responses to Tanning

As a complement to studies of perceived affective reasons for tanning, other research has examined affective responses to tanning behaviors. In a landmark paper published in 2004, Feldman and colleagues sought to explore whether there was a physiologic reinforcing effect of exposure to UV radiation. They used a carefully controlled design to isolate the potential physiologic reinforcing effect of UV exposure from other factors, such as perceived appearance benefits of having a tan. Fourteen young adults who regularly indoor tanned were invited to indoor tan in a laboratory setting three times a week for 6 weeks. Two indoor tanning beds were used in the study, which were identical in all ways except the UV exposure received by users, and participants were blinded to the differences between the beds. One tanning bed was a standard bed that had a filter allowing the UV light from the bulbs to pass through it. The second, non-UV tanning bed used an identical looking filter that blocked the bulbs' UV light. Neither filter blocked infrared light, which meant that users felt the same amount of heat in each tanning bed. Each Monday and Wednesday, participants visited the laboratory and spent 15 minutes in each of the tanning beds. Before and after each tanning session, participants completed a measure of mood that included five positive (active, alert, relaxed, enthusiastic, attentive) and five negative (tense, nervous, distressed, irritable, sad) mood states. Results indicated that participants felt more relaxed and less tense after using the UV tanning bed than the non-UV bed. There were no significant differences for the other mood states. Participants also reported liking the UV bed more than the non-UV bed and that they felt better after using it. On Fridays, participants were allowed to access the tanning beds for up to 20 minutes and could choose how to divide that time between the beds (e.g., only using one bed or going back and forth between beds). Of all of the tanning sessions on Fridays, 95% of them were spent mostly in the UV bed, which far exceeds the 50% rate that one would expect by chance. The results of this study suggest that exposure to UV radiation can be detected by regular users of tanning beds, that such exposure is associated with reported changes in mood (increased relaxation and reduced tension), and that UV exposure has a reinforcing effect that contributes to tanning behaviors.

Other studies have used nonexperimental methods to elicit reports of potential mood changes related to tanning behaviors. For example, a survey study of 139 female university students aged 18–25 years used the Positive Affect and Negative Affect Scale (Watson, Clark, & Tellegen, 1988) to measures mood states before and after the most recent indoor tanning session (Heckman, Darlow, Cohen-Filipic, & Kloss, 2016). Participants who experienced a decrease in negative mood following indoor tanning were more likely to be more frequent indoor tanners. This supports previous findings that decreased negative mood is one of the reasons why indoor tanners continue to tan (Feldman et al., 2004; Kourosh, Harrington, & Adinoff, 2010).

Anticipated Affective Responses to Tanning

In view of the fact that indoor tanning is associated with subsequent mood changes, research has also explored the role of anticipated mood changes in predicting tanning behavior. Noar, Myrick, Morales-Pico, and Thomas (2014) created a comprehensive indoor tanning expectations (CITE) scale, which included mood enhancement as one of its 11 subscales. Items in the mood enhancement subscale include expectations that tanning would be enjoyable and relaxing and would reduce stress or tension. In an online survey of 706 young women in sororities at a southeastern United States university, mood enhancement and psychological/physical discomfort subscales emerged as the two factors that most distinguished among current indoor tanners, former indoor tanners, and non–indoor tanners. The CITE scale has been used in a number of further studies, which have consistently found positive mood expectations to be associated with increased frequency of indoor tanning and negative mood expectations to be associated with decreased frequency of indoor tanning in adolescent and young adult women (e.g., Myrick, Noar, Kelley, & Zeitany, 2016; Noar et al., 2015). Collectively, studies of affective outcomes of tanning behaviors indicate that tanning behaviors trigger affective changes, and that the expectation of such changes is also associated with tanning behaviors.

TANNING DEPENDENCE AND ADDICTION

The persistence of tanning behaviors among some subsections of the population, along with evidence of its reinforcing properties, have spurred research to explore potentially addictive features of tanning. There are many documented instances of people engaging in tanning more regularly than is necessary to maintain a tanned appearance, with reports of some frequent tanners attending salons up to 20 times a month (Poorsattar & Hornung, 2007). Some frequent tanners also continue to tan even after experiencing burns from tanning devices (Stapleton et al., 2013). Substance-related and addictive disorders refer to persistent and maladaptive behaviors or substance use that cause harm. Examples of well-established substance-related or addictive disorders include alcohol dependence, nicotine addiction, and pathological gambling.

Numerous frameworks have been applied to the concept of tanning addiction, including social learning and cognitive models, pharmacological models, behavioral models, and diagnostic models (Nolan & Feldman, 2009; Nolan, Taylor, Liguori, & Feldman, 2009). Typically, diagnostic features of behavioral models of addiction include preoccupation with the behavior, positive reinforcing properties, significant time or emotional energy spent engaging in the behavior, neglecting or putting off other activities in order to engage in the behavior or use the substance, and the continuation of the behavior despite adverse effects. Pharmacological models consider the presence of psychological and physical dependence, withdrawal, and tolerance as defining substance addiction. Regardless of the theoretical model used to define tanning dependence or addiction, the role of affective factors in persistent tanning is evident.

Affective Properties of Tanning Dependence and Addiction

Most studies attempting to measure tanning dependence or addiction have used either a modified version of the Cut Down, Annoyed, Guilt, Eye-Opener (CAGE) criteria or modified diagnostic criteria from the DSM-IV-TR or DSM-5 (American Psychiatric Association, 2000, 2013). The CAGE is a tool originally developed to diagnose alcohol addiction, and was subsequently modified to measure tanning addiction (Warthan, Uchida, & Wagner, 2005). The tanning-modified CAGE asks participants whether they have unsuccessfully tried to stop tanning (**C**ut-Down), if they ever get **A**nnoyed when people tell them not to tan, if they ever feel

Guilt about the frequency of their tanning behavior, and if they want to tan when they wake up in the morning (**E**ye-Opener). Individuals who meet tanning-modified CAGE criteria for problematic tanning are significantly more likely to also meet diagnostic criteria for obsessive-compulsive disorder (Ashrafioun & Bonar, 2014) and body dysmorphic disorder (Ashrafioun & Bonar, 2014). They also report more symptoms of anxiety and depression (Mosher & Danoff-Burg, 2010). In a study of 296 college students, those classified by the CAGE as tanning dependent reported higher opiate-like reactions (i.e., tanning leads to feelings of relaxation, pain relief, stress relief, and a sense of well-being or euphoria) to tanning than the lower level dependent category of abuse tanners, who scored higher than those not categorized as dependent or abuse tanners (Hillhouse et al., 2012). Other measures of tanning addiction and studies that measure tanning frequency show similar associations with mood disorders (e.g., Ashrafioun & Bonar, 2014; Blashill et al., 2016; Mosher & Danoff-Burg, 2010). Taken together, this research indicates that not only is there evidence for behavioral tanning addiction and dependence, affective reactions and other mood disorders are related to this addiction and dependence.

Affective Physiological Responses to Tanning

A number of studies have explored the possibility of a biological underpinning to indoor tanning addiction, based on pharmacologic models of addiction that involve both physical and psychological dependence, withdrawal, and tolerance. Physiological responses (such as endorphin release) lead to concomitant changes in affective states. This is supported by evidence that endorphins have a reinforcing role in addictive behaviors. To date, few studies have explored physiological responses to indoor tanning. However, the available evidence suggests that physiological responses are part of a broader affective response to tanning, and such affective responses may help to explain tanning behaviors and even tanning addiction and dependence.

In order to explore the possibility of biological evidence of tanning addiction, Harrington and colleagues (2012) used a similar approach to that used in Feldman and colleagues' landmark study (2004). Seven frequent indoor tanners participated in a blinded experiment where they were given access to UV and non-UV tanning beds while their cerebral blood flow was measured. Compared to the non-UV tanning beds, use of the UV tanning beds caused increased activation in several regions of the brain related to reward experiences, including the dorsal striatum, anterior insula, and medial orbitofrontal cortex. This provides evidence that frequent tanning may involve central nervous system reward, although the study sample size and episodes of UV exposure were both small, limiting generalizability of the findings.

A more commonly used approach to measure biological responses to UV exposure is to assess β-endorphin levels. Endorphins are opiates produced by the body that influence mood and perceptions of pain. Beta-endorphin is an endorphin with both analgesic and addictive properties (Dalayeun, Nores, & Bergal, 1993; Fell, Robinson, Mao, Woolf, & Fisher, 2014). Studies have suggested that exercise triggers the release of β-endorphin that is associated with feelings of well-being (Carr et al., 1981). When the skin is exposed to UV, the reaction includes production of endogenous opioid β-endorphin (Kaur, Liguori, Lang, et al., 2006). Kaur and colleagues (2005) published a research letter describing the fact that one of the participants from Feldman and colleagues' 2004 study reported temporary alleviation of chronic lower back pain that lasted for 5–6 hours after tanning. A possible mechanism for this perceived pain relief is through β-endorphin release.

Levins, Carr, Fisher, Momtaz, and Parrish (1983) were the first to investigate potential β-endorphin responses to UV exposure in a case study of a 22-year-old white man exposed to nine daily 15-minute sessions of UV-A exposure. The UV-A exposure triggered a significant rise in the participant's β-endorphin levels for 30 minutes. Non-UV-A light exposure with the same heat as the UV-A light did not produce a rise in β-endorphin. A number of subsequent studies have used varying methodologies to explore the potential relationship between UV exposure and β-endorphin. Findings from these studies have been mixed. Gambichler and colleagues (2002) found that participants who received six sessions of UV exposure over 3 weeks had no significant differences in β-endorphin before the study, 20 minutes after the first UV exposure, or 24 hours after the sixth exposure, compared to non-UV-exposed participants. No differences in plasma β-endorphin levels before or after UV or non-UV exposure were observed in a small double-blind placebo controlled trial of three frequent and three infrequent tanners (Kaur, Liguori, Fleischer, & Feldman, 2006). However, the tanning exposure schedules were brief and varied between participants (5–9 minutes of exposure depending on the individual's skin tone).

Experimental studies using other approaches have found support for the potentially reinforcing role of cutaneous endorphins in tanning behaviors of frequent tanners (Kaur, Liguori, Fleischer, & Feldman, 2005; Kaur, Liguori, Lang, et al., 2006). Naltrexone is an opioid antagonist drug that reverses the effects of opioids and is thus used to treat opioid and alcohol abuse disorders. Naltrexone is generally well tolerated in non-opioid-dependent individuals, but can cause physiological withdrawal symptoms (e.g., nausea, jitteriness, shaking) in opioid-dependent individuals. Several studies have been conducted to test the presence of opioid-dependent features among frequent tanners. In one study, three female frequent tanners were treated with naltrexone before exposure to UV and non-UV tanning beds (Kaur, Feldman, et al., 2005). In a second study, eight frequent and eight infrequent adult tanners were exposed to UV and non-UV tanning beds in a double-blind, placebo-controlled trial with placebo-controlled administration of an escalating dose of naltrexone (Kaur, Liguori, Lang, et al., 2006). In both studies, administration of naltrexone diminished frequent tanners' preference for UV over non-UV tanning beds. Furthermore, there was evidence that the participants who were frequent tanners exhibited withdrawal-like symptoms after being administered naltrexone, with several participants dropping out from both studies after experiencing such symptoms (Kaur, Liguori, et al., 2005; Kaur, Liguori, Lang, et al., 2006).

Although there is some evidence for physiological addiction to tanning, particularly among high-frequency tanners, additional research is needed to elucidate the relationship between physiology and tanning dependence and addiction. It is clear that affective factors are related to tanning behaviors, and they may also be related to dependence or addiction to tanning. Several factors make it difficult to generalize across the results of physiological tanning addiction studies, including different UV exposure schedules, varying classifications for frequent tanning users, inconsistent inclusion of infrequent tanning participants, and differences in the timing of blood samples relative to UV exposure. Additionally, there are significant individual differences in plasma β-endorphin levels and factors such as anxiety about blood sampling could influence their levels (Kaur, Liguori, Fleischer, et al., 2006).

THE ROLE OF AFFECTIVE FACTORS IN IMPROVING SKIN CANCER RISK BEHAVIORS

In view of the link between affective factors and tanning behaviors, and the potential for physiological addiction to tanning, it is important to leverage this knowledge to reduce skin cancer risk behaviors. Evidence from behavioral health interventions outside the context of skin cancer suggest that both immediate negative emotional reactions to health risk messages and negative anticipated mood can predict health-promoting behavioral intentions (see Mahler, 2014). There is a small but growing body of research exploring the effect of mood and emotions on skin cancer risk behaviors. One approach has been to present individuals with varying types of messages that may differentially evoke affective responses and concomitant tanning beliefs, intentions, or behaviors. For example, in a study of university students in Belgium, participants who received narrative, affect-laden messages subsequently engaged in more health-promotion behaviors related to skin cancer than individuals who received no message (Lemal & Van den Bulck, 2010). A similar effect was found for participants who were exposed to nonaffective, factual messages. However, rates of engaging in the behaviors did not differ between individuals who received the affect-laden versus the factual messages.

Perceived risk is typically included as a determinant in health behavior theories. Research exploring risk perceptions as a determinant of skin cancer risk and prevention behaviors has evolved to distinguish cognitive beliefs (about true likelihood) and affective beliefs (intuitive feelings about the likelihood) (Janssen, van Osch, de Vries, & Lechner, 2011; Kiviniemi & Ellis, 2014; Morales-Sánchez, Peralta-Pedrero, & Domínguez-Gómez, 2014). Higher levels of affective perceived risk are associated with increased sun protection benefits (Manne, Coups, & Kashy, 2016), explain more variance in sunscreen use and intentions than cognitive perceived risk (Janssen, Waters, van Osch, Lechner, & de Vries, 2014), and fully mediate the relation between cognitively based risk and sunscreen use (Kiviniemi & Ellis, 2014). Risk-related affect has also been assessed using measures of skin cancer worry. A higher level of skin cancer worry is associated with higher skin self-examination intentions (Cameron, 2008), having ever had a full body skin examination from a health professional (Coups et al., 2013), and lower reported levels of sunburn among study participants' children (Tripp et al., 2016). Together, these results suggest that affective risk beliefs may be more strongly associated with skin cancer risk and prevention behaviors than cognitively oriented risk beliefs.

Experimental studies have reported that participants' negative affective response to skin cancer risk information is associated with an increase in skin cancer prevention intentions. Morris, Cooper, Goldenberg, Arndt, and Gibbons (2014) conducted a sun exposure intervention experiment based on the terror management health model (Goldberg & Arndt, 2008), a theory that posits that when thoughts of death are accessible, people become motivated to improve their health-related behaviors in order to psychologically protect against mortality concerns. In an online experiment with 475 young female indoor tanners, Morris and colleagues found that activating thoughts of death and mortality concerns led to an increase in sun protection behavioral intentions. Mays and Zhao (2016) extended this research and included explicit measures of affective response. In an experiment with 682 women aged 18–30 years, participants were exposed to a gain- or loss-framed UV exposure health message in an effort to impact intention to either avoid or quit indoor tanning (Mays & Zhao, 2016). The gain-framed message showed a picture of a woman's face with healthy skin and included text regarding the benefits of avoiding indoor tanning. The loss-framed message showed an image of a woman's face after skin cancer surgery and text about the risks of indoor tanning. Participants who viewed the loss-framed message had significantly lower intentions to engage in indoor tanning and greater intentions to quit indoor tanning. Importantly, the effect of the loss-framed message on indoor tanning intentions was mediated by increased fear.

The preceding examples focused on immediate affective reactions to health risk information. Other studies have explored the role of expected emotions or anticipated mood on health-related behaviors. Negative anticipated mood has been found to be a predictor of increased intentions to engage in health to protective behaviors, including increased contraceptive use and avoiding smoking and drug use (Mahler, 2014). In two studies that examined the role of affect, relative to cognition, in predicting sun protection intentions and behaviors, both immediate and anticipated negative emotional reactions predicted increased UV protective behavior and intentions, independent of cognitive factors (Mahler, 2014). In a study of 257 college students, participants were more inclined to avoid viewing a photograph showing the UV damage to their face if they believed this would lead to negative anticipated responses, such as feeling bad or appearing ugly in the photograph (Dwyer, Shepperd, & Stock, 2015). Thus, although there is some demonstrated potential for affect-laden images and text to promote sun protection behaviors, it is important to recognize that some people may be motivated to avoid such messages.

CONCLUSIONS AND FUTURE DIRECTIONS

Skin cancer is the most commonly diagnosed cancer. It is well known that UV radiation exposure increases the risk of skin cancers, yet tanning behaviors remain pervasive. Much of the research seeking to understand and influence individuals' tanning behaviors has focused on social cognitive factors. However, there has been a gradual and growing focus on affective determinants of tanning behaviors. Studies have shown that positive affective attitudes (e.g., relaxation, improved mood) are associated with increased frequency of tanning behaviors and greater self-reported difficulty to quit indoor tanning. Research has also demonstrated that engaging in tanning behaviors results in positive changes in mood, and that anticipating such mood changes is also associated with such behaviors.

Many theoretical frameworks have been applied to the concept of tanning addiction, a concept that has emerged due to the high prevalence and persistence of tanning behaviors exhibited by certain subsections of the population. Regardless of the theoretical model used to define tanning dependence or addiction, affective determinants are evident in persistent problematic tanning behaviors. Additionally, there is some evidence that affective physiological reactions to tanning behavior may have reinforcing properties. Finally, research exploring the effect of mood and emotions on skin cancer risk prevention behaviors suggests promising avenues for intervention.

There are a number of future directions for this field. First, systematic integration of affective factors into tanning behavior research is needed. There is a lack of robust conceptual models that consider social cognitive factors and affective determinants together to explain tanning behaviors. Second, heterogeneous measurement approaches hinder our understanding of the role of affective determinants of tanning behaviors. Future empirical research should use reliable, validated measures that clearly delineate affective determinants of behavior from social, cognitive, and other factors. Finally, given that affective skin cancer risk beliefs may be more strongly associated with tanning behaviors than cognitive risk beliefs, interventions that address affective factors may be more effective than existing interventions that fail to address affective risk belief factors.

ACKNOWLEDGMENTS

We thank Ryan Goydos for valuable assistance with literature reviews and reviewing articles.

REFERENCES

Ajzen, I. (1991). The theory of planned behavior. *Organizational Behavior and Human Decision Processes, 50*, 179–211. doi: 10.1016/0749-5978(91)90020-T

American Psychiatric Association. (2000). *Diagnostic and statistical manual of mental disorders* (4th ed., text rev.). Washington, DC: Author. doi: 10.1176/appi.books.9780890423349

American Psychiatric Association. (2013). *Diagnostic and statistical manual of mental disorders* (5th ed.). Washington, DC: Author.

Ashrafioun, L., & Bonar, E. E. (2014). Tanning addiction and psychopathology: Further evaluation of anxiety disorders and substance abuse. *Journal of the American Academy of Dermatology, 70*, 473–480. doi: 10.1016/j.jaad.2013.10.057

Blashill, A. J., Oleski, J. L., Hayes, R., Scully, J., Antognini, T., Olendzki, E., & Pagoto, S. (2016). The association between psychiatric disorders and frequent indoor tanning. *JAMA Dermatology, 152*, 577–579. doi: 10.1001/jamadermatol.2015.5866

Cameron, L. D. (2008). Illness risk representations and motivations to engage in protective behavior: The case of skin cancer risk. *Psychology and Health, 23*, 91–112. doi: 10.1080/14768320701342383

Carr, D. B., Bullen, B. A., Skrinar, G. S., Arnold, M. A., Rosenblatt, M., Beitins, I. Z., . . . McArthur, J. W. (1981). Physical conditioning facilitates the exercise-induced secretion of beta-endorphin and beta-lipotropin in women. *New England Journal of Medicine, 305*, 560–563. doi: 0.1056/NEJM198109033051006

Carter, S. (2007). *Rise and shine: Sunlight, technology and health*. New York, NY: Berg.

Chen, S. T., Geller, A. C., & Tsao, H. (2013). Update on the epidemiology of melanoma. *Current Dermatology Reports, 2*, 24–34. doi: 10.1007/s13671-012-0035-5

Cormac, H. D. (1929). Light therapy in mental hospitals. *Proceedings of the Royal Society of Medicine, 22*, 455–468.

Coups, E. J., Stapleton, J. L., Hudson, S. V., Medina-Forrester, A., Rosenberg, S. A., Gordon, M., . . . Goydos, J. S. (2013). Skin cancer surveillance behaviors among US Hispanic adults. *Journal of the American Academy of Dermatology, 68*, 576–584. doi: 10.1016/j.jaad.2012.09.032

Dalayeun, J. F., Nores, J. M., & Bergal, S. (1993). Physiology of beta-endorphins: A close-up view and a review of the literature. *Biomedicine and Pharmacotherapy, 47*, 311–320. doi: 10.1016/0753-3322(93)90080-5

Dennis, L. K., Lowe, J. B., & Snetselaar, L. G. (2009). Tanning behavior among young frequent tanners is related to attitudes and not lack of knowledge about the dangers. *Health Education Journal, 68*, 232–243. doi: 10.1177/0017896909345195

Dwyer, L. A., Shepperd, J. A., & Stock, M. L. (2015). Predicting avoidance of skin damage feedback among college students. *Annals of Behavioral Medicine, 49*, 685–695. doi: 10.1007/s12160-015-9703-6

Feldman, S. R., Liguori, A., Kucenic, M., Rapp, S. R., Fleischer, A. B., Lang, W., & Kaur, M. (2004). Ultraviolet exposure is a reinforcing stimulus in frequent indoor tanners. *Journal of the American Academy of Dermatology, 51*, 45–51. doi: 10.1016/j.jaad.2004.01.053

Fell, G. L., Robinson, K. C., Mao, J., Woolf, C. J., & Fisher, D. E. (2014). Skin beta-endorphin mediates addiction to UV light. *Cell, 157*, 1527–1534. doi: 10.1016/j.cell.2014.04.032

Ferlay, J., Soerjomataram, I., Dikshit, R., Eser, S., Mathers, C., Rebelo, M., . . . Bray, F. (2015). Cancer incidence and mortality worldwide: Sources, methods and major patterns in GLOBOCAN 2012. *International Journal of Cancer, 136*, 359–386. doi: 10.1002/ijc.29210

Findlay, G. M. (1979). Ultra-violet light and skin cancer. *CA: A Cancer Journal for Clinicians, 29*, 169–171.

Gambichler, T., Bader, A., Vojvodic, M., Avermaete, A., Schenk, M., Altmeyer, P., & Hoffmann, K. (2002). Plasma levels of opioid peptides after sunbed exposures. *British Journal of Dermatology, 147*, 1207–1211. doi: 10.1046/j.1365-2133.2002.04859.x

Goldberg, J. L., & Arndt, J. (2008). The implications of death for health: A terror management health model for behavioral health promotion. *Psychological Review, 115*, 1032–1053. doi: 10.1037/a0013326

Harrington, C. R., Beswick, T. C., Graves, M., Jacobe, H. T., Harris, T. S., Kourosh, S., . . . Adinoff, B. (2012). Activation of the mesostriatal reward pathway with exposure to ultraviolet radiation (UVR) vs. sham UVR in frequent tanners: A pilot study. *Addiction Biology, 17*, 680–686. doi: 10.1111/j.1369-1600.2010.00312.x

Heckman, C., Darlow, S., Cohen-Filipic, J., & Kloss, J. (2016). Mood changes after indoor tanning among college women: Associations with psychiatric/addictive symptoms. *Health Psychology Research, 4*, 5453. doi: 10.4081/hpr.2016.5453

Hillhouse, J. J., Adler, C. M., Drinnon, J., & Turrisi, R. (1997). Application of Ajzen's theory of planned behavior to predict sunbathing, tanning salon use, and sunscreen use intentions and behaviors. *Journal of Behavioral Medicine, 20*, 365–378. doi: 10.1023/A:1025517130513

Hillhouse, J. J., Baker, M. K., Turrisi, R., Shields, A., Stapleton, J. L., Jain, S., & Longacre, I. (2012). Evaluating a measure of tanning abuse and dependence. *Archives of Dermatology, 148*, 815–819. doi: 10.1001/archdermatol.2011.2929

Janssen, E., van Osch, L., de Vries, H., & Lechner, L. (2011). Measuring risk perceptions of skin cancer: Reliability and validity of different operationalizations. *British Journal of Health Psychology, 16*, 92–112. doi: 10.1348/135910710X514120

Janssen, E., Waters, E. A., van Osch, L., Lechner, L. & de Vries, H. (2014). The importance of affectively-laden beliefs about health risks: The case of tobacco use and sun protection. *Journal of Behavioral Medicine, 37*, 11–21. doi: 10.1007/s10865-012-9462-9

Janz, N. K., & Becker, M. H. (1984). The health belief model: A decade later. *Health Education Quarterly, 11*, 1–47. doi: 10.1177_109019818401100101

Kaur, M., Feldman, S. R., Liguori, A., & Fleischer, A. B., Jr. (2005). Indoor tanning relieves pain. *Photodermatology Photoimmunology and Photomedicine, 21*, 278. doi: 10.1111/j.1600-0781.2005.00169.x

Kaur, M., Liguori, A., Fleischer, A. B., Jr., & Feldman, S. R. (2005). Side effects of naltrexone observed in frequent tanners: Could frequent tanners have ultraviolet-induced high opioid levels? *Journal of the American Academy of Dermatology, 52*, 916. doi: 10.1016/j.jaad.2005.02.026

Kaur, M., Liguori, A., Fleischer, A. B., Jr., & Feldman, S. R. (2006). Plasma beta-endorphin levels in frequent and infrequent tanners before and after ultraviolet and non-ultraviolet stimuli. *Journal of the American Academy of Dermatology, 54*, 919–920. doi: 10.1016/j.jaad.2006.01.062

Kaur, M., Liguori, A., Lang, W., Rapp, S. R., Fleischer, A. B., Jr., & Feldman, S. R. (2006). Induction of withdrawal-like symptoms in a small randomized, controlled trial of opioid blockade in frequent tanners. *Journal of the American Academy of Dermatology, 54*, 709–711. doi: 10.1016/j.jaad.2005.11.1059

Keesling, B., & Friedman, H. S. (1987). Psychosocial factors in sunbathing and sunscreen use. *Health Psychology, 6*, 477–493. doi: 10.1037/0278-6133.6.5.477

Kiviniemi, M. T., & Ellis, E. M. (2014). Worry about skin cancer mediates the relation of perceived cancer risk and sunscreen use. *Journal of Behavioral Medicine, 37*, 1069–1074. doi: 10.1007/s10865-013-9538-1

Knight, J. M., Kirincich, A. N., Farmer, E. R., & Hood, A. F. (2002). Awareness of the risks of tanning lamps does not influence behavior among college students. *Archives of Dermatology, 138*, 1311–1315. doi: 10.1001/archderm.138.10.1311

Kourosh, A. S., Harrington, C. R., & Adinoff, B. (2010). Tanning as a behavioral addiction. *American Journal of Drug and Alcohol Abuse, 36*, 284–290. doi: 10.3109/00952990.2010.491883

Lemal, M., & Van den Bulck, J. (2010). Testing the effectiveness of a skin cancer narrative in promoting positive health behavior: A pilot study. *Preventive Medicine, 51*, 178–181. doi: 10.1016/j.ypmed.2010.04.019

Lessin, S. R., Perlis, C. S., & Zook, M. B. (2012). How ultraviolet radiation tans skin. In C. J. Heckman & S. L. Manne (Eds.), *Shedding light on indoor tanning* (pp. 87–94). doi: 10.1007/978-94-007-2048-0_5, New York: Springer.

Levins, P. C., Carr, D. B., Fisher, J. E., Momtaz, K., & Parrish, J. A. (1983). Plasma beta-endorphin and beta-lipotropin response to ultraviolet radiation. *Lancet, 2*, 166.

Lomas, A., Leonardi-Bee, J., & Bath-Hextall, F. (2012). A systematic review of worldwide incidence of nonmelanoma skin cancer. *British Journal of Dermatology, 166*, 1069–1080. doi: 10.1111/j.1365-2133.2012.10830.x

Mahler, H. I. (2014). The role of emotions in UV protection intentions and behaviors. *Psychology, Health and Medicine, 19*, 344–354. doi: 10.1080/13548506.2013.802359

Manne, S. L., Coups, E. J., & Kashy, D. A. (2016). Relationship factors and couples' engagement in sun protection. *Health Education Research, 31*, 542–554. doi: 10.1093/her/cyw027

Mawn, V. B., & Fleischer, A. B., Jr. (1993). A survey of attitudes, beliefs, and behavior regarding tanning bed use, sunbathing, and sunscreen use. *Journal of the American Academy of Dermatology, 29*, 959–962. doi: 10.1016/0190-9622(93)70274-W

Mays, D., & Zhao, X. (2016). The influence of framed messages and self-affirmation on indoor tanning behavioral intentions in 18- to 30-year-old women. *Health Psychology, 35*, 123–130. doi: 10.1037/hea0000253

McMichael, T., Prüss-Üstün, A., Smith, W., Lucas, R., Armstrong, B. K., & World Health Organization. (2006). *Solar ultraviolet radiation: Global burden of disease from solar ultraviolet radiation*. Geneva Switzerland: World Health Organization Press.

Miyamura, Y., Coelho, S. G., Schlenz, K., Batzer, J., Smuda, C., Choi, W., . . . Hearing, V. J. (2011). The deceptive nature of UVA tanning versus the modest protective effects of UVB tanning on human skin. *Pigment Cell and Melanoma Research, 24*, 136–147. doi: 10.1111/j.1755-148X.2010.00764.x

Morales-Sánchez, M. A., Peralta-Pedrero, M. L., & Domínguez-Gómez, M. A. (2014). Design and validation of a questionnaire for measuring perceived risk of skin cancer. *Actas Dermo-Sifiliográficas, 105*, 276–285. doi: 10.1016/j.adengl.2013.10.006

Morris, K. L., Cooper, D. P., Goldenberg, J. L., Arndt, J., & Gibbons, F. X. (2014). Improving the efficacy of appearance-based sun exposure interventions with the terror management health model. *Psychology and Health, 29*, 1245–1264. doi: 10.1080/08870446.2014.922184

Mosher, C. E., & Danoff-Burg, S. (2010). Addiction to indoor tanning relation to anxiety, depression, and substance use. *Archives of Dermatology, 146*, 412–417. doi: 10.1001/archdermatol.2009.385

Myrick, J. G., Noar, S. M., Kelley, D., & Zeitany, A. E. (2016). The relationships between female adolescents' media use, indoor tanning outcome expectations, and behavioral intentions. *Health Education and Behavior*. Advance online publication. doi: 10.1177/1090198116667251

Noar, S. M., Myrick, J. G., Morales-Pico, B., & Thomas, N. E. (2014). Development and validation of the comprehensive indoor tanning expectations scale. *JAMA Dermatology, 150*, 512–521. doi: 10.1001/jamadermatol.2013.9086

Noar, S. M., Myrick, J. G., Zeitany, A., Kelley, D., Morales-Pico, B., & Thomas, N. E. (2015). Testing a social cognitive theory-based model of indoor tanning: Implications for skin cancer prevention messages. *Health Communication, 30*, 164–174. doi: 10.1080/10410236.2014.974125

Nolan, B. V., & Feldman, S. R. (2009). Ultraviolet tanning addiction. *Dermatologic Clinics, 27*, 109–112. doi: 10.1016/j.det.2008.11.007

Nolan, B. V., Taylor, S. L., Liguori, A., & Feldman, S. R. (2009). Tanning as an addictive behavior: A literature review. *Photodermatology, Photoimmunology and Photomedicine, 25*, 12–19. doi: 10.1111/j.1600-0781.2009.00392.x

Poorsattar, S. P., & Hornung, R. L. (2007). UV light abuse and high-risk tanning behavior among undergraduate college students. *Journal of the American Academy of Dermatology, 56*, 375–379. doi: 10.1016/j.jaad.2006.08.064

Randle, H. W. (1997). Suntanning: Differences in perceptions throughout history. *Mayo Clinic Proceedings, 72*, 461–466. doi: 10.1016/S0025-6196(11)64867-2

Rhainds, M., De Guire, L., & Claveau, J. (1999). A population-based survey on the use of artificial tanning devices in the Province of Quebec, Canada. *Journal of the American Academy of Dermatology, 40*, 572–576. doi: 10.1016/S0190-9622(99)70439-1

Rogers, H. W., Weinstock, M. A., Feldman, S. R., & Coldiron, B. M. (2015). Incidence estimate of nonmelanoma skin cancer (keratinocyte carcinomas) in the US population, 2012. *JAMA Dermatology, 151*, 1081–1086.

Stapleton, J. L., Hillhouse, J. J., Turrisi, R., Robinson, J. K., Baker, K., Manne, S. L., & Coups, E. J. (2013). Erythema and ultraviolet indoor tanning: Findings from a diary study. *Translational Behavioral Medicine, 3*, 10–16. doi: 10.1001/jamadermatol.2015.1187

Tripp, M. K., Peterson, S. K., Prokhorov, A. V., Shete, S. S., Lee, J. E., Gershenwald, J. E., & Gritz, E. R. (2016). Correlates of sun protection and sunburn in children of melanoma survivors. *American Journal of Preventive Medicine, 51*, 77–85. doi: 10.1016/j.amepre.2016.02.032

US Department of Health and Human Services. (2014). *Reports of the surgeon general: The surgeon general's call to action to prevent skin cancer*. Washington, DC: Office of the Surgeon General.

Vogue, M. (1929). *Back to sunburn with the mode*. Vogue, July 20, 76–78.

Warthan, M. M., Uchida, T., & Wagner, R. F. (2005). UV light tanning as a type of substance-related disorder. *Archives of Dermatology, 141*, 963–966. doi: 10.1001/archderm.141.8.963

Watson, D., Clark, L. A., & Tellegen, A. (1988). Development and validation of brief measures of positive and negative affect: The PANAS scales. *Journal of Personality and Social Psychology, 54*, 1063–1070. doi: 10.1037/0022-3514.54.6.1063

Wehner, M. R., Chren, M. M., Nameth, D., Choudhry, A., Gaskins, M., Nead, K. T., . . . Linos, E. (2014). International prevalence of indoor tanning: A systematic review and meta-analysis. *JAMA Dermatology, 150*, 390–400. doi: 10.1001/jamadermatol.2013.6896

Zeller, S., Lazovich, D., Forster, J., & Widome, R. (2006). Do adolescent indoor tanners exhibit dependency? *Journal of the American Academy of Dermatology, 54*, 589–596. doi: 10.1016/j.jaad.2005.12.038

17

Emotions and Prosociality

Lessons for Blood Donation

EAMONN FERGUSON AND BARBARA MASSER

Without volunteer behavior, health services would struggle to meet and provide the levels of health care and service they currently do. For example, volunteers provide: (1) organs for transplantation; (2) blood for transfusion; (3) participants for medical trials and experiments; (4) staff for hospital radio, cafes, advice, and so forth; (5) money and time to support medical charities; (6) patient and relative support groups; (7) herd immunity against the flu; and so on. Thus, it is essential to understand the processes that motivate people to volunteer and that maintain their helping. This chapter examines what motivates people to donate blood. Altruism is often simplistically described as the main motivation. However, Ferguson and colleagues (Ferguson, Farrell, & Lawrence, 2008; Ferguson, Taylor, Keatley, Flynn, & Lawrence, 2012; Ferguson, Atsma, de Kort, & Veldhuizen, 2012; Ferguson & Lawrence, 2015), developing the mechanisms of altruism (MOA) approach, have shown that this simple assumption is not tenable for blood donation and maybe also for organ donation. In this chapter we explore how motivations to donate blood can be informed from our understanding of the role played by emotions with respect to prosociality.

BLOOD DONATION: MECHANISMS OF ALTRUISM, PROSOCIALITY, AND EMOTIONS

Behaviorally blood donation can be described as an altruistic act. It is voluntary, benefits another in need, and is costly to the donor (Steinberg, 2010). This may have the effect of enhancing the recipient's future fitness from an evolutionary perspective (i.e., long-term survival and fecundity) by saving their lives (to reproduce) (West, Mouden, & Gardner, 2011). Altruism defined in terms of enhancing future fitness of others, at personal cost, is termed *biological* altruism (Sober & Wilson, 1998). *Psychological* altruism, on the other hand, focuses on motivations for acting altruistically (Sober & Wilson, 1998). These can be combined (see Table 17.1) with pure altruism (Cell D: whereby helping others is driven by concern for others with no personal benefit) contrasted with impure altruism (Cell B: whereby helping others is driven primarily by concern for personal benefit). The debate in the blood donor literature primarily surrounds Cells B and D: that is, does blood donation have a selfish component? While blood donors cite pure altruism as their main motivation (Bednall & Bove, 2011) this does not mean that selfish motivations are not a more fundamental driver of blood donor behavior (see Ferguson, 2015, for a review). That a donation of blood or tissue can have a selfish component is highlighted by the Nuffield Council (2011) in relation to tissue donation, who state that helping others: "can be reckoned as virtuous whether or not founded on the pleasure such action brings to the donor (p. 139)." In the context of blood and organ donation this opens up the possibility of interventions that are not based on pure altruism (e.g., financial incentives; see Ferguson, 2015; Ferguson & Lawrence, 2015).

Given that an altruistic act, such as blood or organ donation, that benefits others (biological altruism) may have many motivations (psychological

TABLE 17.1 THE RELATIONSHIP BETWEEN BIOLOGICAL/EVOLUTIONARY ALTRUISM AND PSYCHOLOGICAL ALTRUISM FOR BLOOD DONATION

		Biological/Evolutionary	
		Selfish	**Altruistic**
Psychological	Selfish	**Donates blood to maximally benefit the self and not others or even to harm other.** · *Donate to find out blood group or get a blood test* · *Donate, because you want to, while knowing you have a blood-borne virus that may infect others* *Frequency of Donation*: One off **CELL A (selfish)**	**Donates blood to benefit others (and increases the groups fitness), but only as it provides the helper with some benefits.** · *Feel good (warm-glow) from the act of donating blood* · *Emotional regulation: Donating blood to manage negative mood states in general or from not donating blood (e.g., guilt, shame)* · *Indirect reciprocity (gaining a good reputation by being a blood donor)* · *Sexual Selection/Costly Signals (donate to indicate you are a person who is fit and healthy enough to donate blood and who can bear the cost of losing blood)* · *Reluctant Altruism (donating blood as others do not to gain warm-glow and reputation and to encourage others to donate to increase available resources).* *Frequency of Donation*: Repeat **CELL B (Impure altruism)**
	Altruistic	**Donates blood to help close others who you are generically related to.** · *Donate to help your children, or close relatives* *Frequency of Donation*: None **CELL C (Kin selection)**	**Donates blood to benefit others (and increases the groups fitness), and do this because you care about the welfare of others** · *Pure altruism—no personal benefit* *Frequency of Donation*: Repeat **CELL D (pure altruism)**

altruism) Ferguson (2015) suggested adopting the MOA approach. This involves mapping the insights about the mechanisms of altruism (both biological and psychological) from psychology, economics, biology, sociology, and philosophy onto blood donor motivations (e.g., Andreoni, 1990; Batson, 1991; Fehr & Fischbacher, 2004a, 2004b; Nowak, 2006). These are highlighted in each cell of Table 17.1. In what follows we draw on the literature relating the emotional process of pure and impure altruism in particular to understanding blood donor motivation and enhancing interventions.

BLOOD DONATION: THE MAIN PROSOCIAL EMOTIONS

The appraisal tendency framework (ATF) for emotions, developed by Lerner and colleagues (see Lerner & Keltner, 2000; Ferrer, Klein, Lerner, Reyna, & Keltner, 2015) is adopted as a primary organizing framework for emotions in relation to blood donor behavior. The ATF approach moves beyond exploring the simple valance of specific emotions to differentiate them in terms of appraisal dimensions such as certainty (e.g., the emotion arises as a consequence of a predictable stimulus) (see Table 17.2). This framework identifies six positive emotions (happiness, pride, relief, gratitude, hope, and surprise) and six negative emotions (anger, disgust, sadness, shame, guilt, and fear) (Ferrer et al., 2015). This framework can be combined with the work by Haidt (2003) defining families of moral emotions that to a greater or less extent have a prosocial tendency (see Table 17.1). These families are the "other condemning emotions" of contempt, anger, and disgust (the CAD triad), "self-conscious emotions" of shame, embarrassment and guilt (the SEG triad), the "other-suffering family" (sympathy, empathy, and compassion), and the "other-praising emotions" of gratitude, awe, and elevation. A number of emotions from the ATF and the moral families relate to prosociality (gratitude, happiness, hope, anger, shame, guilt, fear, and sadness). Table 17.1 links these to their respective MOA.

Positive Prosocial Emotions

Below we examine the links between specific aspects of prosociality and specific positive emotions.

Reciprocity and Gratitude

When another person does something positive to benefit an individual, that individual will feel gratitude toward them, especially if they feel it was *intentional* (Fredrickson, 2004). Thus, in terms of appraisals, gratitude is other-directed and linked to prosociality via indirect reciprocity (Ma, Tunney, & Ferguson, 2014; Tsang, Schulwitz, & Carlisle, 2012).

Reciprocity comes in two main flavors (direct and indirect). Direct reciprocity refers to the expectation that helping someone you expect to see again increases the probability that they will repay the favor. Indirect reciprocity has two flavors (down-stream and up-stream) (Nowak, 2006; Nowak & Sigmund, 2005). Down-stream indirect reciprocity works via the altruist gaining *positive reputation* (either via direct observation or gossip) from helping, which increases the likelihood of being helped by another unrelated person in the future (Milinski, Semmann, & Krambeck, 2002). This mechanism may work to encourage blood donors to donate via two routes: (1) enhancing the donor's *reputation* as a potential sexual partner or (2) the donor being drawn to the transfusion service as a worthy cause (see Ferguson, 2015). This suggests interventions that focus on making the donors' donation visible, such as arm bands, car stickers, and so forth, may be beneficial (see Carpenter & Myers, 2010). Up-stream indirect reciprocity operates via the *gratitude* felt by the person who has been helped energizing them to help another person. A recipient of blood (who cannot donate) may feel gratitude to the transfusion service and persuade others to donate. This is an extension of the donor-recruits-donor campaigns to a recipient-recruits-donor campaigns.

Trust and Hope

Hope refers to a desire for the person to have a better future for themselves and/or others with the belief that this is attainable (Cavabagh, Bettman,

TABLE 17.2 THE PROSOCIAL EMOTIONS, EMOTIONAL FAMILIES, APPRAISAL DIMENSIONS, AND INTERVENTIONS

Valance	**Specific Emotion**	**Haidt Prosocial Tendency/ Disinterestedness**	**Haidt Emotion Families**	**Appraisal Dimensions**					**MOA**	**Suggested Interventions**
				Certainty	**Control**	**Other/Situation**	**Attention**	**Anticipated Effort**		
Positive	Gratitude	High/Medium	OPE	Medium	Low	High	Medium	Low	Reciprocity	Public displays—badges, armbands
Positive	Hope			Low	Medium	High	High	High	Trust	Reinforce trust and hope with feedback and messages about blood helping to create better futures for us all
Positive	Happiness	Low/Low		High	Medium	Medium	Medium	Low	Warm-Glow	Highlight the positive benefits of donation
Positive	Pride	High/Low	SCE	High	High	Low	Medium	Low	Warm-Glow	Highlight the positive benefits of donation

Negative	Shame	High/Medium	SCE	Medium	High	Medium	Medium	Medium	Reparative—public	Highlight the health inequality between the healthy donor and ill recipient
Negative	Guilt	High/High	SCE	Medium	High	Low	Low	Medium	Reparative—private	Highlight the health inequality between the healthy donor and ill recipient
Negative	Sadness	Low/Low		Medium	Low	High	Low	Low	Negative State Relief	Detail the positive benefits of donation
Negative	Anger	High/High	OCE	High	High	High	Medium	Medium	Altruistic Punishment	Highlight issues of normative fairness
Negative	Fear	High/Low		Low	Low	Medium	Medium	High	Altruistic Punishment	Highlight issues of normative fairness

NOTE. **Certainty** (the emotion arises as a consequence of a predictable stimulus), **Control** (e.g., the emotion arises as a consequence of actions/cognition under personal control), **Other/Situation** (the emotion is a consequent of action of another person or a situation), **Attention** (the emotion is a consequence of a situation that demands attention), and **Anticipated Effort** (the degree of effort that the person feels that they will have to expend to deal with the emotion, its elicitor or its consequent).
OPE: Other praising emotions, **SCE**: Self-conscious emotions. **OCE**: Other-condemning emotions. **Prosocial tendency**: Extent to which the emotion actives a prosocial action to an eliciting event (High vs Low). **Disinterestedness**: The extent to which the emotion occurs when good or bad happens to the self (Low) or the elicitation of the emotion does not requires that the self is directly involves (High).

& Luce, 2015). Like gratitude, hope is other-directed. Hope has not been studied in relation to prosociality to any great extent (see Meer & Rosen, 2009 for an exception), but people do help as they hope that their actions will lead to a better future for others. Indeed, hope for a better future is one of the main motives given for volunteering in early stage clinical trials (Catt, Langridge, Fallowfield, Talbot, & Jenkins, 2011). With respect to recruiting donors the implication is to reinforce the hope that their donation will lead to a better future for the recipient. This can be achieved by providing evidence that blood is being used effectively. One way being used in Sweden, Australia, and the United Kingdom to do this is by providing donors with a text message when their donation has been used. Messages emphasizing how blood brings hope to people who are ill are therefore worthy of consideration.

Warm-Glow, Moral Value, and Pride

Warm-glow refers to feeling good following a prosocial act (Andreoni, 1990) and is directly proportional to the amount donated (Ferguson & Flynn, 2016). Indeed, the extent of feeling good after donating blood (Piliavin & Callero, 1991), as well as the expectation of feeling good (Ferguson et al., 2008), increases the likelihood of future donations. Consistent with this behavioral economic data shows that blood donors are motivated by warm-glow and not pure altruism (Ferguson, Atsma, et al., 2012). Ferguson and Flynn (2016) also indicate that warm-glow can also operate as an expectancy, in which case it is akin to the concept of an affective attitude in the prosocial context (Ferguson & Lawrence, 2015).

"Pride" is defined by the *Oxford English Dictionary* as a "feeling of deep pleasure or satisfaction derived from one's own achievement." Pride has often been seen as a "deadly sin" and the "root to all evil." So it may seem strange to link it to prosociality. However, pride can be divided into *hubristic* pride (linked to arrogance and conceit) and *authentic* pride (linked to achievement) (Tracy & Robins, 2007) with authentic pride linked to prosociality (Weiner, 1985). Indeed, recent theoretical models in behavioral economics link the "pride of acting altruistically" to warm-glow (Saito, 2015). People are more likely to be proud of achieving a prosocial act that is high cost (e.g., running a charity marathon, donating blood) than a low cost one (e.g., sending a small amount of money to charity) (Tracy & Robins, 2007). Indeed, plasma donors report feeling pride as a function of giving "more" than whole blood donors (Bove, Bednall, Masser, & Buzza, 2011). There is also evidence that appeals to collective pride promote helping (Van Leeuwen, van Dijk, & Kaynak, 2013). Again, this suggests that providing blood donors with a way to display that they are blood donors may be an effective intervention.

Negative Prosocial Emotions

Below we examine the links between specific aspects of prosociality and specific negative emotions.

Repair: Shame and Guilt

Guilt and shame are moral emotions referring to the self-representation of personal wrongdoing. Guilt is more private and behavior-focused, whereas shame is more public and self-focused (Amodio, Devine, & Harmon-Jones, 2007). People will be motivated to avoid the guilt of not acting prosocially or the shame of acting selfishly (Saito, 2015). Guilt also has a reparative function. Indeed, both increases in guilt and shame lead to increased prosociality (e.g., Allpress, Brown, Giner-Sorolla, Deonna, & Teroni, 2014). Furthermore, when people realize they have been unfair to others, they feel guilt, leading to reparative behavior (Keltner, Haidt, & Shiota, 2006).

In the blood donor context, guilt has been identified as a donor motivation (France, Kawalsky, France, Himawan, Kessler, & Shaz, 2014). Thus, appeals based on guilt could be effective. Indeed, evidence shows that anticipatory guilt (guilt that arises in advance of a future transgression, which can be avoided) rather than reactive guilt (guilt experienced when a transgression takes place) promotes stronger blood donor intentions (Renner, Lindenmeier, Tscheulin, & Drevs, 2013). Guilt appeals, however, can often be seen by recipients as having high manipulative intent ("if people like you do not donate then there will be shortages"), which can lead to anger and reactance (Cotte, Coulter, & Moore, 2005).

However, there may be more subtle ways to engender prosocial guilt based on the models of inequality aversion (Fehr & Schmidt, 1999). These models suggest that people are motivated to *reduce inequality* between themselves and others. When you have more than others, inequality is termed advantageous, leading to *guilt*, which triggers actions to reduce the inequality (Fehr & Schmidt, 1999). As the potential donor is healthy and is able to give blood, the donor is better off than any recipient. This advantageous inequality suggests the following appeal, "Being fit and healthy to give blood, means you have the ability to help those less healthy than you. Please don't miss out on the chance to help those less fortunate than you." Indeed, there is some evidence that this type of message is effective and leads to prosocial guilt (guilt linked to taking action to help others), which leads to taking information about becoming a donor (Ferguson, 2016).

Sadness and Negative State Relief

The negative state relief (NSR) model proposes that distress (usually operationalized as sadness), resulting from observing another in need, motivates the helper to help primarily to reduce their own sadness (Cialdini et al., 1987). In terms of interventions, this suggests that highlighting that donating blood may help you feel good about yourself, or at least less bad, will be beneficial and can be linked to warm-glow appeals.

Anger, Moral Elevation, and Altruistic Punishment: The Reluctant Altruist

One major threat to cooperation is free-riding. That is, people gain a relative advantage by not helping at the expense of others' good deeds. The free-riding rate is high for blood donation at about 96% (Abasolo & Tsuchiya, 2014). One mechanism to reduce free-riding and increase cooperation is known as *altruistic punishment* (i.e., people have the provision to identify and punish free-riders: Fehr & Fischbacher, 2004a). Anger is believed to motivate punishment even if it is merely threatened (Skatova & Ferguson, 2013). The concept of altruistic punishment is embodied theoretically in the model of *strong reciprocity*, which is "a willingness to sacrifice resources for rewarding fair and punishing unfair behavior *even if this is costly and provides neither present nor future material rewards for the reciprocator*" (Fehr, Fischbacher, & Gatcher, 2002, p. 2: their italics). Thus helping is conditional on the perceived positive reputation of the recipient, but crucially not on a future reward from the recipient. Strong reciprocation could motivate blood donors as they (1) do not expect a future reward and (2) are likely to perceive both the recipient of blood and the transfusion service as deserving. This implies that the blood donors would be more likely to punish unfair behavior, than nondonors. However, Ferguson, Taylor, et al. (2012) showed that blood donors were no more likely to punish free-riding than to nondonors.

However, anger also has a more energizing role to play in cooperation via eliciting "moral anger." Moral anger occurs when an individual perceives that an injustice has occurred and the individual is motivated to help to redress the injustice (van Doorn & Zeelenberg, 2014). Moral anger promotes prosociality and victim compensation (Montada & Schneider, 1989) and forms part of the concept of *reluctant altruism* identified by Ferguson, Atsma, et al. (2012) and Ferguson (2015). When faced with free-riding, reluctant altruists have a preference for helping rather than punishing. A key aspect is the moral anger directed toward free-riding, energizing helping. This is linked with two other mechanisms that *increase* cooperation in the face of free-riding: a "*negative view of humanity*" (feelings that society is uncaring and selfish) and "*reduced trust*" in others' willingness to cooperate (see Ferguson, 2015, also). This *reluctant altruist triad* leads the reluctant altruist to act prosocially, when others do not, and to encourage others to also act prosocially. The reluctant altruist, therefore, may also be a source of *moral elevation*. Moral elevation occurs when a person witnesses another uphold the highest moral virtues and leads to prosocial behavior (Schnall, Roper, & Fessler, 2010). Thus the reluctant altruist catalyzes prosociality via moral elevation.

One implication of reluctant altruism is to harness the triad of "*moral anger*," "*negative view of humanity*," and "*reduced trust*" to energize helping. One technique for this is *voluntary reciprocal altruism* (VRA), based on a two-question strategy that activates and aligns norms of fairness and reciprocity with self-interest (Landry, 2006). The first question aligns self-interest, reciprocity and fairness: "I would want a blood transfusion to save *my* life: YES or NO." Answering YES, highlights (1) a *personal* potential future need, and (2) that having sufficient blood is contingent on all of us contributing. The second question asks: "I would be willing to donate blood: YES or NO." If you are willing to receive a transfusion it is only *fair* to also donate and answer YES. However, to answer YES means considering NO. This highlights to the decision-maker that some people will answer YES to question 1 and NO to question 2. If others do not intend to donate, but are happy to receive, then shortages could result. This concern about shortages should motivate the reluctant altruistic.

Other Prosocial Emotions

Below we examine the links between specific aspects of prosociality and emapathy and compassion.

Empathy/Compassion and Compassion Fade

These moral emotions fall under Haidt's (2003) "other-suffering family" of emotions. Feeling compassion/sympathy for others motivates helping (Batson, 1991). However, evidence shows that empathic personality traits are not linked to blood donation (Steele et al., 2008). The concepts of "empathic joy" suggests that empathy should have a stronger link to helping when feedback on the consequences of helping is available (Smith, Keating, & Stotland, 1989). This suggests that text messages that provide feedback should be beneficial for those high in empathic traits (Ferguson, 2016).

Alternatively, recruitment campaigns could focus on the type of people helped by transfusions. However, potential problems due to both *compassion fade* (donation rates decrease as people consider more than one person in need; Vastfjall, Slovic, Mayorga, & Peters, 2014) and the "*identifiable victim effect*" (probability of helping is greater for an identifiable victim versus statistical victim: Kogut & Ritov, 2005; Small, Loewenstein, & Slovic, 2005) need to be avoided. These effects suggest that interventions based on specific cases may be more effective in recruiting blood donors. However, the favoring of a single case is more likely to be effective if the need is immediate and case is a member of the donor's in-group (Ein-Gar & Levontin, 2013). However, Ein-Gar and Levontin (2013) showed that when the donation appeal is targeted at future need (or the out-group) then focusing on the charitable organization results in greater donations than focusing on individual cases. Thus, transfusion services could target appeals at the organizational level, emphasizing the respect the organization has for donors (Boezeman & Ellemers, 2007), and focus on future needs.

Non-Prosocial Emotions: Disgust, Fear, Anxiety, and Regret

The preceding discussion has focused on prosocial emotions and how these may energize helping. However, non-prosocial emotional reactions can also impact donations. A substantial body of literature has considered the role of predonation pathogen disgust (Tybur, Lieberman, & Griskevicius, 2009), fear (of needles, blood draw), and anxiety as potential causes of adverse reactions in blood donors, with these reactions negatively impacting retention. Research implicating bodily disgust in fainting (e.g., Sawchuk, Lohr, Westendorf, Menuler, & Tolin, 2002), led Viar, Etzel, Ciesielski, and Olantunji (2010) to explore the role of disgust, anxiety, and injection fear in predicting adverse reactions in donors. Disgust only played a unique role in predicting fainting symptoms alongside anxiety for nonfearful donors. For those donors who were fearful, only anxiety predicted their fainting symptoms. In the context of blood donation, the affective responses of fear and/or anxiety are often conflated in responses. Fear of blood loss is adaptive (Ditto, Gilchrist, & Holly, 2012) and should motivate avoidance therefore making it unlikely to be seen in those who donate. However, it seems that the feelings of uncertainty that presenting donors may experience as to whether the outcome of donating blood will be good or bad (i.e., anxiety) are often expressed as fear. Indeed, a single-item measure asking about fear of the blood draw is highly effective in identifying those at risk of adverse reactions (France et al., 2014). Further, a number of analyses have found predonation state (Chell, Waller, & Masser, 2016) and trait (Meade, France, & Peterson, 1996) anxiety to be good predictors of adverse reactions to donating.

While disgust, fear, and anxiety deter donor recruitment and retention, anticipated regret at not donating can motivate (Zeelenberg, 1999), and the role of anticipated regret in motivating a variety of behavior, including blood donation, is widely documented. As an addition onto the theory of planned behavior, anticipated regret at not donating emerges as a strong, positive predictor of both intention to donate (e.g., Masser, White, Hyde, Terry, & Robinson, 2009; Godin et al., 2005) and actual donor behavior for experienced donors (Godin et al., 2007). However, it is notable that few analyses have considered anticipated regret in the context of other potential anticipated or anticipatory emotions (Baumgartner, Pieters, & Bagozzi, 2008).

BLOOD DONOR CYCLE, CAREER AND EMOTIONAL DECISIONS

The emotions detailed thus far should not be seen as static, but embedded within a dynamic blood donor career cycle, which traces the donor progress from a nondonor to a first-time donor to a committed donor (Ferguson, 1996). This is important, as the evidence shows that the predictive status of factors associated with blood donor behavior changes as a function of the donor career (e.g., Ferguson, Atsma, et al., 2012). Emotions, emotional processes, and their effective functional outcomes are also likely to be modified by stage of the donor career. Figure 17.1 is designed to set out the simple landscape of the dynamic influence of emotional reasoning across the blood donor career. We use this to describe the key emotional states, processes, and biases associated across the blood donor career.

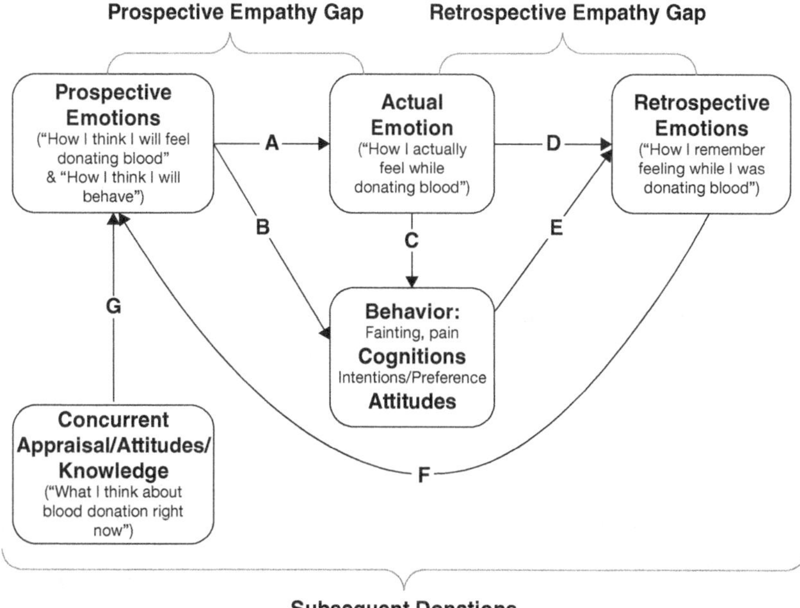

Figure 17.1. Blood donor career, emotions, and memory.

Constructive Episodic Simulation

First and foremost, this model emphasizes the key role of affect in the recall of past events (retrospection) and how these affect-laden recollections are used to predict and simulate future events (prospection). Indeed, autobiographical memory can be used not only to help us make sense of the past and present but to predict (prospection) the future (Schacter & Addis, 2007). Path F reflects this process, which Schacter and Addis (2007) refer to as constructive episodic simulation. But this process is fallible. When we use recalled *past* experiences to simulate imagined *futures* a number of biases (recall, forecasting, empathy gaps) influence this process.

Recall Bias and Affective Forecasting

Schacter and Addis (2007) show consistent support for bias in retrospective recall, with people actively constructing their memories. Paths G plus

A reflect the process of *affective forecasting* bias and in particular what is known as the "impact bias," whereby people overestimate the *duration* and *intensity* of future emotions (see Wilson & Gilbert, 2008; Levine, Lench, & Safter, 2009). It has been shown that this overestimation is linked to people's tendency to pay attention to peak intense emotional episodes during a transaction (Fredrickson & Kahneman, 1993). This overestimation process however, is moderated by personality and current knowledge/ appraisal. For example, Larsen (1992) showed that those high in neuroticism, compared to those low, recalled past symptoms as more intense than they were. Thus those high in trait anxiety may recall negative donation experiences as more intense than they were. People will bias their recall of past emotions with respect to their current level of emotional appraisals (Levine et al., 2009). Further, the intensity of pre-event negative emotions are more likely overestimated following a negative outcome (e.g., exam failure) than a positive outcome (e.g., exam success) (Finenauer, Gallucci, van Dijk & Pollman, 2007). Thus, those who have a negative reaction while donating blood will likely overestimate their predonation anxiety and negative emotions. Also those who experience negative reactions post donation (bruising, feeling faint at home, etc.) may recall experiencing greater negative emotions while donating blood. This overestimated recall of negative emotions may be responsible for reduced return rates. One way to deal with this is to give donors coping skills to deal with their emotional reactions and to reduce episodes of fainting. While applied muscle tension and liquid preloads have shown some initial promise in this context (France et al., 2010), a recent meta-analytic review in the context of blood donation has raised some doubts about their overall effectiveness (Fisher et al., 2016). Playing music may help also for novice donors (Ferguson, Singh, & Cunningham-Snell, 1997).

Empathy Gaps

Another concept important in this temporal patterning is the "empathy gap" (Loewenstein, 2005). This refers to the difficulty people have in predicting how they will act when experiencing an emotional state different to their current one (Loewenstein, 2000). These may be *prospective* (how well people predict their future behavior, when in different emotional states to their current one) or *retrospective* (how well people recall their past behavior that occurred in different emotional states to their current one). Prospective gaps are operationalized as the difference between B and C. That is, how donors *think* they will behave given emotions when donating (B) and how that emotion *actually* influences their behavior (Path C). In the retrospective case the relative difference is between E and C.

Hot-cold and *cold-hot* gaps are also differentiated. Hot-cold gaps are experienced when people in an aroused emotional state underestimate how their current emotions influence their decisions. In cold-hot gaps people underestimate, when in a cold unaroused emotional state, how their emotions in the actual aroused state will influence their behavior. Thus, there are two recurring empathy gaps in the blood donation cycle. The prospective gap examines people's ability to predict whether they will faint or feel pain when donating blood while in their current emotional state prior to donating, and the retrospective gap examines how the donor's current postdonation emotions influence their recall of how they felt they coped or felt pain while donating. The recalled emotion-behavior then drives forward to the prospective memory system. An important development in this area for blood donor research is evidence that potential donor's emotion responses are very different depending on whether or not they can observe images and equipment associated with blood donation (Clowes & Masser, 2012; Masser, France, Himawan, Hyde, & Smith, 2017) with anxiety higher when blood donation paraphernalia is present.

The key take-home message is that memories for emotions and their link to behavior are dynamic, fallible, and influenced by current emotional states (hot or cold). All of which are influenced by context and personality (Ferguson, 2013). Thus research on blood donor emotions needs to adopt a temporal and dynamic approach. Not only measuring emotions as they occur but also tracking how they change and exploring accuracy in emotional recall and how memory for emotion shapes imagined donor futures. The effectiveness of specific interventions that influence memory for emotions needs to be explored in the blood donor context. Thus, the donor cycle offers both a real-world lab context to study emotions, memory, and behavior and addresses the provision of an adequate and safe blood supply.

CONCLUSIONS

Overall, this chapter has set out the complexity and subtlety of the role played by emotions in blood donor behavior. Blood donation provides a "real-world lab" to study altruism and an important area for practical interventions. Indeed, this work has led to new insights in terms of the discovery of reluctant altruism and new potential valuable interventions based on VRA and inequality aversion.

REFERENCES

Abasolo, I., & Tsuchiya, A. (2014). Blood donation as a public good: An empirical investigation of the free rider problem. *European Journal of Health Economics, 15*, 313–321.

Allpress, J. A., Brown, R., Giner-Sorolla, R., Deonna, J. A., & Teroni, F. (2014). Two faces of group-based shame: Moral shame and image shame differentially predict positive and negative orientations to in-group wrongdoing. *Personality and Social Psychology Bulletin, 40*, 1270–1284.

Amodio, D. M., Devine, P. G., & Harmon-Jones, E. (2007). A dynamic model of guilt—Implications for motivation and self-regulation in the context of prejudice. *Psychological Science, 18*, 524–530. doi: 10.1111/J.1467-9280.2007.01933.X

Andreoni, J. (1990). Impure altruism and donations to public goods: A theory of warm glow giving. *Economic Journal, 100*, 464–4877.

Batson, C. D. (1991). *The altruism question: Toward a social-psychological answer.* Hillsdale, NJ: Erlbaum.

Baumgartner, H., Pieters, R., & Bagozzi, R. P. (2008). Future-Oriented Emotions: Conceptualization and Behavioral Effects. *European Journal of Social Psychology, 38*, 685–696. https://doi.org/10.1002/ejsp.467

Bednall, C., & Bove, L. L. (2011). Donating blood: A meta-analytic review of self-reported motivators and deterrents. *Transfusion Medicine Reviews, 25*, 317–334.

Boezeman, E. J., & Ellemers, N. (2007). Volunteering for charity: Pride, respect and the commitment of volunteers. *Journal of Applied Psychology, 92*, 771–785.

Bove, L. L., Bednall, T., Masser, B., & Buzza, M. (2011). Understanding the plasmapheresis donor in a voluntary nonremunerated environment. *Transfusion, 51*, 2411–2424.

Carpenter, J., & Myers., C. K. (2010). Why volunteer? Evidence on the role of altruism, image, and incentives. *Journal of Public Economics, 94*, 911–920.

Cavabagh, L. A., Bettman, J. R., & Luce, M. F. (2015). Feeling Love and Doing More for Distant Others: Specific Positive Emotions Differentially Affect Prosocial Consumption. *Journal of Marketing Research, LII*, 657–673.

Catt, S., Langridge, C., Fallowfield, L., Talbot, D. C., & Jenkins, V. (2011). Reason given by patients for participating, or not, in Phase 1 cancer trials. *European Journal of Cancer, 47*, 1490–1497.

Chell, K., Waller, D., & Masser, B. (2016). The Blood Donor Anxiety scale: A six-item anxiety measure based on the Spielberger State-Trait Anxiety inventory. *Transfusion, 56*, 1645–1653. doi: 10.1111/trf.13520

Cialdini, R. B., Schaller, M., Houlihan, D., Arps, K., Fultz, J., & Beaman, A. L. (1987). Empathy-based helping: Is it selflessly or selfishly motivated? *Journal of Personality and Social Psychology, 52*, 749–758.

Clowes, R., & Masser, B. M. (2012). Right here, right now: The impact of the blood donation context on anxiety, attitudes, subjective norms, self-efficacy, and intention to donate blood. *Transfusion, 52*, 1560–1565. doi: 10.1111/j.1537-2995.2011.03486.x

Cotte, J., Coulter, R. A., & Moore, M. (2005). Enhancing and disrupting guilt: The role of credibility and perceived manipulative intent. *Journal of Business Research, 58*, 361–368.

Ditto, B., Gilchrist, P. T., & Holly, C. D. (2012). Fear-related predictors of vasovagal symptoms during blood donation: It's in the blood. *Journal of Behavioral Medicine, 35*, 393–399. doi: 10.1007/s10865-011-9366-0

Ein-Gar D., & Levontin, L. (2013). Giving from a distance: Putting the charitable organization at the center of the donation appeal. *Journal of Consumer Psychology, 23*, 197–211

Fehr, E., & Schmidt, K. M. (1999). A theory of fairness, competition and cooperation. *Quarterly Journal of Economics, 114*, 817–868.

Fehr, E., & Fischbacher, U. (2004a). Third-party punishment and social norms. *Evolution and Human Behavior, 25*, 63–87.

Fehr, E., & Fischbacher, U. (2004b). Social norms and human cooperation. *Trends in Cognitive Science, 8*, 185–190.

Fehr, E., Fischbacher, U., & Gachter, S. (2002). Strong reciprocity, human cooperation and the enforcement of social norms. *Human Nature, 13*, 1–25.

Ferguson, E. (1996). Predictors of future behaviour: A review of the psychological literature on blood donation. *British Journal of Health Psychology, 1*, 287–308.

Ferguson, E. (2013). Personality is of central concern to understand health: Towards a theoretical model for health psychology *Health Psychology Review, 7*, S32–S70.

Ferguson, E. (2015). Mechanisms of altruism approach to blood donor recruitment and retention: a review and future directions *Transfusion Medicine, 25*, 211–226. doi: 10.1111/tme.12233

Ferguson, E. (2016). *Harnessing altruism in blood donor recruitment and retention.* Paper presented at the European Conference on donor Health and Management. Cambridge, July 13–15.

Ferguson, E., Atsma, F., de Kort, W., & Veldhuizen, I. (2012). Exploring the pattern of blood donor beliefs in first time, novice and experienced donors: Differentiating reluctant altruism, pure altruism, impure altruism and warm-glow. *Transfusion, 52,* 343–355. doi: 10.1111/j.1537-2995.2011.03279.x.

Ferguson, E., Farrell, K., & Lawrence, C. (2008). Blood donation is an act of benevolence rather than altruism. *Health Psychology, 27,* 327–336.

Ferguson, E., & Flynn, N. (2016). Moral Relativism as a Disconnect Between Behavioural and Experienced Warm Glow. *Journal of Economic Psychology, 56,* 163–175. http://dx.doi.org/10.1016/j.jeop.2016.06.002

Ferguson, E., & Lawrence, C. (2015). Blood donation and altruism: The mechanism of altruism approach. *ISBT Science Series, 11*(Suppl. 1), 148–157.

Ferguson, E., Singh, A., & Cunningham-Snell, N. (1997). Stress and blood donation: Effects of music and previous donation experience. *British Journal of Psychology, 88,* 277–294.

Ferguson, E., Taylor, M., Keatley, D., Flynn, N., & Lawrence, C. (2012). Blood donors' helping behavior is driven by warm glow: More evidence for the blood donor benevolence hypothesis. *Transfusion, 52,* 2189–2200. doi. 10.1111/j.1537-2995.2011.03557.x

Ferrer, R., Klein, W., Lerner, J. S., Reyna, V. F., & Keltner, D. (2015). Emotions and health decision-making: Extending the appraisal tendency framework to improve health and healthcare. In C. Roberto & I. Kawachi (Eds.), *Behavioral economics and public health.* Cambridge, MA: Harvard University Press.

Finenauer, C., Gallucci, M., van Dijk, W. W., & Pollman, M. (2007). Investigating the role of time in affective forecasting: Temporal influence on forecasting accuracy. *Personality and Social Psychological Bulletin, 33,* 1152–1166.

Fisher, S., Allan, D., Doree, C., Naylor, J., D'Angelantonio, E., & Roberts, D. (2016). *Interventions to reduce vasovagal reactions in blood donors: A systematic review and meta-analysis.* Poster presented at the European Conference on donor Health and Management. Cambridge, July 13–15.

France, C. R., Ditto, B., Wissel, M. E., France, J. L., Dickert, T., Rader, A., . . . Matson, E. (2010). Pre-donation hydration and applied muscle tension combine to reduce presyncopal reactions to blood donation. *Transfusion, 50,* 1257–1264. doi:10.1111/j.1537-2995.2009.02574.x

France, C. R., Kawalsky, J. M., France, J. L., Himawan, L. K., Kessler, D. A., & Shaz, B. H. (2014). The blood donor identity survey: A multidimensional measure of blood donor motivations. *Transfusion, 54,* 2098–2105.

France, C. R., France, J. L., Carlson, B. W., Himawan, L. K., Stephens, K. Y., Frame-Brown, T. A., . . . Menitove, J. E. (2014). Fear of blood draws, vasovagal reactions, and retention among high school donors. *Transfusion, 54,* 918–924. PMID: 23915025.

Fredrickson, B. L. (2004). Gratitude, like other positive emotions, broadens and builds. In R. A. Emmons & M. E. McCullough (Ed.), *The psychology of gratitude* (pp. 145–166). New York, NY: Oxford University Press.

Fredrickson, B. L., & Kahneman, D. (1993). Duration neglect in retrospective evaluations of affective episodes. *Journal of Personality and Social Psychology, 65*, 45–55.

Godin, G., Conner, M., Sheeran, P., Ariane Bélanger-Grave, A., & Marc Germain, M. (2007). Determinants of repeated blood donation among new and experienced blood donors. *Transfusion, 47*, 1607–1615.

Godin, G., Sheeran, P., Conner, M., Germain, M., Blondeau, D., Gagne, C., . . . Naccache, H. (2005). Factors explain the intention to give blood among the general population. *Vox Sanguinus, 89*, 10–149. doi: 10.1111/j.1423-0410.2005.00674.x

Haidt, J. (2003). The moral emotions. In R. J. Davidson, K. R. Scherer, & H. H. Goldsmith (Eds.), *Handbook of affective sciences* (pp. 852–870). Oxford, UK: Oxford University Press.

Keltner, D., Haidt, J., & Shiota, M. N. (2006). Social functionalism and the evolution of emotions. In M. Schaller, J. A. Simpson & D. T. Kenrick (Eds.), *Evolution and social psychology* (pp. 115–142). Madison, CT: Psychosocial Press.

Kogut, T., & Ritov, I. (2005). The "identifiable victim" effect: An identified group of just a single individual? *Journal of Behavior and Decision Making, 18*, 167–175.

Landry, D. W. (2006). Voluntary reciprocal altruism: A novel strategy to encourage deceased organ donation. *Kidney International, 69*, 957–959.

Larsen, R. J. (1992). Neuroticism and selective encoding and recall of symptoms: Evidence from a combined concurrent-retrospective study. *Journal of Personality and Social Psychology, 62*, 480–488.

Lerner, J. S., & Keltner, D. (2000). Beyond valence: Toward a model of emotion-specific influences on judgment and choice. *Cognition and Emotion, 14*, 473–493.

Levine, L. J., Lench, H. C., & Safter, M. A. (2009). Functions of remembering and misremembering emotion. *Applied Cognitive Psychology, 23*, 1059–1075.

Loewenstein, G. (2005). Hot-cold empathy gaps on medical decision making. *Health Psychology, 24*, S49–S56.

Ma, L. K., Tunney, R. J., & Ferguson, E. (2014). Gratefully received, gratefully repaid: The role of perceived fairness in cooperative interactions. *Plos One*, *9*, doi:10.1371/journal.pone.0114976.

Masser, B. M., France C. R., Himawan, L. K., Hyde, M. K., & Smith, G. (2017). The impact of the context and recruitment materials on nondonors' willingness to donate blood. *Transfusion, 56*, 2995–3003. doi: 10.1111/trf.13805. Epub 201.

Masser, B. M., White, K. M., Hyde, M. K., Terry, D. J, & Robinson, N. G. (2009). Predicting blood donation intentions and behavior among Australian blood donors: Testing an extended theory of planned behavior model. *Transfusion, 49*, 320–329. doi: 10.1111/j.1537-2995.2008.01981.x

Meade, M. A., France, C. R., & Peterson, L. M. (1996). Predicting vasovagal reactions in volunteer blood donors. *Journal of Psychosomatic Research, 40*, 495–501.

Meer, J., & Rosen, H. S. (2009). Altruism and the child cycle of alumni donations. American *Economic Journal, 1*, 258–286.

Milinski, M., Semmann, D., & Krambeck, H. J. (2002). Donor to charity gain in both indirect reciprocity and political reputation. *Proceedings of the Royal Society of London, B, 269*, 881–883.

Montada, L., & Schneider, A. (1989). Justices and emotional reactions to the disadvantaged. *Social Justice Research*, *3*, 313–341.

Nowak, M. A. (2006). Five rules for the evolution of cooperation. *Science*, *314*, 1560–1563.

Nowak, M., & Sigmund, K. (2005). Evolution of indirect reciprocity. *Nature*, *437*, 1291–1298.

Nuffield Council on Bioethics. *Human bodies: Donation for medicine and research.* London, Nuffield Council on Bioethics, 2011.

Piliavin, J. A, & Callero, P. L. (1991). *Giving blood: The development of an altruistic identity*. Baltimore, MD: John Hopkins University Press.

Renner, S., Lindenmeier, J., Tscheulin, D. K., & Drevs, F. (2013). Guilt appeals and prosocial behaviour: An experimental analysis of the effects of anticipatory versus reactive guilt appeals on the effectiveness of blood donor appeals. *Journal of Nonprofit Public Sector and Marketing*, *25*, 237–255.

Saito, K. (2015). Impure altruism and impure selfishness. *Journal of Economic Theory*, *158*, 336–370.

Sawchuk, C. N., Lohr, J. M., Westendorf, D. N., Menuier, S. A., & Tolin, D. F. (2002). Emotional responding to fearful and disgusting stimuli in specific phobics. *Behaviour Research and Therapy*, *40*, 1031–1046.

Schacter, D. L., & Addis, D. R. (2007). The cognitive neuroscience of constructive memory: Remembering the past and imagining the future. *Philosophical Transactions of the Royal Society, B*, *362*, 773–786.

Schnall, S., Roper, J., & Fessler, D. M. T. (2010). Elevation leads to altruistic behaviour. *Psychological Science*, *2*, 315–320.

Skatova, A., & Ferguson, E. (2013). Individual differences in behavioural inhibition explain free riding in the public good games when punishment becomes uncertain. *Behavioral and Brain Functions*, *9*, article 3, doi: 10.1186/1744-9081-9-3.

Small, D. A., Loewenstein, G., & Slovic, P. (2005). Sympathy and callousness: The impact of deliberative thought on donations to identifiable and statistical victims. *Organizational Behavior and Human Decision Process*, *102*, 143–153.

Smith, K. D., Keating, J. P., & Stotland, E. (1989). Altruism reconsidered: The effects of denying feedback on a victim's status to empathically witness. *Journal of Personality and Social Psychology*, *57*, 641–650.

Sober, E., & Wilson, D. S. *Unto others: The evolution and psychology of unselfish behaviour*. Cambridge, MA: Harvard University Press, 1998.

Steele, W. R., Schreiber, G.B., Guiltinan, A., Nass, C., Glynn, S. A., Wright, D. J., . . . Garratty, G. (2008). The role of altruistic behaviour, empathic concern, and social responsibility motivation in blood donation behaviour. *Transfusion*, *48*, 43–54.

Steinberg, D. (2010). Altruism in medicine: Its definition, nature and dilemmas. *Cambridge Quarterly of Healthcare Ethics*, *19*, 249–257. doi: 10.1017/509631801109990521.

Tracy, J. L., & Robins, R. W. (2007). The psychological structure of pride: A tale of two facets. *Journal of Personality and Social Psychology*, *92*, 506–525.

Tsang, J.-A., Schulwitz, A., & Carlisle, R. D. (2012). An experimental test of the relationship between religion and gratitude. *Psychology of Religion and Spirituality*, *4*, 40–55. doi:10.1037/a0025632

Tybur, J. M., Liberman, D., & Griskevicius, V. (2000). Microbes, mating, and morality: Individual differences in three functional domains of disgust. *Journal of Personality and Social Psychology*, *97*, 103–122. doi: 10.1037/a0015474

van Doorn, J., & Zeelenberg, M. (2014). Anger and prosocial behavior. *Emotion Review*, *6*, 261–268.

van Leeuwen, E., van Dijk, W., & Kaynak, U. (2013). Of saints and sinners: How appeals to collective pride and guilt affect outgroup helping. *Group Processes and Intergroup Relations*, *16*, 781–796.

Vastfjall, D., Slovic, P., Mayorga, M., & Peters, E. (2014). Compassion fade: Affect and charity are greatest for a single child in need. *PloSOne*, *9*, e100115.

Viar, M. A., Etzel, E. N., Ciesielski, B. G., & Olantunji, B. O. (2010). Disgust, anxiety, and vasovagal syncope sensations: A comparison of injection-fearful and nonfearful blood donors. *Journal of Anxiety Disorder*, *24*, 941–945.

Weiner, B. (1985). An attributional theory of achievement motivation and emotion. *Psychological Review*, *92*, 548–573.

West, S. A., Mouden C. E., & Gardner, A. (2011). Sixteen common misconceptions about the evolution of cooperation in humans. *Evolution and Human Behavior*, *32*, 231–262.

Wilson, T. D., & Gilbert, D. T. (2008). Explaining away a model of affective adaptation. *Perspectives on Psychological Science*, *3*, 370–386. doi:10.1111/j.1745-6924.2008.00085.x

Zeelenberg, M. (1999). Anticipated regret, expected feedback, and behavioral decision making. *Journal of Behavioral Decision Making*, *12*, 93–106.

18

Affect and Clinical Decision-Making

JANE HEYHOE AND REBECCA LAWTON

BACKGROUND

When we make decisions for our own health, such as those described previously in this book, the repercussions of those decisions are primarily felt by the person making those decisions. For example, if I choose to smoke, exercise irregularly, and eat an unhealthy diet, I increase my own risk of dying prematurely. What makes the topic of this chapter quite different is that the decisions that a health professional makes have direct repercussions for another person—the patient, and indirect repercussions for the decision-maker themselves—the team in which they work and the organization.

Health professionals (doctors, nurses, and allied health professionals) work in an emotionally charged setting. The need for urgent response, caring for patients in extreme pain or with life-threatening conditions, and discussing treatments and prognoses with patients and relatives are all features of the working experience of health professionals. However, health professionals vary considerably in the precise nature of the job they perform. For example surgeons require strong technical skills and nurses need to be more concerned with the psychosocial aspects of care. The working environments and hence factors influencing emotion will also vary as a function of the specialty, with do-not-resuscitate conversations being a feature of care of the elderly, and exposure to life-changing and severe injury a feature of the emergency department.

A fundamental characteristic of the jobs of all health professionals is the need to make decisions about delivering the most appropriate care to their patients. The decision-making of health professionals, whether individually or within teams, is generally considered to be a rational process—the weighing up of the costs and the benefits. Work that highlights how cognitive sequences may contribute to both failure and efficiency in clinical judgment (Pani & Chariker, 2004; Parker & Lawton, 2003) still dominates current understanding of the processes involved. For example, cognitive biases and the use of heuristics have been identified as important factors in diagnostic error (Croskerry, 2009a, 2013; Elstein, 1999; Norman, 2009). However, while health professionals and clinical teams may strive to make decisions that are grounded in a systematic appraisal of clinically relevant facts, decision-making is frequently influenced by nonrational, affect-based processes and factors. There is now a growing recognition that this is the case in other fields, but research within health professional performance is still very much in its infancy.

An example from general practice might help to demonstrate the different ways that affect can influence the decision-making of health professionals.

David first visited his general practitioner (GP) after he noticed a bout of diarrhea had continued for a few weeks. At the time he was not too concerned. The GP who had just arrived at work after struggling to park her car because the temporary stand-in GP had taken her usual spot, was 5 minutes late to start the morning session. After listening to David's symptoms, the GP suggests David should buy some over-the-counter medication and monitor his bowel movements. The GP said if things did not improve, David should come back again. Things did not get much better, but David learned to live with it until 2 months later, when he noticed some blood in the toilet. He made an appointment to see the GP again and this time was clearly anxious that something was seriously wrong. The GP, knowing David to be a fit and healthy 35-year-old, was not too worried but recognized that David was anxious and felt that she wanted to reassure him. They chat about some possible explanations and David is asked to return if the problem persists. Three weeks later, David visits the GP again explaining that he is now experiencing stomach pains and that he and his partner are really worried and want to know what is wrong. The GP, knowing that life-threatening conditions such as bowel cancer are rare in younger men, is still not sure whether referral is necessary but David's clear anxiety and frustration that things are not improving are making the GP worried too. When thinking about whether or not to refer, the GP recalls the case of Sarah a few years back who was diagnosed with bowel cancer at the age of 40 and whose symptoms were similar to David's. The GP still feels guilty for not referring Sarah sooner. She refers David for a colonoscopy. A few weeks later David's report comes back and there is no indication of cancer. The GP feels relieved for David but wonders whether the decision to refer was correct.

Reading this scenario, we can see the different ways affect can impact on decision-making and the types of emotion the GP is experiencing both in the moment in response to the patient in front of her and feelings triggered by thoughts of a previous case. We also note that the GP responds to David on both a professional and personal level. Research from outside healthcare (Conner, McEachan, Taylor, O'Hara, & Lawton, 2015; De Vries, Holland, Corneille, Rondeel, & Witteman, 2012; Kuhnen & Knutson, 2011) suggests that different types of affect that are experienced by an individual are important in decision-making. Studies indicate that immediate emotions felt at the time the decision is being made, that is, anticipatory affect (instant reflexive responses) and incidental affect (an affective state that originates from prior events but is experienced while making an unrelated decision) and thoughts of future feelings, for example, anticipated affect, all appear to impact judgment and choice and may help to provide further understanding of how affect influences clinical practice. In the earlier scenario, the GP is influenced in the moment by the feelings of the patient themselves. In other words, the anxiety experienced by the patient causes anxiety in the GP (anticipatory affect). The GP's existing affective state, frustration with the temporary stand-in GPdoctor who has parked in her space also impacts her actions during the consultation—she does not take a full history. The GP also thinks about previous cases and remembers that she felt guilty. This then makes her consider how she might feel if David is later found to have cancer (anticipated affect—the GP is thinking about feelings she might experience in the future). Here we present some examples of the factors that can impact on the transitory affective state of a health professional, but there are many more, including working relationships, stressors, and the working environment (Croskerry, Abbass, & Wu, 2008).

Of course, there are other factors such as the GP's general psychological well-being that will influence performance and decision-making. Indeed if the GP was experiencing, as is not uncommon (Orton, Orton, & Gray, 2012), the chronic exhaustion, reduced efficacy, and cynicism associated with chronic burnout (Leiter, Bakker, & Maslach, 2014) then this too would impact on the quality of the care that patients might receive. Cimiotti, Aiken, Sloane, and Wu (2012) report that hospitals in the United States in which burnout was reduced by 30% had a total of 6,239 fewer infections, for an annual cost saving of up to $68 million. Chronic states such as depression or burnout are known to be related to poorer outcomes in healthcare. The literature addressing health professional well-being reflects an increasing recognition (see Well-Med conference in May 2016) that healthcare services and those working in them are feeling the strain of growing demand, and that this is having an impact on the quality and safety of care. Although relevant and of huge policy significance, the literatures on well-being and burnout (chronic conditions) are beyond the scope of the current chapter, which focuses on more transitory affective states that impact performance.

It is now widely acknowledged that affect plays an important role in clinical performance (Heyhoe et al., 2015). At the individual level, dual process models have already been used to help construct theoretical accounts of the role of affect and cognition in diagnostic reasoning (Croskerry, 2009a, 2009b, 2013; Elstein, 1999, 2009; Elstein & Schwarz, 2002; Norman, 2009). We discuss dual process models and how these explain the individual decisions that health professionals make in the next section. Theoretical models are now beginning to acknowledge that affective factors in team situations have the potential to compromise the sharing of clinical information. For example, in their model of team performance, Annett, Cunningham, and Mathias-Jones (2000), suggest that affective factors involved in team morale and cohesiveness filter into all aspects of team processes, from cognition to communication and coordination, and ultimately shared goals. In models of nontechnical skills in teamwork (Fletcher, Flin, McGeorge, Galvin, Maran, & Patey, 2003; Yule, Flin, Paterson-Brown, & Maran, 2006), there is reference to affect, but at present these models are largely framed within a cognitive tradition and, as such, the role of affect is not explicit. This relatively recent acknowledgment of the role of affect in models of team working and performance means that there is still very little empirical evidence about the types of affect and triggers of affect within teams. One area that we can look to for some understanding of emotion in social groups is in the social psychological literature on emotions as social information. We come to this model later.

In this chapter we draw on theoretical and empirical literature from within and outside healthcare to understand the role of affect in clinical decision-making at the individual and team level. First we recap theories of individual decision-making and illustrate how dual process models, heuristics, and thought-processing speed explain the role of affect in judgment and behavior. A more detailed discussion of how immediate and expected affective states may play a role in different clinical contexts and settings is structured around the three types of affect exemplified earlier: anticipatory affect, incidental affect, and anticipated affect. We highlight gaps in the existing evidence base and, in particular, in the understanding of the role of affect in clinical team situations. We then make suggestions for interventions that might support better decision-making in this context.

HOW DOES AFFECT INFLUENCE OUR DECISIONS?

Dual Process Models

Dual process theories propose that everyday decisional processes can be understood in terms of a complex interplay between two separate but interacting processing and evaluative systems. In decision-making research, it is inferred that system 1 (an affective-based system characterized as being fast, intuitive, pattern-based, and unconscious) and system 2 (a cognitive-based system considered to be slow, reasoned, normative, and conscious) integrate and overlap to varying degrees during decision-making under risky and uncertain conditions (Epstein, 1994; Loewenstein, Weber, Hsee, & Welch, 2001; Smith & DeCoster, 2000; Strack & Deutsch, 2004). One dual process theory, the risk-as-feelings hypothesis (Loewenstein et al., 2001), draws clear distinctions between the determinants of these two systems. It proposes that if the two evaluative systems conflict, feelings experienced during decision-making or while engaging in an action are often the most powerful behavioral determinant. For example, the enthusiasm and confidence felt by a surgeon operating on a patient may drive the decision to try to excise the entire tumor and risk damage to nearby structures, despite knowing that complete removal seldom has additional prognostic benefit. Affect may therefore sometimes guide decisions in favor of risk-taking behavior and judgments that are inconsistent with a preferred course of action, clinical protocols, and guidelines and produce less optimal outcomes.

The Affect Heuristic

Dual process models have already been used to help construct theoretical accounts of the role of affect and cognition in diagnostic reasoning (Croskerry, 2009a, 2009b, 2013; Elstein, 1999, 2009; Elstein & Schwarz, 2002; Norman, 2009). Heuristics operate within system 1. These rapid, pattern-based mental shortcuts based on previous experience are deemed necessary and useful problem-solving strategies that assist in avoiding cognitive overload in demanding and time-limited situations (Tversky & Kahneman, 1974). However, the biases that heuristics may produce are generally considered to play an important role in diagnostic error (Croskerry, 2009a, 2013; Elstein, 1999; Norman, 2009). For example, *confirmatory bias*, focusing only on information that supports your preconceived ideas, may lead health professionals to fixate on an incorrect course of information gathering due to the initial diagnosis generated when first encountering a patient (Klein, 2005), while *hindsight bias*, believing that you knew what the outcome would be after the end result is known, has been implicated in contaminating diagnostic second opinions (Henriksen & Kaplan, 2003). Some theorists argue that in certain situations the *affect heuristic* plays a powerful role in decision-making (Finucane, Alhakami, Slovic, & Johnson, 2000; Slovic, Peters, Finucane, & MacGregor, 2005) by enabling individuals to use their emotional reactions to stimuli as a judgment gauge (Finucane et al., 2000; Slovic et al., 2005). Less is known about the role of the affect heuristic in clinical judgment (Croskerry, Abbass, & Wu, 2008, 2010), but it may be an important component in clinical settings such as emergency care, where clinical decisions often require a rapid reaction to the specific features and characteristics of a patient (Croskerry et al., 2008, 2010). For example, the twinge of concern that an attending emergency care doctor feels when he notices the pallor of the patient just admitted for assessment for a wrist injury leads him to call for the CPR equipment two minutes before the patient unexpectedly goes into cardiac arrest. Here, the doctor's feeling of concern in response to a specific feature of the patient (pallor) leads to him quickly evaluate that the patient may require urgent treatment for a potentially life-threatening event (cardiac arrest) rather than the benign injury (wrist fracture) that she was being assessed for.

As health professionals regularly work in highly emotional environments, under sustained stressful and time-constrained conditions, the affect heuristic may direct judgment when urgent clinical decisions are required (Croskerry, 2002). However, it is unclear when cognitive or affect-based heuristics are advantageous or detrimental in clinical judgment. There is a need for more research that explores the use of, and interplay between, affect-based and cognitive-based heuristics in clinical decision-making. In particular, it is important to identify the clinical circumstances, contexts, for which type of patients they come into play, and the circumstances in which these facilitate or jeopardize clinical reasoning (Croskerry et al., 2010; Elstein, 2009; Norman, 2009).

Affect and Speed of Thought Processing

Research examining affect and decision-making emphasizes that different types of affect have unique roles in judgment that relies on quicker and slower thought processes (Baumeister, DeWall, & Zhang, 2007a; Baumeister, Vohs, DeWall, & Zhang, 2007; Kahneman, 2011). It is suggested that affect can occur outside the context of emotional states (i.e., state affect) as an instantaneous reaction to situations or stimuli that is largely devoid of mindful awareness. Thus, affect-based decision-making is characterized by automaticity and speed. "Emotion" on the other hand, is regarded to be a more gradual, wholly mindful response to situations or stimuli. Emotion-based decision-making is therefore characterized as being reflective and less rapid.

Both state affect and emotion play a role in clinical decision-making, but may be more or less relevant in particular clinical contexts. State affect may be crucial in guiding decisions when quick action is necessary in settings such as emergency care. Emotion, on the other hand, may play a role in decision-making through a more considered reflection of clinical situations (considering decisions that have been made and relating positive or negative feelings to patient outcomes or an aspect of team work) and may be used in learning to guide and improve future decisions (Croskerry, 2013). What is key here is that the clinical context and setting will determine the roles that affect plays in clinical decisions and behavior. We discuss the implications of understanding the impact of affect on judgment in different clinical context and settings when we make suggestions for interventions to improve clinical decision-making later in the chapter.

Now, we take a closer look at affect involved in immediate and expected feelings and focus on three types of affect identified in the risk as feelings model (Lowenstein et al., 2001): anticipatory affect, incidental affect and anticipated affect.

IMMEDIATE AFFECT AND CLINICAL DECISION-MAKING

Anticipatory Affect

Anticipatory affect is an initial and immediate affective reaction to stimuli that produces a strong visceral state in the current moment (e.g., feeling anger when a patient is verbally abusive). The healthcare setting involves interaction with many different people and situations that can trigger anticipatory affect. Health professionals, like all people, demonstrate a strong visceral reaction to horrific events. For most of us this exposure is rare, but for many health professionals, particularly those working in accident and emergency, these are daily occurrences and these affective reactions may influence their clinical behavior. A healthcare provider's immediate visceral reaction to patients, rather than a logical appraisal of their condition or injury, may drive clinical judgment and behavior irrespective of whether these decisions and actions are the most beneficial or adhere to professionally acceptable conduct (Loewenstein, 2005). In a reflective account of her internship in an emergency department, Amato (2007) describes how the disgust she felt when examining a female patient's maggot-infested wound influenced her judgment of the patient, and resulted in her providing care that lacked in compassion. Similarly, the narratives of 24 newly qualified anesthetists in which they reflected on their experiences of clinical practice, demonstrated that horror felt during a specific clinical event *or in response to knowledge of possible catastrophic outcomes* were common occurrences that became embedded in memory and heightened their awareness of uncertainty in the work they do. This influenced future clinical decisions in a number of ways, including implementing verbal checking during procedures or, even more significantly, choosing to continue their careers in a different field of anesthetics (Iedema, Jorm, & Lum, 2009).

Decisions made by health professionals, like those made by anyone, are likely to be affected by the feelings elicited during interactions with others, and the literature supports this notion. Two randomized experiments, one with 63 trainee GPs (Schmidt et al., 2017) and one with 74 trainee hospital doctors (Mamede et al., 2017), presented doctors with one of two versions of clinical scenarios. While the two versions of each scenario were identical in clinical content, they differed in whether the behavior of the patient was designed to elicit a negative (the patient was either a "frequent demander," aggressive, questioned the doctor's competence, ignored the doctor's advice, had low expectations of doctor's support, or was utterly helpless) or neutral affective response from the doctor who was tasked with diagnosing the patient's condition. Half of the scenarios that each doctor received were from the negative affect category and half were from the neutral affect category. Findings revealed that while there was no difference in the amount of time spent to diagnose each case, likability and diagnostic accuracy were significantly lower for patients in the negative affect scenarios when compared to the neutral affect scenarios. This led the authors to imply that the mental resources required to deal with the patient who is behaving negatively might reduce the capacity available to assimilate and interpret the clinical information for diagnosis—possibly an example of ego depletion at work (Baumeister, Bratslavsky, Muraven, & Tice, 1998).

These studies imply that affect may be a key component in the formation of a health professional's perceptions of a particular patient and that the positive and negative feelings health professionals experience in response to a patient influence their decision-making processes. Another example of this can be found with frequent attender patients. General practitioners and those working in emergency care will be familiar with the scenario of a patient who suffers from anxiety and experiences regular panic attacks. On visiting accident and emergency (A&E) for the fifth time in a week reporting chest pains, their slightly new symptoms are not recognized because only a cursory history is taken and they are not then referred for an electrocardiogram (ECG). Later they arrive as an emergency in an ambulance having suffered a myocardial infarction. The positive and negative affect felt toward frequent attender patients has also been shown to impact GPs' clinical decisions and actions (Bellon & Fernandez-Asensio, 2002). It is reasonable to assume that these feelings may have a role in diagnostic error and may account for some inequalities in healthcare (Dovidio & Fiske, 2012).

Incidental Affect

Incidental affect (referred to by many authors as "mood") is also experienced at the time that a decision is made but is a transitory affective state that originates from prior events unrelated to the stimulus requiring immediate judgment (e.g., receiving good news just before attending a patient consultation results in you attending the consultation in a happy mood). Outside healthcare, incidental affect has been found to influence a variety of risk perceptions (Bruyneel, Dewitte, Franses, & Dekimpe, 2009; Caruso & Shafir, 2006). In a review of 34 experimental, quasi-experimental and correlational studies, Waters (2008) found that in general, studies demonstrated that negative mood was related to judging that more negative health hazards and life events would occur, and that positive hazards and events were less likely. On the other hand, positive mood produced optimism, so that more positive and less negative events were judged as being more likely. Research has also found that everyday behavioral choices may be driven by attempts to maintain a positive mood state or regulate negative affect. For example, in one study, Caruso and Shafir (2006) found that when an individual's positive current mood was made salient this tended to result in choices that corresponded with their current positive mood. Alternatively, when the individual's negative mood was made salient, this appeared to cause them to indulge in a behavior that would help to regulate their negative mood. Another study, exploring perception and judgment of others, found that positive affect tended to direct focus to broader, abstract features of the person, while induced negative affect directed focus to more specific, confined details (Avramova & Stapel, 2008). These findings clearly have implications for the behavioral and decisional motivations of health professionals. For example, they suggest that the positive or negative affect that a clinician may bring to a case may influence how much information the clinician gathers in order to make a diagnosis and suggest that mood may have an important role in determining the type of details that become more noticeable when presented with clinical information.

At present there is only limited research in healthcare suggesting that incidental affect may be important in directing clinical decisions and behavior. For example, on days they indicated they were in a negative mood, 188 primary care physicians reported that they talked less to patients and were more likely to refer them for laboratory or diagnostic tests or for consultations with a specialist. On positive mood days the physicians reported inverse behavior (Kushnir, Kushnir, Sarel, & Cohen, 2011). Furthermore, Isen, Rosenzweig, and Young (1991), found a manipulation to increase positive incidental affect in medical students did not produce more accurate diagnosis but did result in significantly faster diagnostic choices and a tendency to show more concern and interest in the case, leading the authors to suggest that positive incidental affect facilitates decision-making by increasing the efficiency of information processing.

As discussed in the previous section, immediate affect may sometimes erroneously direct attention away from the correct focus or produce behavioral responses that may sometimes be inconsistent with health professionals' preferred course of action or clinical protocols and guidelines. It is therefore important to understand the role of anticipatory affect and incidental affect in patient safety incidents that stem from such deviations from protocols and guidelines. However, it should be acknowledged, immediate affect may also assist and support logical appraisal. As such, it is crucial that we understand the type of circumstances in which a health professional's own affective response facilitates or hinders clinical decision-making and performance.

ANTICIPATED AFFECT AND CLINICAL DECISION-MAKING

Decision-making in medicine is often presented as occurring in an emergency or critical care setting where the most optimal outcomes rely on instinctive and rapid judgment and action. However, not all clinical decisions occur in high-pressured and time-critical contexts. In these situations, anticipated affect may play a greater role, with health professionals considering how the outcomes of their decisions and actions may make them feel.

Anticipated affect is not affect per se, but a cognition about affect and refers to an individual's conscious consideration of how their current actions may make them feel in the future. For example, when deciding how to manage a patient presenting to their GP with dizziness and palpitations, the GP might think, "If I don't send the patient away to monitor their heart rate, because I'm fairly certain the patient's racing pulse is due to anxiety, but then discover that it is due to atrial fibrillation, I will regret it later." We focus on interactions with patients and colleagues to illustrate how the consideration of future feelings, for example, guilt, shame, regret, pride, confidence, and self-respect, can have an impact on the decision-making of health professionals.

Affective factors that stem from a health professional's previous clinical experience may influence decision-making in the present. In diagnosis, the feelings experienced by a health professional during a past patient presentation (whether the experience was associated with strong positive or negative emotions or involved particularly unusual or exceptional features) may lead to a current patient presentation that has a similar presentation or requires similar decisions, being guided by consideration of the feelings associated with the past case. For example, 3 months ago the doctor who had earlier discharged a young female patient with instructions to take pain killers for menstrual pain following complaints of a dull pelvic ache had experienced extreme anxiety when she was readmitted to the A&E department with a suspected ectopic pregnancy. When another young female patient presents with similar symptoms, the doctor orders a pelvic ultrasound to avoid experiencing the same feeling of anxiety should he learn later that this patient also had a serious condition that required urgent treatment, even though the patient's history and findings on examination indicate that this is not necessary.

Selecting and discarding choices is a pivotal part of clinical decision-making. The role of regret and, in particular, avoidance of postdecisional regret, appears to play an important role in clinical decisions involving risk and uncertainty. A recent experimental study in which 132 physicians provided treatment decisions in response to a computer-based clinical scenario involving a patient with an abdominal aortic aneurysm, found that physicians who were presented with a bad patient outcome scenario experienced increased levels of anxiety and decision regret, which influenced their choice of treatment strategy for the next patient with the same condition (Hemmerich, Elstein, Schwarze, Ghini Moliski, & Dale, 2012). Guilt and shame are also emotions that are keenly felt by health professionals and feature in the consideration of past clinical decisions and in the aftermath of a patient safety incident for which the clinician feels responsible (Harrison et al., 2015). For example, in a qualitative study of clinicians' emotions (Kolehmainen & McAnuff, 2014), one therapist admits:

> "[the child] really wasn't very easy to like [. . .] and part of me felt a guilt [. . .] because I didn't like [the child] very much and I don't think a lot of other people liked him, and I think if he was nice family, easy to like, didn't have behavioural problems, would his [care] pathway have been different? I think so. And I don't think these factors should come into it so I tried to overcompensate for my personal feeling [by seeing him when I no longer needed to do so]. (. . .) I should have discharged [him] sooner—much, much sooner. But I felt guilty." (p. 5)

In this example, it would be reasonable to suggest that the guilt experienced by the therapist during the case described would be recalled if they were to be involved in another case that included similar features. This experience and the attempt to avoid any anticipated feelings of guilt are likely to influence the decisions they make in future cases. When a health professional anticipates and seeks to avoid experiencing future feelings of guilt, shame, or regret as a result of their decision, hypervigilance and extreme risk aversion may occur.

The previous examples illustrate that considering future feelings while caring for patients can influence the treatment and management decisions for that particular patient. However, affective factors that stem from a health professional's previous clinical encounters with colleagues may also influence the decisions health professionals make. In a clinical setting, whether or not a junior doctor decides to consult a senior colleague about the significance of a patient's vague symptoms, may be influenced by their past experience with this colleague. If their previous experience of consulting the senior colleague was positive (e.g., they felt valued and supported because the senior colleague praised them for their assertiveness), they are more likely to consult the colleague again. If the doctor's previous experience of consulting the senior colleague was negative (e.g., they felt embarrassed because the senior colleague spoke sharply to them for wasting their time), they are more likely to avoid seeking the colleague's opinion. In a survey of 2,950 NHS staff across seven NHS Trusts in the United Kingdom, 20% of respondents reported that they had experienced bullying and 46% reported that they had witnessed bullying in the last 6 months (Carter et al., 2013). As fear is an emotion that has been shown to cause low personal control and withdrawal from situations (Lerner & Keltner, 2000, 2001), this could clearly have implications in situations where a clinician has to urgently seek the advice of an unfriendly colleague in order to provide correct and urgent care. Indeed, the anticipated hostility from his colleague may influence the clinician's decision of whether or not to seek the urgent advice he/she requires. The repercussions of working in teams where colleagues may be unfriendly and intimidating or cheerful and supportive cannot be underestimated in clinical contexts where sharing information is critical to success.

While little is known about the role of anticipated affect in clinical decision-making, these findings have clear implications for medicine, where decisions with uncertain outcomes are routine and where decisions will impact on the health and well-being of another human being. As such, more focused empirical research examining whether clinicians' choices are based on avoiding or experiencing specific future emotions, and whether those choices augment or compromise optimal clinical judgments, would progress understanding of the role of anticipated affect in clinical performance.

In the previous section, we have described how affect elicited through interaction with colleagues can influence clinical decision-making at an individual level. Until recently, research has largely ignored the relational dynamics that come with human interaction and the affect that this produces in a healthcare context where affect becomes distributed and more social.

SOCIAL MOOD

Team Climate

Clear and effective communication of clinical information and patient symptoms and shared cognition within clinical teams is pivotal to efficient decision-making and appropriate case management in healthcare settings (Christensen et al., 2000; Flin, O'Connor, & Crichton, 2008; Greenberg et al., 2007). In a clinical team context, health professionals must share relevant clinical information, their interpretation of patient symptoms, and the desires and feelings of the patient. When breakdowns in communication occur, patient safety is compromised, which can result in negative patient outcomes (Greenberg et al., 2007; Sutcliffe, Lewton, & Rosenthal, 2004).

In recognition of the pivotal role that optimal interprofessional interaction plays in providing safe patient care, programs focusing on teamwork have been developed and introduced into healthcare settings and organizations (Flin et al., 2008). These include simulation-based training using crew resource management (CRM) and behavioral rating tools to assess "nontechnical" skills (NTS) such as communication, decision-making, and situation awareness (Yule et al., 2006), and is reflected in the recent requirement for the WHO Surgical Safety Checklist (Haynes et al., 2009) to be used by surgical teams during all surgical interventions in the NHS in England and Wales (National Patient Safety Agency, 2009). The surgical checklist was introduced as a means of improving team communication and consistency of care and, when evaluated internationally, the impact on mortality was significant (Haynes et al., 2009). However, more recent studies have been unable to replicate these initial findings. A review of 18 qualitative studies that have attempted to understand this phenomenon argue that checklists require new forms of communication between team members and it is only when this happens (and the checklist is not implemented tick-box style) that it has any benefits (Bergs et al., 2015).

These approaches have highlighted the importance of cognitive processes in communication and decision-making in multiprofessional clinical teams. However, very little is known about the specific role of affect in teams involving doctors and nurses or allied health professions, despite research suggesting that affective factors such as emotional climate (Nurok et al., 2011) and feelings of psychological safety (confidence of team members to raise concerns, admit to not knowing, and question seniors) (Edmondson, 1999) may impact individual and team communication behavior.

How and whether important clinical information is shared effectively may be influenced by affect-based responses and reactions of team members to the work climate.

Affective factors such as aggression and disagreement (Coe & Gould, 2007), rudeness (Flin, 2010), intergroup competition (Hewett, Watson, Gallois, Ward, & Leggett, 2009), and tension (Lingard, Reznick, Espin, Regehr, & DeVito, 2002) between health professional groups have been shown to foster a tone of conflict and to negatively impact communication and collaboration. Furthermore, interprofessional boundaries and conflict have been found to contribute to breakdowns in collaborative working and the verbalization of clinical information (Dewitt, Baldwin, & Daugherty, 2008; Finn, 2008; Greenberg et al., 2007; Powell & Davies, 2012). Work that has examined multiprofessional clinical teams has found that strain between team members may be due to differences between professions in their perceptions of roles, responsibilities, hierarchy, and goals (Allen, 1997; Greenberg et al., 2007; Salhani & Coulter, 2009). It is therefore possible those professional boundaries elicit different affective responses in doctors and nurses and allied health professions during teamwork tasks and that these feelings are related to their perception of team communication and effectiveness. In a study involving observations and interviews with operating theater nurses, Timmons and Tanner (2005) found that nurses engaged in behavior and displays that were juxtaposed to actual feelings in order to maintain equanimity in the mood of the surgeons they worked with. In another study involving simulations of critical care incidents during simulations (Heyhoe, 2013), doctors reported higher levels of "alert" and "active" affective states implying a more immediate, transient response state that is required for instantaneous decision-based actions and performance. In contrast, the affective states of "inspired," "determined," "upset," and "ashamed" were experienced more intensely by nurses or allied health professionals, indicating a more considered and emotionally burdensome response during the simulation. Therefore, it is possible that the nurses observed were carrying out the hostess role and that during team scenarios, they were acting as a team affect gauge and were therefore more likely to be more acutely aware of, and report, the affective states they were feeling. This finding supports research on the expected management of both displayed and inward feelings as part of workplace roles known as emotional labor (James, 1989; Smith, 1992). Research should try to establish whether emotional labor assists or hinders nurses' verbalization of information they feel is clinically relevant to the rest of the team.

In our recent work in which we use routinely collected data to identify those teams that provide safe and compassionate care, we have identified that relationships, trust, and knowing each other well are fundamental characteristics of these high-performing teams, and this is most likely in teams that are stable and where the senior medical and nursing leads demonstrate mutual respect (Baxter, 2016). On these wards, one frequently expressed sentiment of staff is that they enjoy coming to work. Thus, the emotional tone of the group can have far-reaching consequences, such as a willingness of staff to cover for one another, continuously improve, and deliver more patient-centered care. Thus a positive affective climate has potential implications for outcomes as diverse as patient experience and safety. Affect can also influence the level of communication between team members (Edmondson, 1999; Kish-Gephart, Detert, Trevino & Edmondson, 2009; Lingard et al., 2002), and information sharing is pivotal in diagnostic and treatment decisions. It is therefore important to identify models that may help us explain the affective "tone" within the team. In order to understand the role of affect in social groups the next section draws on the social psychological literature on emotions as social information.

EASI Model

While dual process theories emphasize the impact of individual feelings on decision-making and behavior, clinical work often involves judgments and actions that stem from a collaborative reaction to, and assessment of, a clinical presentation or situation. As clinical teams involve individuals working together, it is likely that both individual and team affective factors will play a role in how health professionals respond to, and function within, clinical teams. The emotions as social information model (EASI: Van Kleef, 2009; Van Kleef, De Dreu, & Manstead, 2010, see Figure 18.1), posits that as well as individual responses to stimuli, group-based social interaction involves the observation of emotion in others. The emotional display of one or a group of individuals may subsequently influence the judgments and actions of another individual. Van Kleef (2009) argues that this may occur through two different processes; inferential mechanisms (e.g., a registrar's anxiousness alerts you to the fact that they regard the case as urgent, which causes you to collect the blood test results yourself) or affective responses (e.g., a registrar's nervousness about the case makes you anxious and urges you to seek the advice of another senior colleague).

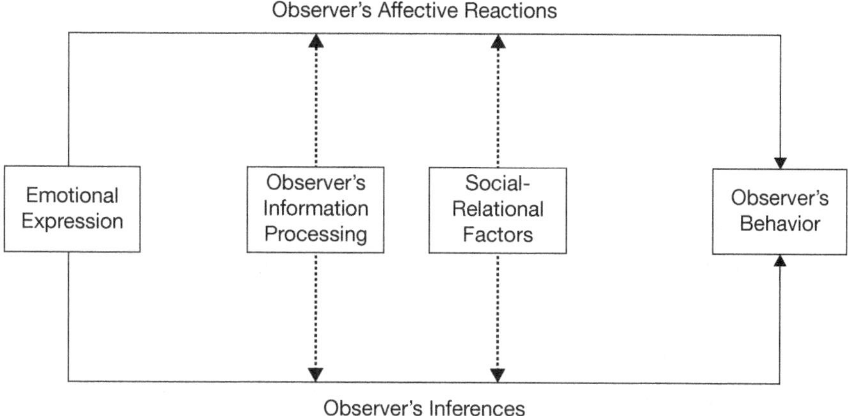

Figure 18.1. Emotion as social information (EASI) model.

Intuitively, health professionals are aware of the importance of expressed emotions in shaping social interactions and decisions. Ask most and they will tell you that they know whether it is going to be a good or bad day the minute they arrive on shift. How? If the grumpy matron or abrupt healthcare assistant are on shift or they know that consultant X is on and they seem to always contradict and anger registrar Y. It is all about social emotion, but rarely are problems expressed in these terms. Rarely is the role of social emotion acknowledged in either the research that is conducted or the interventions that are delivered to improve teamwork, decision-making, patient safety, and so forth.

The model proposed by Van Kleef sets out a clear set of testable hypotheses and emphasizes the difference between the perception of expressed emotions in predominantly cooperative or competitive settings. There is also a strong argument proposed for the role of leaders in setting the emotional tone of the group/team. Finally, Van Kleef and colleagues reflect on the way we use affect to make sense of uncertainty—so called "fuzzy situations." Our actions are then driven, at least in part, and more so when there is uncertainty, by the expressed emotions of others. That social emotion is largely ignored within the healthcare literature may have serious implications for a workforce who are under immense pressure, who work with uncertainty, and whose actions have serious consequences for the lives of others.

Heyhoe (2013) interviewed 16 anesthetists and emergency care doctors about how emotion influenced critical decisions they had made in the past. Many of these doctors placed great importance on working with supportive colleagues and recalled that this was crucial for gaining feedback and reassurance for diagnosis and case management decisions, as well as the building of trust in the undertaking of clinical roles and responsibilities. In contrast, when doctors felt there was conflict between colleagues, this was perceived to be unhelpful to delivering safe and optimal care for the patient and resulted in negative emotions that on some occasions caused hesitant behavior. These findings support literature that suggests cooperation is important for the fostering of effective team communication and behavior and implies that social as well as individual affect influences perceptions of team communication and performance (Van Doorn, Heerdink, & Van Kleef, 2012; Van Kleef, 2009).

RECOMMENDATIONS FOR FUTURE RESEARCH, CLINICAL PRACTICE AND PATIENT SAFETY

The literature on affect and clinical decision-making is still in its infancy. This means that despite evidence from the more general literature on affect and decision-making that negative mood states appear to increase the tendency to take more risks, but in some instances to be more risk averse (Hockey, Maule, Clough, & Bdzola, 2000; Pezza Leith & Baumeister, 1996), we still know little about the role of discrete emotions in clinical decision-making. Lerner and Keltner (2000) propose "a model of emotion-specific influences on judgement and choice" (p. 473) that we could draw on to underpin this research. They emphasize the importance of establishing and identifying not only how positive and negative affect influence decision-making under different situations but also how specific emotions impact judgment and choice. Lerner and Keltner (2000, 2001) propose that different negative emotions lead to different appraisal tendencies. So, while anger can cause individuals to consider they have more control over a situation, which leads to more risk-taking, anxiety can lead to feelings of low personal control, and therefore an aversion to risk. This suggests that the relationship between positive and negative affect and information gathering may not be simple. Furthermore, Pezza Leith and Baumeister (1996) conclude that because anger (an emotion that is likely to induce high arousal in an individual) appears to increase risk-taking, while sadness (an emotion associated with low arousal) appears to produce a decrease in risky choice, that high arousal may be a contributing factor to risk-taking. These ideas emphasize the importance of establishing and identifying not only how positive and negative affect influence clinical decision-making under different situations but also how specific emotions impact judgment and choice.

Further work is also needed to understand whether the errors implicated in the unconscious, fast, and effortless nature of system 1 can be overcome through educational and debiasing strategies (Croskerry, 2002, 2013; Graber, 2009). It cannot be assumed that simply knowing about human fallibility in reasoning can actually help to prevent it. However, this assumes that in all clinical situations, rapid, affect-based decision-making is inferior to slower, cognitive-based reasoning and would involve developing strategies that would train system 2 to override system 1. As it is currently not known whether system 2 processing always produces better diagnostic decision-making, further testing is required before moving forward with this idea.

As both anxiety and fear have been associated with low personal control and aversive behavior (Lerner & Keltner, 2000, 2001), increased nervousness and fear in health professionals may reduce the level of communication within a team context (Kish-Gephart et al., 2009). In a clinical team context, this could hinder or delay the sharing of important clinical information. Further research should examine differences in the expression of anxiety and fear in multiprofessional clinical teams and assess how quickly and accurately these emotions are gauged by other members of the team. This would aid the development of team strategies to mitigate omissions or errors caused by emotion-based avoidance behavior. These findings further support the need to develop a better understanding of the role that specific emotions play in decisions and behavior in applied settings (Van Kleef, Homan, & Chesin, 2012).

The evidence presented in this chapter makes a strong case for the role of affect in decision-making in healthcare—what are the implications then for clinical practice? The first suggestion perhaps is to develop innovations that are designed to support better decision-making (Graber, Gordon, & Franklin, 2002; Newman-Toker & Pronovost, 2009) such as computerized decision prompts and decision-making tools to improve diagnosis (Graber et al., 2002; Newman-Toker & Pronovost, 2009; Ramnarayan et al., 2006). However, while such approaches may assist and support the diagnostic process, unique patient presentations and evolving clinical contexts mean that health professionals will, to some extent, always have to make decisions using their own reasoning strategies. It is neither desirable nor possible to completely eliminate the role of the clinician in decision-making.

As we have illustrated, emergency care doctors work in an affectively charged environment and affect can provide information that may both hinder and assist clinical judgment. Therefore, it is recommended that doctors should adopt "mindfulness" strategies during practice (Croskerry, 2013). A diagnostic decision-making checklist that includes items that prompt doctors to consider their feelings when making key judgments about a case presentation should be developed. This would facilitate the consideration and management of nonrational information that may be hindering or delaying judgment and action, or may alert doctors to the need to pursue a "gut instinct" and to gather further diagnostic information.

Similarly, affect-based items should also be added to and trialed in the current checklists used by clinical teams (Haynes et al., 2009). The addition of items that foster the open discussion of feelings about clinical cases, treatment strategies, and roles and responsibilities, before, during, and after emergency admissions or surgical procedures, or at handover, may prompt individuals to share potentially vital clinical information. It may also encourage members of the team to be more open about how confident they feel in undertaking clinical tasks and responsibilities, which may lead to improved support, an increased sense of team cooperation, and safer patient care.

Clinicians could also engage in reflective practice (Bradley, 2005; Epstein, 1999; Mamede, Schmidt, & Rikers, 2007) in order to learn how affect influences diagnostic decision-making at both an individual and team level. Reflection on the role of affect in decision-making and patient safety should become part of professional training practice and continuing professional development. Another strategy would be to use counterfactual thinking (Kahneman & Miller, 1986; Kahneman & Tversky, 1982). Reflective practice could incorporate both upward and downward counterfactual thinking (Markman, Gavanski, Sherman, & McMullen, 1993). The discussion of upward counterfactual thinking (e.g., If I/we had made that decision, the outcome would have been better) and downward counterfactual thinking (e.g., If I/we had made that decision, the outcome would have been worse) could be used to compare instances of negative and positive clinical outcomes and would enable individuals and teams to identify key decisions and any individual or social affect that was associated with the decision. This may help individuals and teams to understand the types of affect and the circumstances in which they might be most relevant to their practice, and would also encourage a positive practice approach to diagnosis and case management.

Another approach might be to use video reflexivity, pioneered by Jessica Mesman (Iedema, Mesman, & Carroll, 2013) to support safe practice in neonatal units in the Netherlands by bringing the team together to reflect not only on the role of their technical skills but also on the influence of emotion on their group performance. Leaders and mentors are also critical to fostering a culture in which the discussion of emotion and its impact on practice is actively encouraged. The increasing use of Schwartz Rounds (Schwartz Centre for Compassionate Care, 2016) in healthcare organizations suggests that there is a growing recognition of the value of reflective practice initiatives that allow health professionals to do this. However, more explicit training for leaders that focuses on the importance of recognizing and influencing the emotional tone of their team so as to support cooperation rather than competition would also be justified based on the findings we report.

These different strategies could also be used in undergraduate and postgraduate medical education programs that use simulated clinical scenarios. These strategies, combined with affective cues and carefully designed decision points, would enable teams of healthcare students and multiprofessional healthcare teams to participate in, and then review, whether and how affect influenced team communication and discuss the implications for diagnostic and case management decision-making. This would encourage interprofessional lifelong learning about the role of affect in clinical team performance

CONCLUSION

Current knowledge from inside and outside healthcare has highlighted that the role of affect in clinical decision-making is still relatively unexplored (Croskerry et al., 2008, 2010; Iedema et al., 2009; Ubel, 2005). Empirical research is beginning to emerge, but so far, progress has mainly been theoretical or based on anecdotal evidence. It is now important to extend knowledge of clinical decision-making processes beyond a cognitive approach and to understand how and why affect influences clinical performance. In order to make progress, current models explaining how system 1 and system 2 processing interacts during decision-making must be further refined. One way of achieving this is by identifying the triggers of affect (other than patients and relationships with our colleagues) and types of affect that influence decision-making, establishing the mechanisms involved in the processing of affective factors, and assessing how they affect clinical outcomes.

This chapter helps to inform health professionals of the complex psychological processes involved in the nonrational influences of clinical decision-making and may go some way to helping shift the skepticism in the notion that decision-making is anything other than a judgment based purely on a rational consideration of the options. This work may contribute to a wider acceptance that affect has direct implications for clinical performance, and the progress in knowledge may assist in improving the clinical decision-making of health professionals across a range of clinical contexts.

Recent reports on patient safety (Berwick et al., 2013; Francis et al., 2013) have emphasized the pivotal role that professionalism, responsibility, and a culture of "openness" play in the provision of optimal care. With this comes a moral obligation to acknowledge and foster discussion about, and incorporate into clinical practice, new evidence of factors that may hinder or facilitate safe patient care. This should include the role of affect in clinical decision-making.

REFERENCES

Allen, D. (1997). The nursing-medical boundary: A negotiated order? *Sociology of Health and Illness*, *19*, 498–520.

Amato, T. (2007). Respecting the power of denial. *Academic Emergency Medicine*, *14*, 184.

Annett, J., Cunningham, D., & Mathias-Jones, P. (2000). A method for measuring team skills. *Ergonomics*, *43*, 1076–1094.

Avramova, Y. R., & Stapel, D. A. (2008). Mood as spotlights: The influence of mood on accessibility effects. *Journal of Personality and Social Psychology*, *95*, 542–554.

Baumeister, R. F., Bratslavsky, E., Muraven, M., & Tice, D. M. (1998). Ego depletion: Is the active self a limited resource? *Journal of Personality and Social Psychology*, *74*(5), 1252–1265.

Baumeister, R. F., DeWall, C. N., & Zhang, L. (2007). Do emotions improve making process? In K. D. Vohs, R. F. Baumeister, & G. Loewenstein (Eds.), *Do emotions help or hurt decision making? A hedgefoxian perspective* (pp. 11–31). New York, NY: Russell Sage Foundation.

Baumeister, R. F., Vohs, K. D., DeWall, C., & Zhang, L. (2007). How emotion shapes behaviour: Feedback, anticipation, and reflection, rather than direct causation. *Personality and Social Psychology Review*, *11*, 167–203.

Baxter, R. M. (2016). *Learning from positive deviants to improve the quality and safety of healthcare*. PhD thesis, University of Leeds.

Bellon, J. A., & Fernandez-Asensio, M. E. (2002). Emotional profile of physicians who interview frequent attenders. *Patient Education and Counseling*, *48*, 33–41.

Bergs, J., Lambrechts, F., Simons, P., Vlayen, A., Marneffe, W., Hellings, J., . . . Vandijck, D. (2015). Barriers and facilitators related to the implementation of surgical safety checklists: A systematic review of the qualitative evidence. BMJ Qual Saf 2015 Jul 21. doi:bmjqs-2015-004021.

Berwick, D., et al., National advisory group on the safety of patients in England. (2013). *A promise to learn—a commitment to act: Improving the safety of patients in England*. London: Department of Health.

Bradley, C. P. (2005). Commentary: Can we avoid bias? *British Medical Journal, 330*, 784.

Bruyneel, S. D., Dewitte, S., Franses, P. H., & Dekimpe, M. G. (2009). I felt low and my purse feels light: Depleting mood regulation attempts affect risk decision making. *Journal of Behavioral Decision Making, 22*(2), 153–170. doi: 10.1002/bdm.619.

Carter, M., Thompson, N., Crampton, P., Morrow, G., Burford, B., Gray, C., & Illing, J. (2013). Workplace bullying in the UK NHS: A questionnaire and interview study on prevalence, impact and barriers to reporting. *BMJ Open, 3*(6), e002628.

Caruso, E. M., & Shafir, E. (2006). Now that I think about it, I'm in the mood for laughs: Decisions focused on mood. *Journal of Behavioral Decision Making, 19*, 155–169.

Christensen, C., Larson, J. R., Abbott, A., Ardolino, A., Franz, T., & Pfeiffer, C. (2000). Decision making of clinical teams: Communication patterns and diagnostic error. *Medical Decision Making, 20*, 45–50.

Cimiotti, J. P., Aiken, L. H., Sloane, D. M., & Wu, E. S. (2012). Nurse staffing, burnout, and health care-associated infection. *American Journal of Infection Control, 40*, 486–490.

Coe, R., & Gould, D. (2007). Disagreement and aggression in the operating theatre. *Journal of Advanced Nursing, 61*, 609–618.

Conner, M., McEachan, R., Taylor, N., O'Hara, J., & Lawton, R. (2015). Role of affective attitudes and anticipated affective reactions in predicting health behaviors. *Health Psychology, 34*, 642–652.

Croskerry, P. (2002). Achieving quality in clinical decision making: Cognitive strategies and detection of bias. *Academic Emergency Medicine, 9*, 1184–1204.

Croskerry, P. (2009a). Clinical cognition and diagnostic error: Applications of a dual process model of reasoning. *Advances in Health Sciences Education, 14*, 27–35.

Croskerry, P. (2009b). A universal model of diagnostic reasoning. *Academic Medicine, 84*, 1022–1028.

Croskerry, P., Abbass, A. A., & Wu, A. W. (2008). How doctors feel: Affective issues in patients' safety. *Lancet, 372*, 1205–1206.

Croskerry, P., Abbass, A. A., & Wu, A. W. (2010). Emotional influences in patient safety. *Journal of Patient Safety, 6*, 199–205.

Croskerry, P. (2013). From mindless to mindful practice—Cognitive bias and clinical decision making. *New England Journal of Medicine, 368*, 2445–2448.

De Vries, M., Holland, R. W., Corneille, O., Rondeel, E., & Witteman, C. L. M. (2012). Mood effects on dominated choices: Positive mood induces departures from logical rules. *Journal of Behavioral Decision Making, 25*, 74–81.

Dewitt, C., Baldwin, J. R., & Daugherty, S. R. (2008). Interprofessional conflict and medical errors: Results of a national multi-specialty survey of hospital residents in the US. *Journal of Interprofessional Care, 22*, 573–586.

Dovidio, J. F., & Fiske, S. T. (2012). Under the radar: How unexamined biases in decision-making processes in clinical interactions can contribute to health care disparities. *American Journal of Public Health, 102*, 945–952.

Edmondson, A. (1999). Psychological safety and learning behaviour in work teams. *Administrative Science Quarterly, 44*, 350–383.

Elstein, A. S. (1999). Heuristics and biases: Selected errors in clinical reasoning. *Academic Medicine, 74*, 791–794.

Elstein, A. S. (2009). Thinking about diagnostic thinking: A 30-year perspective. *Advances in Health Science Education, 14*, 7–18.

Elstein, A. S., & Schwarz, A. (2002). Clinical problem solving and diagnostic decision making: Selective review of the cognitive literature. *British Medical Journal, 324*, 729–732.

Epstein, R. M. (1999). Mindful practice. *Journal of the American Medical Association, 282*, 833–839.

Epstein, S. (1994). Integration of the cognitive and the psychodynamic unconscious. *American Psychologist, 49*, 709–724.

Finn, R. (2008). The language of teamwork: Reproducing professional divisions in the operating theatre. *Human Relations, 61*, 103–130.

Finucane, M. L., Alhakami, A., Slovic, P., & Johnson, S. M. (2000). The affect heuristic in judgments of risks and benefits. *Journal of Behavioral Decision Making, 13*, 1–17.

Fletcher, G., Flin, R., McGeorge, P., Galvin, R., Maran, N., &Patey, R. (2003). Anaesthetists' non-technical skills (ANTS): Evaluation of a behavioural marker system. *British Journal of Anaesthesia, 90*, 580–588.

Flin, R. (2010). Rudeness at work: A threat to patient safety and quality of care. *BMJ, 340*, c2480. doi:10.1136/bmj/.c2480.

Flin, R., O'Connor, P., & Crichton, M. (2008). *Safety at the sharp end. A guide to non-technical skills.* Surrey: Ashgate Publishing Limited.

Francis, R., et al. (2013). *The Mid Staffordshire NHS Foundation Trust public inquiry. Report of the Mid Staffordshire NHS Foundation Trust public inquiry—Executive summary*. London: The Stationary Office.

Graber, M. (2009). Educational strategies to reduce diagnostic error: Can you teach this stuff? *Advances in Health Science Education, 14*, 63–69.

Graber, M., Gordon, R., & Franklin, N. (2002). Reducing diagnostic errors in medicine: What's the goal? *Academic Medicine, 77*, 981–992.

Greenberg, C. C., Regenbogen, S. E., Studdert, D. M., Lipsitz, S. R., Rogers, S. O., Zinner, M. J., & Gawande, A. A. (2007). Patterns of communication breakdowns resulting in injury to surgical patients. *Journal of the American College of Surgeons, 204*, 533–540.

Harrison, R., Lawton, R., Perlo, J., Gardner, P., Armitage, G., & Shapiro, J. (2015). Emotion and coping in the aftermath of medical error: A cross-country exploration. *Journal of Patient Safety, 11*(1), 28–35.

Haynes, A. B., Weiser, T. G., Berry, W. R., Lipsitz, S. R., Breizat, A.-H. S., Pratchen Dellinger, E., . . . Gawande, A. A. (2009). A surgical safety checklist to reduce morbidity and mortality in a global population. *New England Journal of Medicine, 360*, 491–499.

Hemmerich, J. A., Elstein, A. S., Schwarze, M. L., Ghini Moliski, E., & Dale, W. (2012). Risk as feelings in the effect of patient outcomes on physicians' future treatment decisions: A randomized trial and manipulation validation. *Social Science and Medicine, 75*, 367–376.

Henriksen, K., & Kaplan, H. (2003). Hindsight bias, outcome knowledge and adaptive learning. *Quality and Safety in Health Care, 12* (Suppl II), ii46–ii50.

Hewett, D. G., Watson, B. M., Gallois, C., Ward, M., & Leggett, B. A. (2009). Intergroup communication between doctors: Implications for quality of patient care. *Social Science and Medicine, 69*, 1732–1740.

Heyhoe, J. (2013). *Affective and cognitive influences on decision making in healthcare.* (Unpublished doctoral thesis), University of Leeds.

Heyhoe, J., Birks, Y., Harrison, R., O'Hara, J. K., Cracknell, A., & Lawton, R. (2015). The role of emotion in patient safety: Are we brave enough to scratch beneath the surface? *Journal of the Royal Society of Medicine*, 0141076815620614.

Hockey, G. R. J., Maule, A. J., Clough, P. J., & Bdzola, L. (2000). Effects of negative mood states on risk in everyday decision-making. *Cognition and Emotion, 14*, 823–855.

Iedema, R., Jorm, C., & Lum, M. (2009). Affect is central to patient safety: The horror stories of young anaesthetists. *Social Science and Medicine, 69*, 1750–1756.

Iedema, R., Mesman, J., & Carroll, K. (2013). *Visualising health care practice improvement: Innovation from within.* London: Radcliffe Publishing Ltd.

Isen, A. M., Rosenzweig, A. S., & Young, M. J. (1991). The influence of positive affect on clinical problem solving. *Medical Decision Making, 11*, 221–227.

James, N. (1989). Emotional labour: Skill and work in the regulation of feelings. *Sociological Review, 37*, 18–33.

Kahneman, D., & Miller, D. T. (1986). Norm theory: Comparing reality to its alternatives. *Psychological Review, 93*, 136–153.

Kahneman, D., & Tversky, A. (1982). The simulation heuristic. In D. Kahneman, E. Slovic, & A. Tversky (Eds.), *Judgment under uncertainty: Heuristics and biases.* New York, NY: Cambridge University Press.

Kahneman, D. (2011). *Thinking, fast and slow.* London: Allen Lane.

Kish-Gephart, J. J., Detert, J. R., Trevino, J. K., & Edmondson, A. C. (2009). Silenced by fear: The nature, sources, and consequences of fear at work. *Research in Organizational Behavior, 29*, 163–193.

Klein, J. G. (2005). Five pitfalls in decisions about diagnosis and prescribing. *British Medical Journal, 330*, 781–783.

Kolehmainen, N., & McAnuff, J. (2014). "I should have discharged him but I felt guilty": A qualitative investigation of clinicians' emotions in the context of implementing occupational therapy. *Implementation Science, 9*, 141.

Kuhnen, C. M., & Knutson, B. (2011). The influence of affect on beliefs, preferences, and financial decisions. *Journal of Financial Quantitative Analysis, 46*, 605–626.

Kushnir, T., Kushnir, J., Sarel, A., & Cohen, A. H. (2011). Exploring physician perceptions of the impact of emotions on behaviour during interactions with patients. *Family Practice, 28*, 75–81.

Leiter, M. P., Bakker, A. B., & Maslach, C. (2014). *Burnout at work: A psychological perspective.* Hove: Psychology Press.

Lerner, J. S., & Keltner, D. (2000). Beyond valence: Toward a model of emotion-specific influences on judgement and choice. *Cognition and Emotion, 14*, 473–493.

Lerner, J. S., & Keltner, D. (2001). Fear, anger, and risk. *Journal of Personality and Social Psychology, 81*, 146–159.

Lingard, L., Reznick, R., Espin, S., Regehr, G., & DeVito, I. (2002). Team communications in the operating room: Talk patterns, sites of tension, and implications for novices. *Academic Medicine, 77*, 232–237.

Loewenstein, G. (2005). Projection bias in medical decision making. *Medical Decision Making, 25*, 96–105.

Loewenstein, G., Weber, E. U., Hsee, C. K., & Welch, N. (2001). Risk as feelings. *Psychological Bulletin, 127*, 267–286.

Mamede, S., Schmidt, H. G., & Rikers, R. (2007). Diagnostic errors and reflective practice in medicine. *Journal of Evaluation in Clinical Practice, 13*(1), 138–145.

Mamede, S., Van Gog, T., Schuit, S. C. E., Van den Berge, K., Van Daele, P. L. A., Bueving H., . . . Schmidt, H. G. (2017). Why patients' disruptive behaviours impair diagnostic reasoning: A randomised experiment. *BMJ Quality and Safety, 26*(1), 13–18. doi:10.1136/bmjqs-2015-005065

Markman, K. D., Gavanski, I., Sherman, S. J., & McMullen, M. N. (1993). The mental simulation of better and worse possible worlds. *Journal of Experimental Social Psychology, 29*, 87–109.

National Patient Safety Agency. *WHO surgical safety checklist: Patient safety alert.* National Patient Safety Agency. January 2009. Retrieved December 19, 2017 from www.nrls.npsa.nhs.uk/alerts

Newman-Toker, D. E., & Pronovost, P. J. (2009). Diagnostic errors—The next frontier for patient safety. *Journal of the American Medical Association, 301*, 1060–1062.

Norman, G. (2009). Dual processing and diagnostic errors. *Advances in Health Science Education, 14*, 37–49.

Nurok, M., Evans, L. A., Lipsitz, S., Satwicz, P., Kelly, A., & Frankel, A. (2011). The relationship of the emotional climate of work and threat to patient outcome in a high-volume thoracic surgery operating room team. *BMJ Quality and Safety, 20*, 237–242.

Orton, P., Orton, C., & Gray, D. P. (2012). Depersonalised doctors: A cross-sectional study of 564 doctors, 760 consultations and 1876 patient reports in UK general practice. *BMJ Open, 2*(1), e000274.

Pani, J. R., & Chariker, J. H. (2004). The psychology of error in relation to medical practice. *Journal of Surgical Oncology, 88*, 130–142.

Parker, D., & Lawton, R. (2003). Psychological contribution to the understanding of adverse events in health care. *Quality and Safety in Health Care, 12*, 453–457.

Pezza Leith, K., & Baumeister, R. F. (1996). Why do bad moods increase self-defeating behavior? Emotion, risk taking, and self-regulation. *Journal of Personality and Social Psychology, 71*, 1250–1267.

Powell, A. E., & Davies, H. T. O. (2012). The struggle to improve patient care in the face of professional boundaries. *Social Science and Medicine, 75*, 807–814.

Ramnarayan, P., Winrow, A., Coren, M., Nanduri, V., Buchdahl, R., Jacobs, B., et al. (2006). Diagnostic omission errors in acute paediatric practice: Impact of a reminder system on decision-making. *BMC Medical Informatics and Decision Making, 6*, 37. doi: 10.1186/1472-6947-6-37.

Salhani, D., & Coulter, I. (2009). The politics of interprofessional working and the struggle for professional autonomy in nursing. *Social Science and Medicine, 68*, 1221–1228.

Schmidt, H. G., van Gog, T., Schuit, S. C. E., Van den Berge, K., Van Daele, P. L. A., Bueving, H., . . . Mamede, S. (2017). Do patients' disruptive behaviours influence the accuracy of a doctor's diagnosis? A randomised experiment. *BMJ Quality and Safety*, *26*(1), 19–23. doi:10.1136/bmjqs-2015-004109

Schwartz Centre for Compassionate Care. (2015). Schwartz Center rounds. Retrieved July 1, 2016 from: http://www.theschwartzcentre.org/supporting-caregivers/schwartz-center-rounds/

Slovic, P., Peters, E., Finucane, M. L., & MacGregor, D. G. (2005). Affect, risk, and decision making. *Health Psychology*, *24*, S35–S40.

Smith, P. *The emotional labour of nursing*. 1992. London: Macmillan.

Smith, E. R., & DeCoster, J. (2000). Dual-process models in social and cognitive psychology: Conceptual integration and links to underlying memory systems. *Personality and Social Psychology Review*, *4*, 108–131.

Strack, F., & Deutsch, R. (2004). Reflective and impulsive determinants of social behavior. *Personality and Social Psychology Review*, *8*, 220–247.

Sutcliffe, K. M., Lewton, E., & Rosenthal, M. M. (2004). Communication failures: An insidious contributor to medical mishaps. *Academic Medicine*, *79*, 186–194.

Tversky, A., & Kahneman, D. (1974). Judgment under uncertainty: Heuristics and biases. *Science*, *185*, 1124–1131.

Ubel, P. A. (2005). Emotions, decisions, and the limits of rationality: Symposium introduction. *Medical Decision Making*, *25*, 95–96.

Van Doorn, E. A., Heerdink, M. W., & Van Kleef, G. A. (2012). Emotion and the construal of social situations: Inferences of cooperation versus competition from expressions of anger, happiness and disappointment. *Cognition and Emotion*, *26*, 442–461.

Van Kleef, G. A. (2009). How emotions regulate social life: The emotions as social information (EASI) model. *Current Directions in Psychological Science*, *18*, 184–188.

Van Kleef, G. A., De Dreu, C. K. W., & Manstead, A. S. R. (2010). An interpersonal approach to emotion in social decision making: The emotions as social information model. *Advances in Experimental Psychology*, *42*, 45–96.

Van Kleef, G. A., Homan, A. C., & Chesin, A. (2012). Emotional influence at work. *Organizational Psychology Review*, *2*, 311–339.

Waters, E. A. (2008). Feeling good, feeling bad, and feeling at-risk: A review of incidental affect's influence on likelihood estimates of health hazards and life events. *Journal of Risk Research*, *11*, 569–595.

Well-Med. (2016). 2nd International Meeting on Well-Being and Performance in Clinical Practice, Greece, May, 2016.

Yule, S., Flin, R., Paterson-Brown, S., & Maran, N. (2006). Development of a rating system for surgeons' non-technical skills. *Medical Education*, *40*, 1098–1104.

19

Emotions, Delay, and Avoidance in Cancer Screening

Roles for Fear, Embarrassment, and Disgust

NATHAN S. CONSEDINE, LISA M. REYNOLDS, AND CHARMAINE BORG

THE ORIGINS OF DELAY AND AVOIDANCE IN CANCER SCREENING—A POTTED HISTORY

Delay and avoidance are major foci in cancer screening research, in part because population screening reduces morbidity and mortality. Delays and avoidance are, however, common and occur at multiple points, from delays in evaluating symptoms as potentially dangerous or in need of examination to delays in making appointments, screening, deciding on a course of treatment, or filling prescriptions. Delay can lead to worsening conditions, later stage diagnoses, and restricted treatment options, thus compounding the health, social, and economic costs of cancer.

Unsurprisingly, delay and avoidance are heavily overdetermined. Work has considered a range of predictors, from age, marital status, and income to culture and masculinity. Studies have evaluated system factors, geography, education, sexual orientation, race, and minority status. However, while such factors may *predict* screening, they are limited in several ways. First, they typically explain a small portion of the variance; screening remains suboptimal even where it is free and convenient (Von Wagner, Good, Whitaker, & Wardle, 2013). While demographics are descriptively useful, they fail to explain *why* individuals delay or avoid and may be difficult to change (Consedine, Magai, Horton, Neugut, & Gillespie, 2005).

Such limitations have increased the focus on the psychological predictors of delay. Much work has been cognitively focused, examining knowledge (Weinrich, Weinrich, Boyd, & Atkinson, 1998), risk (Kunkel et al., 2004), and screening (Myers, Hyslop, Jennings-Dozier, et al., 2000) or treatment efficacy (Myers, Hyslop, Wolf, et al., 2000) perceptions. This psychological approach has tended to view people as "rational" decision-makers (Brock & Wartman, 1990) despite it being increasingly clear that decision-making of this kind does not often occur in practice (Broadstock & Michie, 2000).

THE ORIGINS OF DELAY AND AVOIDANCE—AN EMOTIONS THEORY PERSPECTIVE

In our view, emotions are integral to the processes by which people delay and avoid most experiences, including cancer screening. In this view, emotions constitute the primary, in-built motivational systems underpinning human behavior (Izard, 1991). Delay and avoidance are no different from other behaviors insofar as they are built on the actions of these same systems. More to the point, because some emotions evolved *precisely because* they motivate the avoidance of their elicitors and these elicitors are frequently present in cancer screening contexts, avoidance and delay are commensurately common. In what follows, we describe this approach more fully, concentrating on three emotions—fear, embarrassment, and disgust—that have documented or likely links to low screening.

In evolutionary-functionalist views, each emotion represents an adaptation that evolved to deal with a specific class of adaptive challenge or opportunity. So, for example, anger evolved to facilitate responding to goal blockages, sadness to situations involving current loss, guilt to situations in which reparation was needed, regret to possible future losses, and so on. Emotions were selected to adjust our responses to these situational "classes" in ways that, on average, offered an adaptive advantage (Johnson-Laird & Oatley, 1992; Lazarus, 1991). Importantly, emotions may not always be "helpful" vis-à-vis current challenges (including cancer screenings). Emotions evolved in environments that likely differed from those encountered today, meaning that while the general pattern of changes has, on average, been advantageous, emotions may or may not promote behaviors that look "adaptive" now.

So, emotions evolved to facilitate adaptation to a *class* of situations rather than to specific stimuli (Johnson-Laird & Oatley, 1992). Fear facilitates adaptation to physical dangers by urging us to flee (Spoor & Kelly, 2004), while anxiety is useful for less immediate or overt threats (Marks & Nesse, 1994). Disgust aids adaptation to health threats through ejection and withdrawal (Reynolds, Consedine, Pizarro, & Bissett, 2013), and embarrassment motivates behaviors that reduce the chance of social exclusion (Consedine, Krivoshekova, & Harris, 2007). Importantly, the manifestations of emotions—in experience, physiology, cognition, signals, and behaviors—are similar despite variations in the elicitor. It does not matter whether embarrassment is elicited by genital inspections or something as mundane as forgetting a name. We blush (signaling an awareness of norm violation), feel a desire to hide or escape, and may plan future avoidance. Hence, although the "direction" of the response varies depending on what is being responded to, the components of the response are generic.

This commonality noted, *each* time we get emotional, the response occurs as a reaction to a specific situation, event, or elicitor. Responses are not "sourceless" but are "about something in particular" (Consedine, Adjei, Ramirez, & McKiernan, 2008; Consedine, Ladwig, Reddig, & Broadbent, 2011); behaviors, including those that are avoidant, occur vis-à-vis this something. There are specific aspects of cancer screenings that elicit avoidance-producing emotions, and it is these specific aspects we are motivated to avoid. In some senses, avoidance of the *entire* screening context may be epiphenomenal to the function of the emotion in motivating avoidance of specific fear, embarrassment, or disgust elicitors.

Importantly in terms of screening, emotions motivate avoidance both immediately and in anticipation (Consedine & Moskowitz, 2007); anticipating experientially aversive emotion is a key driver of avoidance in health (Chapman & Coups, 2006; Sussner et al., 2009). Immediate responses facilitate the minimization of immediate harm, while anticipating that certain stimuli or behavior will increase or decrease the odds of certain feelings facilitates learning and future avoidance. The fact that the anticipation of emotion motivates behavior is important because it helps explain why screens that have never been experienced may be actively avoided (Reynolds et al., 2013).

In sum, while most emotions did not evolve to fulfill health-related functions per se (Consedine, 2008)—disgust being the exception—several emotions' core functions involve the immediate or anticipated avoidance of certain stimuli. These stimuli—threats to bodily integrity, nudity, norm violations, bodily products, and the like—are common in cancer screening. Thus, while emotions did not evolve to promote screening avoidance, they did evolve to promote avoidance. Differences between the situations emotions were "designed" to remedy and modern environments suggest "misfits" will occur and avoidance will be common.

FEAR, EMBARRASSMENT, AND DISGUST PREDICT DELAY AND AVOIDANCE IN CANCER SCREENING

Historically, the literature linking emotions with cancer has concentrated on fear and embarrassment (Consedine & Moskowitz, 2007) but, until recently, has overlooked other avoidance-producing emotions such as disgust. Each of these emotions is discussed in this section.

Embarrassment and Its Links to Cancer Screening

Embarrassment evolved to help humans navigate social interactions by preventing norm violations and/or amending social relations after transgressions (Keltner & Buswell, 1997). Embarrassment is characterized by our feeling awkward, foolish, and highly self-aware (Keltner & Anderson, 2000; Miller, 1992). It has a range of normative elicitors and follows norm violations (Keltner & Anderson, 2000) and/or negative social evaluation. Expressions signal awareness of the violation (Semin & Manstead, 1982) and reduce social judgment (Dijk, de Jong, & Peters, 2009); anticipated embarrassment motivates subsequent avoidance of behaviors or situations likely to elicit it (Consedine et al., 2011).

Embarrassment's normative elicitors are common in cancer screening—perceptions of physical ineptness or inadequacy (Keltner & Buswell, 1996), such as excess weight (Amy, Aalborg, Lyons, & Keranen, 2006) or the loss of control or poise (Miller, 1992) as with flatulence. Embarrassment is common when "failures" at privacy regulation occur (Keltner & Anderson, 2000); having genitals touched (Gascoigne, Mason, & Roberts, 1999) or discussing sexual issues (Ansong, Lewis, Jenkins, & Bell, 1998) in the presence of strangers or with observers present routinely elicit this feeling (Consedine, Krivoshekova, et al., 2007).

The threat of embarrassment may deter care-seeking for sexual examinations, even when symptoms are serious and patients know behaviors are important. Much of what is known is based on qualitative studies (e.g., Forrester-Anderson, 2005; Shaw, Williams, Assassa, & Jackson, 2000) that offer a conflicted picture. Of note, while physicians see embarrassment as important (Klabunde et al., 2005), patients may or may not. One study found that only 8% (fecal stool) and 7% (colonoscopy) reported embarrassment as a barrier (Nicholson & Korman, 2005). Such studies may tell us as much about reporting bias and implicit models as they do about the role of embarrassment in screening.

Survey-based studies suggest that actual or anticipated embarrassment predicts lower screening. Embarrassment predicts lower screening for prostate (Consedine, Horton, et al., 2007; Myers et al., 1996; Shelton, Weinrich, & Reynolds, 1999), breast (Consedine, Magai, & Neugut, 2004; Lerman, Rimer, Trock, Balshem, & Engstrom, 1990), testicular (Gascoigne et al., 1999), and colon/rectum (Consedine et al., 2011; Harewood, Wiersema, & Melton, 2002; Hou, 2005) cancers. Often, it does so even when demographics (Shelton et al., 1999) and/or system factors (Consedine et al., 2011) are controlled.

However, while embarrassment predicts lower screening, several issues remain unclear. First, the specific aspects of screening that are embarrassing are unknown. Such aspects might include staff interactions, privacy or nudity, exposure to feces (Consedine et al., 2011) or penetration and homophobic concerns (Winterich et al., 2009). While it is the experiential aspect of emotions that the individual is motivated to avoid, the functional "aim" of the response is to avoid the elicitor. This critical issue is discussed more fully later. Second, as will become clear, cross-sectional designs predominate. One study found that induced embarrassment *caused* help-seeking delays for embarrassment elicitors (e.g., physical exams) (McCambridge & Consedine, 2014). Experimental designs are uncommon, however, and the interpretative limits of correlational designs coupled with heavy covariation among avoidance-producing emotions present an issue for fear, embarrassment, and disgust research.

Disgust and Its Links to Cancer Screening

Disgust is a health-related emotion (Consedine & Moskowitz, 2007; Curtis, Aunger, & Rabie, 2004), with disease or contamination avoidance functions (Davey, 2011; Oaten, Stevenson, & Case, 2009; Reynolds, Bissett, & Consedine, 2015). Originating in the need to avoid pathogen ingestion (Rozin & Fallon, 1987), disgust is a core part of the behavioral immune system (Schaller & Park, 2011). It is elicited by body envelope violations (e.g., internal exams, insertions), bodily products and waste (e.g., feces, blood), poor hygiene, and contamination threats (e.g., con tact with strangers) (Curtis & Biran, 2001). Such stimuli are common in cancer screening, creating a prima facie case for the involvement of disgust.

Like fear and embarrassment, disgust evolved to facilitate adaptation through avoidance and withdrawal (Reynolds, Bissett, Porter, & Consedine, 2016); it does so at both immediate and anticipatory levels (Reynolds et al., 2013). Immediate responses include withdrawal, gaze aversion, nose plugging, tongue protrusion and gagging, and increased salivation (Rozin, Haidt, & McCauley, 1999). Second, and despite evidence that our ability to forecast emotions is poor (discussed later), disgust motivates anticipatory avoidance, enabling us to deal with potential health threats preventatively (Schaller & Duncan, 2007).

Empirical studies of disgust in cancer screening are uncommon. A review of disgust in colorectal cancer (CRC) screening identified only nine disgust-related studies (Reynolds et al., 2013); disgust was almost always a barrier to screening. Reluctance to complete a fecal occult blood test (FOBT) is linked to the aversiveness of handling stools, storing samples at home (Jones et al., 2010), or posting them (Chambers, Callander, Grangeret, & O'Carroll, 2016). One large study of 60,000 adults from the Scottish National program showed that the "ick" factor predicted FOBT kit return over and above intentions (O'Carroll, Chambers, Brownlee, Libby, & Steele, 2015). Another found that a 4-item "ick" factor predicted FOBT intention better than either propensity or sensitivity (Chambers et al., 2016) and disgust predicts avoidance in chemotherapy patients (Reynolds, Bissett, Porter, & Consedine, 2016).

Again, however, cancer-screening research evaluating disgust is mostly cross-sectional and thus plagued by the same third variable issue confronting most research of this type. Immediate avoidance when disgusted is well documented. Less clear is whether induced disgust impacts decisions regarding health events that have yet to occur. One study had participants read vignettes highlighting disgust elicitors in CRC screening and treatment. Manipulated and trait disgust both predicted immediate avoidance and interacted in predicting *anticipated* avoidance; delay was greater among trait sensitive persons when disgusted (Reynolds, McCambridge, Bissett, & Consedine, 2014). A second study found that disgust predicted greater socially avoidant health decisions (Reynolds, Lin, Zhou, & Consedine, 2015). A final study found that disgust caused delays in sexual healthcare when seeking help would involve exposure to disgust elicitors (e.g., collecting genital discharge), but only among persons reporting poorer health (McCambridge & Consedine, 2014). Although these data are complex, an evidence base consistent with disgust deterring screening is emerging, although the specific cancer screens that are impacted and possible interventions remain unclear.

Fear and Anxiety and Their Links to Cancer Screening

Fear and anxiety are among the most studied emotions, have been consistently linked to screening, and have been leveraged in health messaging for more than 60 years (Janis & Feshbach, 1953; Ruiter, Abraham, & Kok, 2001; Witte & Allen, 2000). Multiple aspects of cancer screening elicit fear, from the possibility of internal damage, disease, or a positive diagnosis, to the threat of invasive, painful, or intimate examinations. When a threat is detected and a person becomes fearful or anxious, cognitive processes shift to assess the threat's source and physiological changes provide physical resources. In addition to encouraging immediate flight, fear and anxiety also guide behavior by motivating the subsequent avoidance of elicitors (Consedine, Magai, Krivoshekova, Ryzewicz, & Neugut, 2004). Importantly, the core response—immediate withdrawal or future avoidance—is similar notwithstanding whether elicitors are present or anticipated or whether they involve heights, animals, darkness, separation, or, we suspect, screening.

A huge literature implicates fear, anxiety, or worry in cancer screening (Consedine, Magai, Krivoshekova, et al., 2004; Dale, Bilir, Han, & Meltzer, 2005; Hay, Buckley, & Ostroff, 2005). The findings are complex, with links to both greater and lower screening. Work has converged on a view in which fear/anxiety predicts screening differently depending on the source of the fear (Consedine, Magai, Krivoshekova, et al., 2004). Greater cancer worry (an emotionally laden cognitive process) predicts greater screening (Consedine, Magai, & Neugut, 2004; Hay, McCaul, & Magnan, 2006) and intentions to screen (Vrinten, Waller, Von Wagner, & Wardle, 2015), while fear of screening predicts less (Consedine et al., 2008).

Interim Remarks

Overall, the literatures reviewed thus far are sufficiently developed to permit a few interim remarks. First, fear, embarrassment, and disgust all evolved to promote the avoidance of elicitors and they do so for both immediate and anticipated events. Second, the prototypical elicitors for these emotions are common in cancer screening contexts; examinations and interactions “map” onto prototypical elicitors. Thus, it seems likely that experienced or anticipated fear, embarrassment, and disgust are etiologically implicated in health-related avoidance. There is, however, an ongoing failure to directly assess avoidance, a lack of experimental data, uncertainty around the specific aspects of intimate cancer screens that elicit avoidance-promoting emotion, and the problem of covariance. In the next section, we consider these issues more fully, concluding by offering directions for interventions and future study.

AREAS FOR FUTURE DEVELOPMENT IN EMOTION-SCREENING RESEARCH

First, to substantiate the hypothesized avoidance-promoting role of emotions, researchers need to begin manipulating them and assessing screening. Studies routinely assume that the *absence* of screening (or a lower frequency) is indicating avoidance. For example, reports of greater embarrassment predict less frequent screening, a fact that is taken to indicate that embarrassment is causing lower screening. However, avoidance and delay are not directly assessed and causal proof is lacking. People cannot be assumed to be avoiding merely because they are not behaving. In addition to using objective measures, asking about delay/avoidance and the reasons for it seems an obvious solution to this problem. However, avoiding socially mandated behaviors is undesirable and likely prone to reporting biases. Our suspicion here is that such biases are more likely to skew reports regarding the *reasons* for avoidance rather than the fact of it per se. Patients may report delay or avoidance but be reluctant (or unable) to report that they avoided a mammogram, digital rectal exam (DRE), or FOBT *because* they were afraid, embarrassed, or disgusted. Normalizing affectively based avoidance in the research “dialogue,” perhaps by noting that such avoidance is common, may be useful.

Identifying the Source of Embarrassment, Fear, and Disgust

A second area in need of development involves designing studies that delineate the *specific* aspects of cancer-screening contexts that elicit emotion and are thus avoided. Because the fear literature is among the best developed in emotion-screening research, it is also a useful context in which to consider how delineating the *source* of emotions in health (their specific elicitors) may help. In brief, fear/anxiety data have been scattered, with findings showing positive, negative, or no links between fear-type constructs and screening. A decade ago, a review suggested that the association between fear/anxiety and screening is determined, in part, by the source of the fear and thus the extent to which the behavior will alleviate or increase felt emotion (Consedine, Magai, Krivoshekova, et al., 2004). A later study found that cancer worry predicted greater screening while screening fear predicted less screening *at the same time* (Consedine et al., 2008), perhaps suggesting that cancer worry predicts screening because people anticipate lower anxiety after screening. Because *cancer* is the source of fear in cancer worry, people engage in behaviors that subjectively reduce the threat—they screen. However, the threat in "fear of screening" is the screening context itself. Again, fear-based avoidance motivates the avoidance of the fear's source—people avoid screening (Consedine et al., 2008). Similar arguments have been put forth in embarrassment research:

> [I]t is insufficient to understand that people are embarrassed . . . and thus may not screen . . . we must know whether they are. . . . embarrassed by the prospect of having something inserted into their rectum, whether it is about being touched, whether it relates to obesity or their having poor skin, whether they worry about the thoughts the technician has during the procedure, about their response to possible pain . . . and so forth. (Consedine et al., 2007, p. 442)

Data suggest that embarrassment may predict greater care-seeking, at least when patients are embarrassed by symptoms (Consedine et al., 2011). For example, men with more severe urinary symptoms report greater embarrassment, but it is those who were bothered by *socially observable* symptoms (e.g., wet pants, dribbling), that were more likely to visit a doctor. Thus, although it may lead to avoidance, embarrassment may not lead to the avoidance of screening. Where symptoms create embarrassment in daily life, persons will engage in behaviors they see as likely to reduce symptoms; screening should be greater. However, where embarrassment regards aspects of the examination process itself, screening should be deterred.

Findings consistent with this view in disgust are yet to be reported. One study of 200 Scottish adults found that a 4-item "ick" factor predicted FOBT intention better than either dispositional disgust propensity or sensitivity (Chambers et al., 2016), presumably because the items captured variance associated with the specific elicitors that were being avoided. Comparatively, however, the fear and embarrassment literatures provide good examples of how important it may be to identify the specific (affective) elements in screening contexts because it is these elements (rather than "the situation" per se) that the emotions are motivating us to avoid.

The Problem with Sex

A further point is that, insofar as they involve the examination of sexual characteristics, most screenings are fundamentally *sexual*; sexual stimuli are core sources of anxiety, embarrassment, and disgust. In many ways, this is not surprising. The body parts and secretions at the core of human sexuality (e.g., penis, saliva, vagina) are easily infected, carry disease risk, and are (thus) potent disgust elicitors (Rozin & Fallon, 1987). Because many screenings require contact with these stimuli (e.g., collecting stools) or body parts (genitals, anus, mouth), avoidance-promoting emotions are common. Contamination fears and disgust increase as a function of proximity (Rozin, Nemeroff, Horowitz, Gordon, & Voet, 1995) and sexual stimuli are neurally processed like disgust in the absence of arousal (Borg et al., 2014).

Furthermore, cancer screens may elicit fears regarding any consequential treatments, many of which are detrimental to sexual functioning or body image. The possibility of disfigurement or damage to an erotic zone (e.g., mastectomy) or a treatment that weakens sexual functioning (e.g., lowered testosterone) may all contribute to disgust or embarrassment, triggering avoidance and delay. Perhaps particularly when people have restrictive moral values regarding sexuality, stranger-based contact with erotic zones or sexual body parts may increase the intensity of avoidance-driving negative emotions (Borg, de Jong, & Weijmar Schultz, 2011). Behaving in ways that are inconsistent with strongly held principles may both exaggerate emotional responses (and thus avoidance) and further shape moral values. Screening researchers need to remember that many common screens are sexual in nature, a fact that increases the likelihood of strong emotional responses and thus avoidance.

THE COVARIATION PROBLEM

Research at the emotions-screening intersection faces a singular challenge insofar as a single test or context can engender multiple emotions, any, some, or all of which may promote avoidance; this issue reflects "covariation" among negative emotions (Consedine & Moskowitz, 2007). Disgust and embarrassment co-occur (Rozin, Haidt, McCauley, Dunlop, & Ashmore, 1999), as do fear and disgust (Olatunji et al., 2009). Equally, given links between embarrassment and social anxiety (Jowett & Ryan, 1985; Miller, 1995; Sabini, Siepmann, Stein, & Meyerowitz, 2000), embarrassment likely shares elicitors with fear as well.

Although covariation is a problem for emotions-health research in general, it is a particular problem for those studying avoidance for the simple reason that fear, embarrassment, and disgust all evolved to promote avoidant responses. Most studies assess a single emotion and/or aggregate multiple emotional responses within "barrier" constructs (Menon et al., 2003;

Rawl et al., 2001). Summating discrete emotions makes it difficult to evaluate each emotion's relevance or address questions of necessity and specificity. Screening research needs to assess multiple emotions and evaluate their unique contributions. Without this specificity, we cannot be sure which responses promote avoidance for which type of screen and, thus, which specific emotions our interventions should target.

Actual and Anticipated Emotions

Research in emotions and screening would benefit from greater clarity in the measurement of felt emotions versus emotions that are (cognitively) seen as likely to arise (anticipated emotions). Both forms of emotion are recursively linked to one another as well as to future behavior (Van der Schalk, Bruder, & Manstead, 2013). Although some longitudinal data suggest that prior experience only weakly predicts future screening (Drossaert, Boer, & Seydel, 2002, 2003), theory is clear in suggesting that while emotional factors predict behavior they also change in response to screening (Consedine, Christie, & Neugut, 2009). For example, women reporting a prior embarrassing cervical smear are more deterred from future smears (Orbell, 1996), suggesting that prior emotional experiences may shape both anticipated emotions as well as future behavior.

In theory, current emotional state may serve as an "affective cue" that makes particular aspects of a decision more salient (Peters, Lipkus, & Diefenbach, 2006). Elicited disgust, embarrassment, or fear may thus trigger individuals to be more attentive to relevant cues. A recent study found that manipulated disgust produced greater anticipated delay in response to bowel symptoms, and the possibility of disgusting symptoms is more likely to deter adherence, at least among persons high in trait disgust (Reynolds et al., 2014). Other work has noted that the effect of emotion on behavior may be stronger where patients have no recent frame of reference (Wong & Kwong, 2007); emotions may "fill the gap" when knowledge is incomplete.

Importantly, the fact that people are routinely inaccurate in anticipating the affective consequences of behavior (or not behaving) does not prevent anticipated emotion from influencing decisions. We may overestimate the aversive emotion we expect to experience in screening contexts and behave accordingly. Regardless of whether affective forecasting is accurate or not, anticipation of aversive emotion is a key driver of avoidant behavior in health (Chapman & Coups, 2006; O'Carroll, Foster, McGeechan, Sandford, & Ferguson, 2011), although this distinction remains poorly investigated in cancer screening work.

Emotional Responses and Avoidance Among Physicians

Finally, disgust, embarrassment, and fear are not only relevant to avoidance and delay among patients; they also impact physician behavior. Anticipated regret influences physician decision-making (Sorum et al., 2004), and embarrassment may deter the taking of full sexual histories (Merrill, Laux, & Thornby, 1990) or error disclosure (Allman, 1998). Anxiety may lead physicians to request additional investigations, initiate referrals, and overuse resources (Anderson, 1999; Katz et al., 2005). Despite the nature of medical contact, disgust is infrequently studied among medical professionals. A few reports allude to disgust when caring for obese patients (Poon & Tarrant, 2009), in anal health (Hardy, 2010), and in medical career choice (Consedine, Yu, & Windsor, 2013). However, because disgust plays a key role in the stigmatization and avoidance of persons with detectable diseases (Park, Faulkner, & Schaller, 2003), its influence may be far more pervasive.

Although data are lacking, the elicitation (or anticipation) of embarrassment, fear, and disgust may influence clinicians' decisions and behavior in ways that are likely to reduce or prevent these affective states. Physicians may become decisionally, interpersonally, or behaviorally avoidant in ways that are detrimental to their capacity to deliver optimal care. Future work should clarify the areas of clinical decision-making, judgment, and behavior that are impacted by embarrassment, fear, and disgust and develop interventions that "cue" physicians to the possibility that they become avoidant in some areas of their practice.

CONCLUDING REMARKS

Delay and avoidance are widespread problems in cancer screening and are associated with a range of negative health, social, and economic consequences. The approach put forward here suggests that people avoid disgust-, embarrassment- and fear-inducing cancer screens precisely because they are innately motivated to avoid these experiences. To an extent then, this view suggests that delay and avoidance of medical *situations* is a byproduct of the motivated desire to avoid certain emotional experiences. Because emotions constitute the primary motivational substrate for most human behavior, understanding their evolved design, normative elicitors, and associated behavioral tendencies has the potential to illuminate at least some of the causes of avoidance and delays in cancer-screening contexts.

REFERENCES

Allman, J. (1998). Bearing the burden or baring the soul: Physicians' self-disclosure and boundary management regarding medical mistakes. *Health Communication, 10*, 175–197.

Amy, N. K., Aalborg, A., Lyons, P., & Keranen, L. (2006). Barriers to routine gynecological cancer screening for White and African-American obese women. *International Journal of Obesity, 30*, 147–155.

Anderson, R. E. (1999). Billions for defense: The pervasive nature of defensive medicine. *Archives of Internal Medicine, 159*, 2399–2402.

Ansong, K. S., Lewis, C., Jenkins, P., & Bell, J. (1998). Help-seeking decisions among men with impotence. *Urology, 52*, 834–837.

Borg, C., de Jong, P. J., & Weijmar Schultz, W. (2011). Vaginismus and dyspareunia: Relationship with general and sex-related moral standards. *Journal of Sexual Medicine, 8*, 223–231.

Borg, C., Georgiadis, R. J., Renken, R. J., Spoelstra, K., Weijmar Schultz, W., & de Jong, P. J. (2014). Brain processing of sexual penetration versus core and animal-reminder disgust pictures in women with genito-pelvic pain/penetration disorders. *PLoS ONE, 9*, e84882.

Broadstock, M., & Michie, S. (2000). Processes of patient decision making: Theoretical and methodological issues. *Psychology and Health, 15*, 191–204.

Brock, D. W., & Wartman, S. A. (1990). When competent patients make irrational choices. *New England Journal of Medicine, 322*, 1595–1599.

Chambers, J. A., Callander, A. S., Grangeret, R., & O'Carroll, R. E. (2016). Attitudes towards the Faecal Occult Blood Test (FOBT) versus the Faecal Immunochemical Test (FIT) for colorectal cancer screening: Perceived ease of completion and disgust. *BMJ Cancer, 16*. doi:10.1186/s12885-016-2133-4

Chapman, G. B., & Coups, E. J. (2006). Emotions and preventive behavior: Worry, regret, and influenza vaccination. *Health Psychology, 25*, 82–90.

Consedine, N. S. (2008). The health-promoting and health-damaging effects of emotions: The view from developmental functionalism. In M. Lewis, J. Haviland-Jones, & L. F. Barrett (Eds.), *Handbook of emotions* (3rd ed., pp. 676–690). New York, NY: Guilford.

Consedine, N. S., Adjei, B. A., Ramirez, P. M., & McKiernan, J. (2008). An object lesson: Differences in source determine the relations that trait anxiety, prostate cancer worry, and fear of screening hold with prostate screening frequency. *Cancer Epidemiology Biomarkers and Prevention, 17*, 1631–1639.

Consedine, N. S., Christie, M. A., & Neugut, A. I. (2009). Physician, affective, and cognitive variables differentially predict "initiation" versus "maintenance" PSA screening profiles in diverse groups of men. *British Journal of Health Psychology, 14*, 303–322.

Consedine, N. S., Horton, D., Ungar, T., Joe, A., Ramirez, P., & Borrell, L. (2007). Fear, knowledge and efficacy beliefs differentially predict the frequency of DRE versus PSA screening in ethnically diverse samples of older men. *American Journal of Men's Health, 1*, 29–43.

Consedine, N. S., Krivoshekova, Y. S., & Harris, C. R. (2007). Bodily embarrassment and judgment concern as separable factors in the measurement of medical embarrassment: Psychometric development and links to treatment-seeking outcomes. *British Journal of Health Psychology, 12*, 439–462.

Consedine, N. S., Ladwig, I., Reddig, M. K., & Broadbent, E. A. (2011). The many faeces of colorectal cancer screening embarrassment: Preliminary psychometric development and links to screening outcome. *British Journal of Health Psychology, 16*, 559–579.

Consedine, N. S., Magai, C., Horton, D., Neugut, A. I., & Gillespie, M. (2005). Health belief model factors in mammography screening: Testing for interactions among subpopulations of Caribbean women. *Ethnicity and Disease, 15*, 444–452.

Consedine, N. S., Magai, C., Krivoshekova, Y. S., Ryzewicz, L., & Neugut, A. I. (2004). Fear, anxiety, worry, and breast cancer screening behavior: A critical review. *Cancer Epidemiology, Biomarkers and Prevention, 13*, 501–510.

Consedine, N. S., Magai, C., & Neugut, A. I. (2004). The contribution of emotional characteristics to breast cancer screening among women from six ethnic groups. *Preventive Medicine, 38*, 64–77.

Consedine, N. S., & Moskowitz, J. T. (2007). The role of discrete emotions in health outcomes: A critical review. *Applied and Preventive Psychology, 12*, 59–75.

Consedine, N. S., Yu, W., T.-C., & Windsor, J. (2013). Nursing, pharmacy, or medicine? Disgust sensitivity predicts career interest among trainee health professionals. *Advances in Health Sciences Education, 18*, 997–1008.

Curtis, V., Aunger, R., & Rabie, T. (2004). Evidence that disgust evolved to protect from risk of disease. *Proceedings of the Royal Society Biological Sciences: Series B, 271*, S131–S133.

Curtis, V., & Biran, A. (2001). Dirt, disgust, and disease: Is hygiene in our genes? *Perspectives in Biology and Medicine, 44*, 17–31.

Dale, W., Bilir, P., Han, M., & Meltzer, D. (2005). The role of anxiety in prostate carcinoma. *Cancer, 104*, 467–478.

Davey, G. C. L. (2011). Disgust: The disease-avoidance emotion and its dysfunctions. *Philosophical Transactions of the Royal Society B: Biological Sciences, 366*, 3453–3465.

Dijk, C., de Jong, P. J., & Peters, M. L. (2009). The remedial value of blushing in the context of transgressions and mishaps. *Emotion, 9*, 287–291.

Drossaert, C. H. C., Boer, H., & Seydel, E. R. (2002). Monitoring women's experiences during three rounds of breast cancer screening: Results from a longitudinal study. *Journal of Medical Screening, 9*, 168–175.

Drossaert, C. H. C., Boer, H., & Seydel, E. R. (2003). Prospective study of the determinants of repeat attending and attendance patterns in breast cancer screening using the theory of planned behavior. *Psychology and Health, 18*, 551–565.

Forrester-Anderson, I. T. (2005). Prostate cancer screening perceptions, knowledge, and behaviors among African American men: Focus group findings. *Journal of Health Care for the Poor and Underserved, 16*, 22–30.

Gascoigne, P., Mason, M. D., & Roberts, E. (1999). Factors affecting presentation and delay in patients with testicular cancer: Results of a qualitative study. *Psycho-Oncology, 8*, 144–154.

Hardy, D. (2010). *When we dare not speak its name: Anal taboo, anal health and affect theory* (Ed. dissertation). Widener University, Pennsylvania.

Harewood, G. C., Wiersema, M. J., & Melton, L. J. (2002). A prospective, controlled assessment of factors influencing acceptance of screening colonoscopy. *American Journal of Gastroenterology, 97*, 3186–3194.

Hay, J. L., Buckley, T. R., & Ostroff, J. S. (2005). The role of cancer worry in cancer screening: A theoretical and empirical review of the literature. *Psycho-Oncology, 14*, 517–534.

Hay, J. L., McCaul, K. D., & Magnan, R. E. (2006). Does worry about breast cancer predict screening behaviors? A meta-analysis of the prospective evidence. *Preventive Medicine, 42*, 401–408.

Hou, S.-I. (2005). Factors associated with intentions for colorectal cancer screenings in a Chinese sample. *Psychological Reports, 96*, 159–162.

Izard, C. E. (1991). *The psychology of emotions*. New York, NY: Plenum Press.

Janis, I. L., & Feshbach, S. (1953). Effects of fear-arousing communications. *Journal of Abnormal and Social Psychology, 48*, 78–92.

Johnson-Laird, P. N., & Oatley, K. (1992). Basic emotions, rationality, and folk theory. *Cognition and Emotion, 6*, 201–223.

Jones, R. M., Woolf, S. H., Cunningham, T. D., Johnson, R. E., Krist, A. H., Rothermich, S. F., & Vernon, S. W. (2010). The relative importance of patient-reported barriers to colorectal cancer screening. *American Journal of Preventive Medicine, 38*, 499–507.

Jowett, S., & Ryan, T. (1985). Skin disease and handicap: An analysis of the impact of skin conditions. *Social Science and Medicine, 20*, 425–429.

Katz, D. A., Williams, G. C., Brown, R. L., Aufderheide, T. P., Bogner, M., Rahko, P. S., & Selker, H. P. (2005). Emergency physicians' fear of malpractice in evaluating patients with possible acute cardiac ischemia. *Annals of Emergency Medicine, 46*, 525–533.

Keltner, D., & Anderson, C. (2000). Saving face for Darwin: The functions and uses of embarrassment. *Current Directions in Psychological Science, 9*, 187–192.

Keltner, D., & Buswell, B. N. (1996). Evidence for the distinctiveness of embarrassment, shame, and guilt: A study of recalled antecedents and facial expressions of emotion. *Cognition and Emotion, 10*, 155–171.

Keltner, D., & Buswell, B. N. (1997). Embarrassment: Its distinct form and appeasement functions. *Psychological Bulletin, 122*, 250–270.

Klabunde, C. N., Vernon, S. W., Nadel, M. R., Breen, N., Seeff, L. C., & Brown, M. L. (2005). Barriers to colorectal cancer screening: A comparison of reports from primary care physicians and average-risk adults. *Medical Care, 43*, 939–944.

Kunkel, E. J. S., Meyer, B., Daskalakis, C., Cocroft, J., Jennings-Dozier, K., & Meyers, R. E. (2004). Behaviors used by men to protect themselves against prostate cancer. *Cancer Epidemiology Biomarkers and Prevention, 13*, 78–86.

Lazarus, R. S. (1991). *Emotion and adaptation*. New York, NY: Oxford University Press.

Lerman, C., Rimer, B. K., Trock, B., Balshem, A., & Engstrom, P. F. (1990). Factors associated with repeat adherence to breast cancer screening. *Preventive Medicine, 19*, 279–290.

Marks, I. M., & Nesse, R. M. (1994). Fear and fitness—An evolutionary analysis of anxiety disorders. *Ethology and Sociobiology, 15*, 247–261.

McCambridge, S. A., & Consedine, N. S. (2014). For whom the bell tolls: Experimentally-manipulated disgust and embarrassment cause sexual health avoidance among some people. *Emotion, 14*, 407–415.

Menon, U., Champion, V. L., Larkin, G. N., Zollinger, T. W., Gerde, P. M., & Vernon, S. W. (2003). Beliefs associated with fecal occult blood test and colonoscopy use at a worksite colon cancer screening program. *Journal of Occupational and Environmental Medicine, 45*, 891–898.

Merrill, J. M., Laux, L. F., & Thornby, J. I. (1990). Why doctors have difficulty with sex histories. *Southern Medical Journal, 83*, 613–617.

Miller, R. S. (1992). The nature and severity of self-reported embarrassing circumstances. *Personality and Social Psychology Bulletin, 18*, 190–198.

Miller, R. S. (1995). On the nature of embarrassability: Shyness, social evaluation, and social skill. *Journal of Personality, 63*, 315–339.

Myers, R. E., Hyslop, T., Jennings-Dozier, K., Wolf, T. A., Burgh, D. Y., Diehl, J. A., . . . Chodak, G. W. (2000). Intention to be tested for prostate cancer risk among

African-American men. *Cancer Epidemiology Biomarkers and Prevention, 9,* 1323–1328.

Myers, R. E., Hyslop, T., Wolf, T. A., Burgh, D., Kunkel, E. J. S., Oyesanmi, O. A., & Chodak, G. J. (2000). African-American men and intention to adhere to recommended follow-up for an abnormal prostate cancer early detection examination result. *Urology, 55,* 716–720.

Myers, R. E., Wolf, T. A., McKee, L., McGrory, G., Burgh, D. Y., Nelson, G. T., & Nelson, G. A. (1996). Factors associated with intention to undergo annual prostate cancer screening among African American men in Philadelphia. *Cancer, 78,* 471–479.

Nicholson, F. B., & Korman, M. G. (2005). Acceptance of flexible sigmoidoscopy and colonoscopy for screening and surveillance in colorectal cancer prevention. *Journal of Medical Screening, 12,* 89–95.

Oaten, M. J., Stevenson, R. J., & Case, T. I. (2009). Disgust as a disease-avoidance mechanism. *Psychological Bulletin, 135,* 303–321.

O'Carroll, R. E., Chambers, J., Brownlee, L., Libby, G., & Steele, R. (2015). Anticipated regret to increase uptake of colorectal cancer screening (ARTICS): A randomised controlled trial. *Social Science and Medicine, 142,* 118–127.

O'Carroll, R. E., Foster, C., McGeechan, G., Sandford, K., & Ferguson, E. (2011). The "ick" factor, anticipated regret, and willingness to become an organ donor. *Health Psychology, 30,* 236–245.

Olatunji, B. O., Wolitzky-Taylor, K. B., Ciesielski, B. G., Armstrong, T., Etzel, E. N., & David, B. (2009). Fear and disgust processing during repeated exposure to threat-relevant stimuli in spider phobia. *Behaviour Research and Therapy, 47,* 671–679.

Orbell, S. (1996). Cognition and affect after cervical screening: The role of previous test outcome and personal obligation in future uptake expectations. *Social Science and Medicine, 43,* 1237–1243.

Park, J. H., Faulkner, J., & Schaller, M. (2003). Evolved disease-avoidance processes and contemporary anti-social behavior: Prejudicial attitudes and avoidance of people with physical disabilities. *Journal of Nonverbal Behavior, 27,* 65–87.

Peters, E., Lipkus, I., & Diefenbach, M. A. (2006). The functions of affect in health communications and in the construction of health preferences. *Journal of Communication, 56,* S140–S162.

Poon, M.-Y., & Tarrant, M. (2009). Obesity: Attitudes of undergraduate student nurses and registered nurses. *Journal of Clinical Nursing, 18,* 2355–2365.

Rawl, S. M., Champion, V. L., Menon, U., & Skinner, C. S. (2001). Validation of scales to measure beliefs and barriers to colorectal cancer screening: Scale development. *Journal of Psychosocial Oncology, 19,* 47–63.

Reynolds, L. M., Bissett, I. P., & Consedine, N. S. (2015). Predicting the patients that will struggle with anal incontinence: sensitivity to disgust matters. *Colorectal Disease, 17,* 73–80.

Reynolds, L. M., Bissett, I. P., Porter, D., & Consedine, N. S. (2016). The "ick" factor matters: Disgust prospectively predicts avoidance in chemotherapy patients. *Annals of Behavioral Medicine, 935–945,* 1–11. http://link.springer.com/article/10.1007/s12160-016-9820-x

Reynolds, L. M., Consedine, N. S., Pizarro, D. A., & Bissett, I. P. (2013). Disgust and behavioral avoidance in colorectal cancer screening and treatment: A systematic review and research agenda. *Cancer Nursing, 36*, 122–130.

Reynolds, L. M., Lin, Y.-S., Zhou, E., & Consedine, N. S. (2015). Does a state mindfulness induction moderate disgust-driven social avoidance and decision-making? An experimental investigation. *Journal of Behavioral Medicine, 38*, 98–109.

Reynolds, L. M., McCambridge, S. A., Bissett, I. P., & Consedine, N. S. (2014). Trait and state disgust: An experimental investigation of disgust and avoidance in colorectal cancer decision scenarios. *Health Psychology, 33*, 1495–1506.

Rozin, P., & Fallon, A. E. (1987). A perspective on disgust. *Psychological Review, 94*, 23–41.

Rozin, P., Haidt, J., McCauley, C., Dunlop, L., & Ashmore, M. (1999). Individual differences in disgust sensitivity: Comparisons and evaluations of paper-and-pencil versus behavioral measures. *Journal of Research in Personality, 33*, 330–351.

Rozin, P., Haidt, J., & McCauley, C. R. (1999). Disgust: The body and soul emotion. In. T. Dalgleish & M. Power (Eds.), *Handbook of Cognition and Emotion* (pp. 429–445). Chichester, England. John Wiley & Sons.

Rozin, P., Nemeroff, C., Horowitz, M., Gordon, B., & Voet, W. (1995). The borders of the self: Contamination sensitivity and potency of the body apertures and other body parts. *Journal of Research in Personality, 29*, 318–340.

Ruiter, R. A. C., Abraham, C., & Kok, G. (2001). Scary warnings and rational precautions: A review of the psychology of fear appeals. *Psychology and Health, 16*, 613–630.

Sabini, J., Siepmann, M., Stein, J., & Meyerowitz, M. (2000). Who is embarrassed by what? *Cognition and Emotion, 14*, 213–240.

Schaller, M., & Duncan, L. A. (2007). The behavioural immune system: Its evolution and social psychological implications. In J. P. Forgas, M. G. Haselton, & W. von Hippel (Eds.), *Evolution and the social mind: Evolutionary psychology and social cognition* (pp. 293–307). New York, NY: Psychological Press.

Schaller, M., & Park, J. H. (2011). The behavioral immune system (and why it matters). *Current Directions in Psychological Science, 20*, 99–103.

Semin, G. R., & Manstead, A. S. R. (1982). The social implications of embarrassment displays and restitution behaviour. *European Journal of Social Psychology, 12*, 367–377.

Shaw, C., Williams, K., Assassa, P. R., & Jackson, C. (2000). Patient satisfaction with urodynamics: A qualitative study. *Journal of Advanced Nursing, 32*, 1356–1363.

Shelton, P., Weinrich, S., & Reynolds, W. A. (1999). Barriers to prostate cancer screening in African American men. *Journal of the National Black Nurses Association, 10*, 14–28.

Sorum, P. C., Mullet, E., Shim, J., Bonnin-Scaon, S., Chasseigne, G., & Cogneau, J. (2004). Avoidance of anticipated regret: The ordering of prostate-specific antigen tests. *Medical Decision Making, 24*, 149–159.

Spoor, J. R., & Kelly, J. R. (2004). The evolutionary significance of affect in groups: Communication and group bonding. *Group Processes and Intergroup Relations, 7*, 398–412.

Sussner, K. M., Thompson, H. S., Jandorf, L., Edwards, T. A., Forman, A., Brown, K., . . . Valdimarsdottir, H. B. (2009). The influence of acculturation and breast cancer-specific distress on perceived barriers to genetic testing for breast cancer among women of African descent. *Psycho-Oncology, 18*, 945–955.

Van der Schalk, J., Bruder, M., & Manstead, A. (2013). Regulating emotion in the context of interpersonal decisions: The role of anticipated pride and regret. *Frontiers in Psychology, 3*, art. no. 513.

Von Wagner, C., Good, A., Whitaker, K. L., & Wardle, J. (2013). Psychosocial determinants of socioeconomic inequalities in cancer screening participation: A conceptual framework. *Epidemiologic Reviews, 33*, 135–147.

Vrinten, C., Waller, J., Von Wagner, C., & Wardle, J. (2015). Cancer fear: Facilitator and deterrent to participation in colorectal cancer screening. *Cancer Epidemiology Biomarkers and Prevention, 24*, 400–405.

Weinrich, S. P., Weinrich, M. C., Boyd, M. D., & Atkinson, C. (1998). The impact of prostate cancer knowledge on cancer screening. *Oncology Nursing Forum, 25*, 527–534.

Winterich, J. A., Quandt, S. A., Grzywacz, J. G., Clark, P. E., Miller, D. P., Acuna, J., & Arcury, T. A. (2009). Masculinity and the body: How African American and White men experience cancer screening exams involving the rectum. *American Journal of Men's Health, 3*, 300–309.

Witte, K., & Allen, M. (2000). A meta-analysis of fear appeals: Implications for effective public health campaigns. *Health Education and Behavior, 27*, 565–591.

Wong, K. F. E., & Kwong, J. Y. Y. (2007). The role of anticipated regret in escalation of commitment. *Journal of Applied Psychology, 92*, 545–554.

20

Decision Making in Cancer Prevention and Control

Insights from Affective Science

ERIN M. ELLIS AND REBECCA A. FERRER

Each day, individuals make a variety of decisions that guide their behaviors, and they are often unable to articulate the reasoning behind these choices. It often seems that deliberative explanations fail to explain many choices, and that emotionally laden inputs (e.g., imagery, affective evaluations, anecdotes) often overwhelm more calculated, purposeful, or intentional inputs. Emotion is a particularly relevant decision-making input in the context of cancer, where human behavior and decision making plays a central role (Klein, et al., 2014; Willett, 2002), and where emotions permeate decisions about treatment, clinical trial participation, palliative care, and end-of-life (Ferrer, Klein, Lerner, Reyna, & Keltner, 2016; Ferrer & Padgett, 2015; Ferrer, Padgett, & Ellis, 2016; Padgett & Ferrer, 2015). Indeed, cancer is considered to be a disease feared beyond others (Barraclough, 1999; Stanton, Danoff-burg, & Huggins, 2002; Stanton & Snider, 1993), "involving a range of affectively-laden issues such as symptom and pain management; reactions such as anxiety, sadness, and anger; social and family concerns; and existential questions about life and death" (Holland, 2003, p. 253). That cancer is affectively laden can be explained by a variety of mechanisms, including media depictions of cancer that foster uncertainty and related affective reactions (Gottlieb, 2001; Niederdeppe, Fowler, Goldstein, & Pribble, 2010) as well as perceptions that cancer is unpredictable, uncontrollable, and randomly occurring (Hay, Baser, & Weinstein, 2014; Hay, Shuk, Cruz, & Ostroff, 2005).

The role of emotions in general decision making has been studied extensively, and recent advances in affective science[1] have changed our understanding of how humans make decisions. For example, we now know that emotion, often considered a hindrance to decision making, is often necessary for individuals to make choices that are in their own best interest, and to efficiently use their cognitive resources in the decision-making process (e.g., Damasio, 1994; Lerner & Keltner, 2000, 2001; Loewenstein & Lerner, 2003). Taken together, the state of the science suggests that emotions are powerful and have predictable effects on decision making, motivations, and behavior, which are systematically deleterious or beneficial depending on other decision-making inputs, and can therefore be reliably identified and intervened on as appropriate (Lerner, Li, Valdesolo, & Kassam, 2015). Note that the influence of emotion is highly dependent on the decision-making context (Lerner et al., 2015), underscoring the importance of examining emotion's influence on cancer-specific contexts in order to be able to use this knowledge to develop effective interventions to improve cancer decision making and outcomes (Ferrer, Green, & Barrett, 2015).

Academic fields like social and affective neuroscience, marketing, education, and consumer science—as well as industry (e.g., advertising agencies)—have been quick to capitalize on advances in affective science to produce basic knowledge with important real-world implications. For example, in consumer psychology, findings suggest that sadness facilitates reward-seeking behavior, even when delaying reward would result in substantial benefit and when there are real financial stakes (Lerner & Weber, 2013). These findings have largely not been translated to yield parallel advances in cancer control contexts. This research deficit also exists despite knowledge that medical decisions are more affect-rich than financial decisions, which has implications for the processing and use of different types of information in medically relevant decisions (Buechel, Zhang, Morewedge, & Vosgerau, 2014; Luce, Payne, & Bettman, 1999; Pachur, Hertwig, & Wolkewitz, 2014; Rottenstreich & Hsee, 2001). Several recent syntheses have underscored the importance of examining emotions in health-related judgment and decision making (DeSteno, Gross, & Kubzansky, 2013; Ferrer, Klein, et al., 2016; Williams & Evans, 2014), including as it relates to cancer (Ferrer, Green, et al., 2015). Fundamental knowledge regarding how affect influences cancer-related decision making could be leveraged to develop interventions to optimize decisions about treatment, clinical trial participation, and palliative care among cancer patients and survivors, thereby improving cancer-related outcomes (Ferrer, Green, et al., 2015).

A cancer diagnosis introduces the need to make countless high-stakes decisions that are affectively laden themselves and occur within affectively laden environments. These decisions include single-event decisions (e.g., whether to have a lumpectomy or mastectomy, what chemotherapy regimen to begin; whether to enroll in clinical trial studies); sequential decisions (e.g., moving from first-line chemotherapy to second-line when first-line is ineffective; integrating palliative care into a treatment plan to augment or in lieu of curative treatment); and adherence/maintenance decisions (e.g., adhering to a self-administered oral chemotherapy or hormone therapy regimen; attending multiple medical chemotherapy or radiation administration sessions). In what follows, we outline some specific ways in which affect/emotion influences these and other decisions faced by cancer patients, and how emotions are relevant to the interpersonal context in which these decisions occur.

PATIENT DECISION MAKING

What Treatment Should I Choose?

Cancer treatment decisions often take place at critical transitions in care that are likely to elicit emotional responses from patients, such as immediately after diagnosis with cancer or when previously selected treatment options have failed or stopped working. The many emotions that patients (as well as physicians and loved ones/informal caregivers) experience at the time of the decision, including anger, sadness, fear, and hope, are likely to influence treatment decision making. Each of these discrete emotions (i.e., feeling states that differ on dimensions beyond simply positive/negative valence) is characterized by cognitive tendencies or appraisal dimensions (Smith & Ellsworth, 1985) as well as core appraisal themes or mental schemas (Lazarus, 1991), which can trigger emotion-specific action tendencies (Frijda, 1986) that shape predictable patterns of judgment, decision making, and behavior (Han, Lerner, & Keltner, 2007; Lerner & Keltner, 2000, 2001).

For instance, anger is associated with cognitive appraisals of certainty and control and a core appraisal theme of being transgressed against, all of which trigger action tendencies associated with active attempts to rectify the situation. Consequently, anger is associated with optimistic risk perceptions and greater risk-taking, particularly among men (Ferrer, Maclay, Litvak, & Lerner, 2017; Lerner & Keltner, 2001), as well as more implemental/ action-oriented mindsets (Maglio, Gollwitzer, & Oettingen, 2013). Although the role of anger in cancer treatment decisions remains largely unexplored, theory and research in other domains suggests that anger would lead to a riskier course of action. This may mean that anger could lead to perceptions that a given treatment is likely to be effective (i.e., optimistic risk perceptions), and motivate greater acceptance of more experimental treatment options (i.e., greater risk-taking). Anger can also reduce or reverse the reliance on defaults (Garg, Inman, Mittal, 2005), which may mean that cancer patients are more likely to deviate from status quo treatments, resulting in either more positive or negative outcomes, depending on the known effectiveness of the status quo treatment.

Conversely, fear is associated with low certainty and control and a core appraisal theme of existential threat, which triggers action tendencies associated with avoiding or mitigating the threat (Lerner et al., 2015). As such, fear triggers pessimistic risk perceptions, leading to risk-averse choices (Lerner & Keltner, 2000, 2001), and promotes a more deliberative information-processing mindset (Maglio et al., 2013). In cancer treatment decision making, this may translate to more pessimistic risk perceptions regarding whether a treatment will be effective, and less willingness to accept experimental treatment options. However, because of the core appraisal theme of existential threat, fear may also motivate willingness to try any therapy with promise of extending life, and thus contribute to decisions to accept third- and fourth-line therapies that are unlikely to be effective. Indeed, patients experiencing exaggerated hope (as well as fear) may decide to pursue treatments with low likelihood of efficacy (Aronowitz, 2010). Additional research is necessary to examine these competing hypotheses.

Discrete emotions may also influence cancer treatment decision making through their effects on risk perceptions related to side effects. Treatment decisions often involve the understanding and weighing of complex risk or probability estimates, related not only to likelihood of therapeutic benefit but also to risk for side effects or increasing risk for comorbid conditions. Emotions can influence the interpretation of numeric probability information (Peters, Dieckmann, Västfjäll, Mertz, Slovic, & Hibbard, 2009), perceived risk (Peters, Lipkus, & Diefenbach, 2006), and the weight given to affectively laden potential outcomes, including death, cancer recurrence, and immediately experienced side effects that increase risk for comorbid infection (e.g., immunocompromisation; Collins et al., 2011; Earle & Deevy, 2013; Hurria et al., 2011; Monsuez, Charniot, Vignat, & Artigou, 2010; Vanneman & Dranoff, 2012). Many patients express a particularly strong desire to avoid side effects. "Side effect aversion" is a prominent example of how emotional reactions to a potential threat can override objective estimates of risk and probability and lead to a decision that relies almost exclusively on one's affective reactions (e.g., Waters, Weinstein, Colditz, & Emmons, 2007a, 2007b, 2009). Such tendencies may be exacerbated by temporal discounting, in which the short-term avoidance of side effects is valued or prioritized over health benefits that take longer to be realized (Chapman, 1996; Chapman & Elstein, 1995; Critchfield & Kollins, 2001).

In addition to their main effects on cancer decisions or components of the decision-making process, discrete emotions may also interact in complex ways with other decision-making factors, including message framing, (i.e., whether a treatment's benefit is communicated in terms of benefit to the patient—gain-framed—or risk to the patient—loss-framed). For instance, whether an oncologist presents prognostic information in terms of survival estimates or mortality risks has been shown to influence patients' preference for a hypothetical toxic cancer treatment (O'Connor, Boyd, Tritchler, Kriukov, Sutherland, & Till, 1985). These framing effects may interact with emotional state to either augment or amplify their effects on decision making. For instance, research in other domains suggests that emotion can modify ways in which individuals respond to material presented, such that framed messages matched to affect (e.g., positive affective state matched with gain-framed messages) are most persuasive (DeSteno, Petty, Rucker, Wegener, & Braverman, 2004; Keller, Lipkus, & Rimer, 2003; Wegener, Petty, & Klein, 1994). Emotions may also interact with goal salience to shift attentional focus, preferences, and decisions (Reyna, 2008, 2012). Empirical evidence from cancer and other health domains also suggest that emotions, such as worry about getting cancer, may either interact with (see Ferrer & Klein, 2015) or mediate (Kiviniemi & Ellis, 2014) the relations between objective risk estimates and preventive behaviors. Knowledge of how emotions interact with factors, such as message framing or perceived risk, may improve our ability to leverage emotions as a means of improving the effectiveness of interventions targeting these other constructs to improve treatment decisions (DeSteno et al., 2004; Keller et al., 2003; Wegener et al., 1994).

Not only does the affect/emotion experienced at the time of the decision influence cancer treatment decision making but also how people anticipate or forecast they will feel following a decision or engaging in a behavior is important (Connolly & Reb, 2005). In particular, people tend to be poor forecasters of their future emotions and ability to cope with adversity. In fact, there is a systematic tendency to underestimate one's ability to cope and to overestimate the severity and duration of the negative emotions that will ensue. These inaccuracies can undermine cancer-related decision-making. For example, people anticipate the experience of fasting and using a laxative prior to a colonoscopy will be worse than it actually is, and that the procedure will be more disgusting than it actually is, which deters adherence to colorectal cancer screening guidelines (Dillard, Fagerlin, Cin, Zikmund-Fisher, & Ubel, 2010; Kiviniemi, Jandorf, & Erwin, 2014). Efforts to improve the accuracy of these and related forecasts have resulted in greater screening uptake (Dillard et al., 2010; Ferrer, Klein, Zajac, Land, & Ling, 2012) and genetic testing for cancer risk factors (Diefenbach et al., 2008). Intervening to improve forecasting abilities remains a promising intervention target in the context of cancer prevention and treatment. For instance, individuals could be asked to "pre-live" their emotional states following a treatment decision in order to improve the accuracy of their forecasts (see Ferrer et al., 2012). Similarly, asking patients to express their fears regarding treatment can lead to more informed and accurate decision making (Catania et al., 2013). As we discuss later, palliative care may be a particularly important context in which to target and improve affective forecasting.

Following a treatment decision, patients' emotions may influence their adherence to treatment recommendations. For instance, meta-analytic evidence suggests that clinical levels of negative affect (e.g., anxiety, depression) can lead to suboptimal adherence to self-administered chemotherapy regimens (DiMatteo, Lepper, & Croghan, 2000). However, nonclinical negative affect can also be functional and motivate goal-pursuit; thus, research should examine whether there are "optimal" levels or types of negative affect that may facilitate treatment adherence. For example, worry about or fear of cancer may actually motivate medication adherence rather than deter it (see Leventhal, Diefenbach, & Leventhal, 1992). Indeed, research suggests that worry about recurrence is associated with treatment initiation decisions (Friese et al., 2013). Moreover, little is known about how positive affective associations may motivate treatment adherence, although research suggests that attaching positive affect to diagnosis may result in greater intentions to adhere to treatment recommendations (Schuettler & Kiviniemi, 2006).

Should I Enroll in a Clinical Trial?

Clinical trials are necessary to assess the efficacy and safety of cancer treatments. Despite this, enrollment of patients in cancer clinical trials is suboptimal (Collyar, 2000; Cox & McGarry, 2003). The decision whether to enroll in a clinical trial for a new cancer drug is affectively laden for a number of reasons (Mellon, Kershaw, Northouse, & Freeman-Gibb, 2007; Mullens, McCaul, Erickson, & Sandgren, 2004; Stanton & Snider, 1993). Often these trials are offered following a series of ineffective courses of treatment when alternative options are limited and prognosis is grim. Fear of treatment side effects and ineffectiveness is mixed with hope for new-found treatment efficacy (e.g., Daugherty et al., 1995; Jansen et al., 2011; Penman et al., 1984; Rodenhuis et al., 1984), and these conflicting emotions permeate the decision-making process. Moreover, these trials are aimed at increasing the scientific knowledge about the treatment's efficacy, and while the patient may experience direct benefits, there are no guarantees (Jansen et al., 2011). The uncertainty surrounding possible but not guaranteed benefits, elicits its own set of emotions. Indeed, patients may be reluctant to enroll in clinical trials because they are anxious about side effects or the uncertain benefit of the treatment (Cox & McGarry, 2003; Cox & Avis, 1996; Kelly, Ghazi, & Caldwell, 2002; Quinn et al., 2012), or because they are fearful that enrolling in a clinical trial reflects or implies that they have no hope for improvement on traditional therapies (Catania et al., 2013). Positive affective evaluations that a therapy is likely to be effective, conversely, are associated with greater trial participation (Yang et al., 2010).

Enrollment in a clinical trial begins by administering a potentially complicated and extensive informed consent process (Brody, McCullough, & Sharp, 2005). Reflective of the complexity of the information, patients often misunderstand facets of what their participation involves (Leroy, Christophe, Penel, Clisan, & Antoine, 2011), or even mistakenly hold the belief that the treatment will certainly benefit them or that they are more likely to benefit than other trial volunteers (Appelbaum, Lidz, & Grisso, 2004; Bergenmar, Johansson, & Wilking, 2011; Bergenmar, Molin,

Wilking, & Brandberg, 2008; Daugherty et al., 1995; Jansen et al., 2011). Patients' current emotional state may serve to facilitate (or aid in) the accurate interpretation and use of this information. For instance, when patients are provided with information about trials for which they are eligible, their current emotions can influence visual attention to different pieces of information, the depth of processing about the information (systematic versus heuristic), and the ability to accurately recall information (Chaiken & Eagly, 1989; Lerner & Tiedens, 2006; Angie, Connelly, Waples, & Kligyte, 2011; Han et al., 2007). These differences can improve or degrade informed consent for and enrollment in clinical trials (Ferrer, Klein, et al., 2016). For example, one study found that individuals in a fearful state engaged in more systematic information processing (assessed via fixations to the informed consent document) than those in an anger state, and that fear was associated with less willingness to participate in a hypothetical trial (Ferrer, Stanley, et al., 2016). Future work should examine whether affective influences can be leveraged to aid patients in their comprehension of clinical trial informed consent, increase enrollment in trials, improve understanding of risks and benefits of trial participation (conveyed via informed consent documentation), or align patients' decisions with their broader preferences and values.

Should I Receive Palliative Care?

Palliative care is defined as any treatment that is intended to provide relief from the symptoms and stress of a serious illness by providing an extra layer of support for both patients and families (Center to Advance Palliative Care [CAPC]). For patients coping with the symptoms and side effects of cancer treatment, palliative care can include the management of pain (Badr Naga, Al-atiyyat, & Kassab, 2013), peripheral neuropathy (Delanian, Lefaix, & Pradat, 2012), nausea and vomiting (Grunberg et al., 2004), hot flashes and night sweats (Carpenter et al., 1998; Couzi, Helzlsouer, & Fetting, 1995), fatigue (Horneber, Fischer, Dimeo, Rüffer, & Weis, 2012), sleep disturbance (Davidson, MacLean, Brundage, & Schulze,

2002), cognitive impairment (Ahles & Saykin, 2002; Nelson & Suls, 2013; Wefel, Saleeba, Buzdar, & Meyers, 2010), and clinical affect (e.g., depression/anxiety/distress; Ng, Boks, Zainal, & de Wit, 2011; Vahdaninia, Omidvari, & Montazeri, 2010). Palliative care is often erroneously equated with hospice or end-of-life care, but it can be administered in conjunction with curative care and has positive effects on quality of life, prognosis (Bakitas et al., 2015; El-Jawahri, Greer, & Temel, 2011; Temel et al., 2010), healthcare costs (Teno, Freedman, Kasper, Gozalo, & Mor, 2015), and caregiver outcomes (Dionne-Odom et al., 2015; El-Jawahri et al., 2011). Despite evidence that palliative care does not interfere with curative care nor increase mortality risk (Novak, Nemeth, & Lawson, 2004; Temel et al., 2010), research suggests that palliative care is desperately underused. There are many ways in which affect and emotion influence and may undermine the complex series of decisions and social transactions needed to effectively implement palliative care (Ferrer, Padgett, et al., 2016; Padgett & Ferrer, 2015).

As already mentioned, the term "palliative care" is often portrayed in the context of end-of-life care, so even prior to any direct experience with it, the term itself elicits an emotional reaction that can deter thoughtful consideration of its benefits by both patients and doctors (Mellon et al., 2007; Mullens et al., 2004; Stanton & Snider, 1993). These affective associations may be particularly consequential, given that research in other domains suggests that individuals are more likely to engage in behaviors with which they have positive feelings or affective associations (Kiviniemi & Bevins, 2007; Ellis, Homish, Parks, Collins, & Kiviniemi, 2015; Ellis, Kiviniemi, & Cook-Cottone, 2014). In addition, patients and physicians have emotional or affective reactions to the uncertainty surrounding a patient's prognosis, which can influence palliative care decision making (Christakis & Lamont, 2000; Parkes, 2000; Smith, 2000).

Emotions are also important in the palliative care context because of their relevance to goal-pursuit. Patients and their doctors may (inaccurately) perceive palliative care and curative goals as conflicting rather than complementary (Gawande, 2014). Patients may fear that expressing a desire for palliative care will cause their physician to abandon goals of a cure (Cohen et al., 2008), and physicians may likewise fear that a palliative care recommendation will be viewed by the patient as a loss of hope and progress toward curative goals (Center to Advance Palliative Care [CAPC], 2011; Gawande, 2014; Keating et al., 2010). In addition to these conflicting goals, palliative care also involves a shift from an achievement focus (i.e., curing cancer) to a relationship focus (i.e., optimizing time with loved ones at end-of-life; Carstensen, Isaacowitz, & Charles, 1999). This may coincide with a greater reliance on affective processing that occurs later in life and illness (Peters, Diefenbach, Hess, & Vastfjall, 2008; Peters, Hess, Vastfjall, & Autman, 2007). Taken together, these shifts in goal pursuit and reliance on affective processing have implications for palliative care decision making, given that emotions motivate goal-fulfillment (Keltner & Gross, 1999). Emotions may be an important factor shaping the salience of different goals and facilitating shifts between goals throughout treatment. For instance, some emotions, such as sadness, are associated with more reward-seeking behavior than others, such as anxiety (Raghunathan & Pham, 1999), happiness (Chuang & Lin, 2007; Ifcher & Zarghamee, 2015), and disgust (Cryder, Lerner, Gross, & Dahl, 2008; Han, Lerner, & Zeckhauser, 2010; Lerner, Small, & Loewenstein, 2004; Lerner, Li, & Weber, 2013). Thus, sadness may lead to the pursuit of either curative or palliative care goals depending on which have the greatest potential to change one's situation. Future work is needed to more fully elucidate the role of affect and emotion when a patient's own goals are conflicting, and when they conflict with the goals of the doctor and/or family members.

Future Directions

Incidental Versus Integral Affect

Historically, discrete emotions have been delineated as either integral or incidental (e.g., Lerner et al., 2015; Loewenstein & Lerner, 2003; Williams & Evans, 2014). Integral affect is normatively relevant to the decision at hand, whereas incidental affect is normatively not relevant but has been shown to influence the decision nonetheless (e.g., Lerner & Keltner, 2000;

2001; Lerner & Tiedens, 2006). For example, anxiety about the side effects of a cancer treatment is an integral emotion—elicited by the treatment decision at hand—that may lead to a decision to avoid that treatment option. Anxiety about an upcoming job interview may likewise influence this treatment decision, despite being elicited outside the cancer treatment decision-making context and normatively irrelevant to the decision (see Ferrer, Klein, et al., 2016).

Importantly, most experimental evidence of the role of affect and emotions in decision making has relied on a manipulation of *incidental* affect because it provides greater experimental control and rigor. Integral and incidental affect are assumed to behave similarly, thus allowing these findings to be generalized to integral affect as well (e.g., Ferrer, Klein, et al., 2016; Persky, Ferrer, & Klein, 2016). However, this remains a largely untested hypothesis and there is some evidence to suggest that the effects of integral affect may have different, more complex, or stronger effects compared to incidental affect (Lerner, Han, & Keltner, 2007). For example, health communications may elicit fear about a consequence of a risky behavior, and to the extent that people react defensively, it may actually increase engagement in the risky behavior (de Hoog, Stroebe, & de Wit, 2007). Alternatively, worry about a consequence of a behavior has also been shown to predict health-protective behaviors (Kiviniemi & Ellis, 2014). In other words, very similar integral emotions (fear and worry) have been shown to have very different effects on behavioral risk factors for cancer. Future research is needed to more systematically examine whether integral and incidental affect do indeed generate similar patterns of influence, particularly within the cancer treatment domain (e.g., Han et al., 2007).

Complex or Blended Emotions

Future work is also needed to better understand the way in which affect influences cancer treatment decision making when the emotions are more complex. Many complex emotions contribute to affective experiences at any given time (e.g., Wilson & Gilbert, 2003), and patients' emotions may conflict (e.g., feeling hopeful and scared) and evolve over time from diagnosis through treatment and beyond. Indeed, feeling complex emotions such as hope and fear may trigger decisions to pursue treatments with little chance of success (Aronowitz, 2010). Particularly in palliative care, patients and doctors may be experiencing a complex blend of emotions, such as anger and sadness, as well as peace, hope, and comfort, and these emotions may be in direct conflict at times (Peters et al., 2004). These conflicting affective states may influence behavior concurrently or interactively (Lerner & Tiedens, 2006). However, laboratory research inducing blended emotional states has been largely unsuccessful (Winterich, Han, & Lerner, 2010), and little is known about how blended or conflicting emotional states influence cancer-related decisions (Ferrer, Klein, et al., 2016). For instance, when do discrete emotions matter, and when is it the arousal or valence of the emotion that is driving its effect on decision making (Gross & Feldman Barrett, 2011; Larsen, McGraw, Mellers, & Cacioppo, 2004)?

Risk Tradeoffs

Although research has examined how individuals navigate decisions that involve tradeoffs between therapeutic benefit and risk of side effects, little work has examined how such tradeoff decisions are made when a particular treatment increases the risk of another disease. For example, and as previously stated, some cancer therapies weaken the immune system and as such increase risk for opportunistic or secondary infections. As these examples illustrate, few medical decisions are equivocally good or bad, but rather, reflect complex tradeoffs of both costs and benefits. Research suggests that these types of medical tradeoffs may be more affectively laden than other risky tradeoffs, such as those involving monetary loss (Chapman, 1996; Suter, Pachur, & Hertwig, 2015). More work is needed to fully understand the scope of affective influences in these continually evolving affect-rich high-stakes medical decisions (Cavanaugh, Bettman, Luce, & Payne, 2007; Lerner et al., 2007). For instance, features of these medical trade-off decisions may interact with incidental emotion to influence decision making (Cavanaugh et al., 2007).

Positive Emotions

Another area for future work involves the role of positive emotions (Fredrickson & Branigan, 2005; Fredrickson, Tugade, Waugh, & Larkin, 2003; Moskowitz, 2003). Research suggests that positive emotions can bolster resilience (Fredrickson et al., 2003), including to traumatic or stressful experiences such as diagnosis of metastatic or advanced cancer (Algoe & Stanton, 2012; Stanton, Danoff-burg, & Huggins, 2002). However, little is known about how positive emotions influence decision making in the cancer context, including related to cancer treatments. In other domains, positive emotion can influence choices where a tradeoff is involved. Positive emotion also facilitates broader attentional scope (Fredrickson & Branigan, 2005) and more efficient decision-making, especially when choosing between several options (Isen & Means, 1983). Thus, it is possible that positive emotions may facilitate more informed and effective decision making surrounding treatment choices and other decisions faced by cancer patients and their physicians (Ferrer, Padgett, et al., 2016). Positive emotions, perhaps via their influence on resilience, may also allow individuals to shift their goals and preferences to be more in line with their prognosis. For example, individuals may be better able to focus on relationship goals in the context of poor prognosis (see Carstensen, Isaacowitz, & Charles, 1999), thus facilitating decisions to avoid overly aggressive treatment in favor of quality of life.

BEYOND THE PATIENT

As alluded to in the prior section, cancer treatment decisions are not made by individuals in isolation. Decisions are contextualized within families and patient–provider interactions where emotions are shared, transmitted, interpreted, masked, and possibly conflicting. Patients may have competing treatment goals for which they may have very different affective associations, and these goals may also be in conflict with their doctors' and loved ones' goals. The interpersonal transmission of emotion and mood states between individuals may also influence the discrete emotions experienced at the time of the decision (De Vignemont & Singer, 2006; Parkinson & Simons, 2009). This underscores the importance of extending our understanding of blended and complex emotions, as well as the interindividual perception, disclosure, coregulation, and transmission of emotions in cancer treatment contexts.

Informal Caregivers

Caregivers of cancer patients may have different emotional needs and feelings about treatment options than patients, particularly as prognosis worsens and end-of-life draws near (Clayton, Hancock, Butow, Tattersall, & Currow, 2007; Hoerger et al., 2013). For instance, compared to the patients themselves, caregivers often report more guilt and anxiety over giving up on loved ones when moving from curative to hospice care (Keating et al., 2010). Caregivers responsible for clinical decisions report greater feelings of depression and dejection when they make these decisions while actively thinking about their loved ones (Barnato & Arnold, 2013). Future work is needed to more fully understand how decisions are made when patients' feelings do not align with those of their loved ones. For example, if a patient is fearful and her caretaker is angry, which emotion drives decisions?

Caregivers are also important as an opportunity for emotional disclosure, (co)regulation, and coping. Studies suggest that cancer patients who engage in emotional disclosure conversations with their spouses report better adjustment and well-being (Robbins, Lopez, Weihs, & Mehl, 2014), and social proximity improves health outcomes, particularly through the social regulation of emotions (Beckes & Coan, 2011). Caregivers also play a role in the coregulation of emotions with patients. Coregulation facilitates emotional stability by creating a system whereby partners can dynamically adjust to changes in arousal and dampening in order to maintain an optimal emotional state (Butler et al., 2003; Butler & Gross, 2009). For instance, romantic partners can regulate each other's worrying through calming and alerting attempts (Parkinson, Simons, & Niven, 2016). Given the psychosocial toll that a cancer diagnosis takes on both the patient and caregivers (Dionne-Odom et al., 2015), effective coregulation of emotions may be particularly important throughout the diagnosis and treatment process.

Healthcare Providers

Treatment decisions require buy-in from all levels of healthcare personnel (Clayton et al., 2007; Hoerger et al., 2013; Parker et al., 2007; see also chapter 18 in this volume), but little is known about how emotion influences the decision making of doctors and other experts (Ferrer, Green, et al., 2015; Ferrer, Klein, et al., 2016). We know that affect can influence problem-solving in medical practice (Estrada, Isen, & Young, 1994), and that experts are vulnerable to decision bias (Reyna, Chick, Corbin, & Hsia, 2014), but our understanding of emotions' effects on decision making of experts in real-world contexts remains limited.

Providers' emotions are particularly important in the palliative care context. Doctors may be reluctant to recommend palliative care because it threatens their medical identity, particularly when it is administered in lieu of curative treatment (CAPC, 2011; Gawande, 2014; Keating et al., 2010). Doctors also dread giving bad news (Fallowfield & Jenkins, 2004; Mitchell, 2007; Panagopoulou, Mintziori, Montgomery, Kapoukranidou, & Benos, 2008) and worry it will deprive patients of hope (McCahill, et al., 2003). According to the appraisal tendency framework (Lerner & Keltner, 2001), these emotions may influence a physician's ability to empathize with her/his patient. For instance, feeling guilt should enhance empathy, whereas shame should attenuate it (Ferrer, Klein, et al., 2016). Providers may also have difficulty understanding or anticipating that patients may value palliative and curative goals equally (Fried et al., 2002), owed in part to the interpersonal hot-cold empathy gap (Loewenstein, 2005). Closing the interpersonal hot-cold empathy gap could facilitate some perspective-taking and allow physicians to better calibrate preferences, shifting to palliative goals for care when necessary (see Kim, Kaplowitz, & Johnston, 2004).

Although research on clinician decision making is in early stages, several preliminary studies suggest that there are many ways in which affect/emotion may influence a doctor's treatment recommendations and patient interactions. For instance, oncologists' negative affect is associated with patient outcomes, such that clinicians who report greater trait-level negative affect have more patients who also report negative affective outcomes, including clinical depression (Pirl et al., 2015). On the other hand, patients are more likely to comply with a physician's treatment recommendations when she/he is perceived as compassionate (Kim et al., 2004). Moreover, physician tolerance of uncertainty has been associated with physician decision making, such that physicians with less tolerance for uncertainty are more likely to endorse paternalistic recommendations for patients (Portnoy et al., 2013). Moreover, anger is known to reduce trust (Dunn & Schweitzer, 2005), so angry patients may have less trust or confidence in the treatment recommendations of their doctors. The detrimental effects of anger on trust and the patient–provider relationship may be exacerbated by providers' tendency, however unintentional, to attribute blame or stigma to the patient (e.g., blaming a patient for her/his cancer because she/he smoked, was obese, and so forth; Cegala & Broz, 2003), particularly among minority patients (Persky et al., 2016). Taken together, these studies provide preliminary support for how treatment decisions are influenced by physicians' current emotions (Gawande, 2014; Ofri, 2014), although many of these theoretical and anecdotal claims have not been examined systematically or empirically.

Future Directions

Goals for Care

While there are many models of shared decision making in medical contexts (Kon, 2010), few explicitly integrate the role of emotions as an important factor that may facilitate or undermine shared decision making goals.

Future work is needed to understand the interplay between patients' and providers' feelings about treatment and palliative care as it relates to their goals for care, as well as how these emotions are coregulated, transferred, and interpreted in a clinical setting. For instance, people are quite able to notice the discrete emotions communicated by others (Frijda, 1986), and patients may try to use their oncologists' or caregivers' emotional expressions as evidence or information to help them arrive at a treatment-related decision (e.g., van Kleef, 2010). Extending our understanding of how others' emotions influence decision making can help inform efforts to leverage emotions in interventions in order to facilitate desired decisional outcomes.

Emotional Communication

Most social psychological research on affect and emotion focuses on intraindividual processes, but emotions occur within a social context and as a social process (e.g., Parkinson & Simons, 2009). For example, emotion suppression is a relatively common regulatory technique that involves purposely containing one's emotional reaction or expression in a social context (Gross & John, 2003). Suppression has negative consequences for social relationships (Butler & Gross, 2004; Gross, 2002; Gross & John, 2003; John & Gross, 2004), which may influence cancer-related decisions. For example, one study found that individuals who tend to suppress emotional displays from others are less likely to enroll in clinical trials (Leroy et al., 2011), possibly because suppression disrupts the rapport between patients and their physicians (see Richards, Butler, & Gross, 2003). Research suggests that clinical trials are more likely to be offered when the patient–provider interactions are characterized by higher levels of trust and mutual positive regard (Albrecht et al., 2008). Both of these may be inhibited by emotion suppression, thus reducing the likelihood that physicians will provide a clinical trial recommendation.

Research in other domains suggests that suppression leads to lower levels of rapport and affiliation (Richards et al., 2003; Tackman & Srivastava, 2016) and decreased social support and social connection (English, John, Srivastava, & Gross, 2012; Labott, Martin, Eason, & Berkey, 1991;

Srivastava et al., 2009). While each of these consequences is conceptually relevant to patient, caregiver, and clinician decision making, more work is needed to examine the consequences of emotion suppression within the context of patients' relationships with informal caregivers and their clinicians. Moreover, future work is needed to fully elucidate the ways in which the regulation, expression, and transmission of emotion influences cancer treatment decision making.

Emotion Coregulation

The coregulation of emotions and emotional states within dyads or social groups is also an important area warranting future research, particularly when these emotions are mixed or conflicting. These coregulation efforts may be enacted in order to improve one's own mood (e.g., seeking consolation from others when feeling sad or anxious), or to change another person's emotions (e.g., trying to stop a loved one from feeling anxious). More work is needed to understand how caregivers and patients coregulate each other's emotions, and whether patients and their physicians also engage in emotion coregulation. For example, many breast cancer patients who are offered the opportunity to take part in clinical trials have unexpressed fears, which can lead them to deny participation. When a clinician discusses fears with patients, patients report greater deliberative engagement in the decision-making process (Catania et al., 2013). Relatedly, research suggests that an oncologist's empathy improves patient-reported outcomes, such as distress (Lelorain et al., 2012), but more work is needed to elucidate the mechanisms driving these effects.

CONCLUSION

Given the importance of emotion in cancer contexts and cancer-related decisions, it is critically important to facilitate research on emotion and decision making in this context (Ferrer, Green, et al., 2015). Emotions are important inputs into decisions about treatment, clinical trial participation, palliative care, and end-of-life (Ferrer, Klein, et al., 2016; Ferrer

& Padgett, 2015; Ferrer, Padgett, et al., 2016; Padgett & Ferrer, 2015). Moreover, cancer is a uniquely affectively laden context, given that it is perceived to be unpredictable, uncontrollable, and randomly occurring, producing sadness, anger, fear, hope, and other complex emotions among patients, informal caregivers, and clinicians (Barraclough, 1999; Gottleib, 2001; Hay et al., 2005; Hay et al., 2014; Holland, 2003; Niederdeppe et al., 2010; Stanton, Danoff-burg, & Huggins, 2002; Stanton & Snider, 1993). Emotion has powerful influences on decision making that can be deleterious or advantageous depending on the context (Lerner et al., 2015), further underscoring the need for research situated firmly in cancer contexts. This work would help to elucidate the specific mechanisms through which emotions influence decision making, thereby informing more strategic, tailored, and effective interventions aimed at improving the decision making and health outcomes of cancer patients.

NOTE

1. *Affective science* refers to the scientific study of emotions, such as fear, anger, or happiness, as well as other types of affective states, such as positive and negative mood. *Emotion* refers to a relatively brief affective reaction to a specific person, situation, or sensory stimulus. Generally, emotion is considered to be different from other affective states (e.g., mood, stress) in that it is (1) relatively fleeting, and (2) directed at specific targets.

REFERENCES

Ahles, T. A., & Saykin, A. J. (2002). Breast cancer chemotherapy-related cognitive dysfunction. *Clinical Breast Cancer, 3*, S84–S90.

Albrecht, T. L., Eggly, S. S., Gleason, M. E., Harper, F. W., Foster, T. S., Peterson, A. M., & Ruckdeschel, J. C. (2008). Influence of clinical communication on patients' decision making on participation in clinical trials. *Journal of Clinical Oncology, 26*, 2666–2673.

Algoe, S. B., & Stanton, A. L. (2012). Gratitude when it is needed most: Social functions of gratitude in women with metastatic breast cancer. *Emotion, 12*, 163–168.

Angie, A. D., Connelly, S., Waples, E. P., & Kligyte, V. (2011). The influence of discrete emotions on judgement and decision-making: A meta-analytic review. *Cognition and Emotion, 25*, 1393–1422.

Appelbaum, P. S., Lidz, C. W., & Grisso, T. (2004). Therapeutic Misconception in Clinical Research: Frequency and Risk Factors. *IRB: Ethics & Human Research*, *26*, 1–8.

Aronowitz, R. (2010). Decision making and fear in the midst of life. *Lancet*, *375*, 1430–1431

Badr Naga, B. S. H., Al-Atiyyat, N. M. H., & Kassab, M. I. (2013). Pain experience among patients receiving cancer treatment: A review. *Journal of Palliative Care & Medicine* 3, 1–4.

Bakitas, M. A., Tosteson, T. D., Li, Z., Lyons, K. D., Hull, J. G., Li, Z., . . . Azuero, A. (2015). Early versus delayed initiation of concurrent palliative oncology care: Patient outcomes in the ENABLE III randomized controlled trial. *Journal of Clinical Oncology*, *33*, 1438–1445.

Barnato, A. E., & Arnold, R. M. (2013). The effect of emotion and physician communication behaviors on surrogates' life-sustaining treatment decisions: A randomized simulation experiment. *Critical Care Medicine*, *41*, 1686–1691

Barraclough, J. (1999). *Cancer and Emotion: A Practical Guide to Psycho-oncology* (3rd Ed.). Oxford, UK: John Wiley & Sons.

Beckes, L., & Coan, J. A. (2011). Social baseline theory: The role of social proximity in emotion and economy of action. *Social and Personality Psychology Compass*, *5*, 976–988.

Bergenmar, M., Johansson, H., & Wilking, N. (2010). Levels of knowledge and perceived understanding among participants in cancer clinical trials—factors related to the informed consent procedure. *Clinical Trials*, *8*, 77–84.

Bergenmar, M., Molin, C., Wilking, N., & Brandberg, Y. (2008). Knowledge and understanding among cancer patients consenting to participate in clinical trials. *European Journal of Cancer*, *44*, 2627–2633.

Brody, B. A., McCullough, L. B., & Sharp, R. R. (2005). Consensus and controversy in clinical research ethics. *JAMA*, *294*, 1411–1414.

Buechel, E. C., Zhang, J., Morewedge, C. K., & Vosgerau, J. (2014). More intense experiences, less intense forecasts: Why affective forecasters overweight probability specifications. *Journal of Personality and Social Psychology*, *106*(1), 20–36.

Butler, E. A., Egloff, B., Wilhelm, F. H., Smith, N. C., Erickson, E. A., & Gross, J. J. (2003). The social consequences of expressive suppression. *Emotion*, *3*, 48–67.

Butler, E. A., & Gross, J. J. (2004). Hiding feelings in social contexts: Out of sight is not out of mind. In P. Philippot & R. S. Feldman (Eds.), *The regulation of emotion* (pp. 101–126). Mahwah, NJ: Taylor & Francis.

Butler, E. A., & Gross, J. J. (2009). Emotion and emotion regulation: Integrating individual and social levels of analysis. *Emotion Review*, *1*, 86–87.

Carpenter, J. S., Andrykowski, M. A., Cordova, M., Cunningham, L., Studts, J., McGrath, P., . . . Munn, R. (1998). Hot flashes in postmenopausal women treated for breast carcinoma. *Cancer*, *82*, 1682–1691.

Carstensen, L. L., Isaacowitz, D. M., & Charles, S. T. (1999). Taking time seriously: A theory of socioemotional selectivity. *American Psychologist*, *54*, 165–181.

Catania, C., Radice, D., Spitaleri, G., Adamoli, L., Noberasco, C., Delmonte, A., . . . De Pas, T. (2013). The choice of whether to participate in a phase I clinical trial: Increasing the awareness of patients with cancer: An exploratory study. *Psycho-Oncology, 23*, 322–329.

Cavanaugh, L. A., Bettman, J. R., Luce, M. F., & Payne, J. W. (2007). Appraising the Appraisal-Tendency Framework. *Journal of Consumer Psychology, 17*, 169–173.

Cegala, D. J., & Broz, S. L. (2003). Provider and patient communication skills training. In T. L. Thompson, A. Dorsey, R. Parrott & K. Miller (Eds.), *The Routledge Handbook of Health Communication* (pp. 95–119). Mahwah, NJ: Lawrence Erlbaum Assoicates.

Center to Advance Palliative Care. (n.d.). *2011 public opinion research on palliative care: A report based on research by Public Opinion Strategies.* Retrieved from https://media.capc.org/filer_public/18/ab/18ab708c-f835-4380-921d-fbf729702e36/2011-public-opinionresearch-on-palliative-care.pdf

Chaiken, S., & Eagly, A. H. (1989). Heuristic and systematic information processing within and beyond the persuasion context. In J. S. Uleman & J. A. Bargh (Eds.), *Unintended thought* (pp. 212–252). New York, NY: Guilford Press.

Chapman, G. B. (1996). Temporal discounting and utility for health and money. *Journal of Experimental Psychology: Learning, Memory, and Cognition, 22*, 771.

Chapman, G. B., & Elstein, A. S. (1995). Valuing the future temporal discounting of health and money. *Medical Decision Making, 15*, 373–386.

Christakis, N. A., & Lamont, E. B. (2000). Extent and determinants of error in doctors' prognoses in terminally ill patients: Prospective cohort study. *BMJ: British Medical Journal, 320*, 469.

Chuang, S. C., & Lin, H. M. (2007). The effect of induced positive and negative emotion and openness-to-feeling in student's consumer decision making. *Journal of Business and Psychology, 22*, 65–78.

Clayton, J. M., Hancock, K. M., Butow, P. N., Tattersall, M. H. N., & Currow, D. C. (2007). Clinical practice guidelines for communicating prognosis and end-of-life issues with adults in the advanced stages of a life-limiting illness, and their caregivers. *Medical Journal of Australia, 186*, S77–S108.

Cohen, E., Botti, M., Hanna, B., Leach, S., Boyd, S., & Robbins, J. (2008). Pain beliefs and pain management of oncology patients. *Cancer Nursing, 31*, E1–E8.

Collins, K. K., Liu, Y., Schootman, M., Aft, R., Yan, Y., Dean, G., & Jeffe, D. B. (2011). Effects of breast cancer surgery and surgical side effects on body image over time. *Breast Cancer Research and Treatment, 126*, 167–176.

Collyar, D. E. (2000). The Value of Clinical Trials from a Patient Perspective. *The Breast Journal, 6*, 310–314.

Connolly, T., & Reb, J. (2005). Regret in cancer-related decisions. *Health Psychology, 24*, S29–S34.

Couzi, R. J., Helzlsouer, K. J., & Fetting, J. H. (1995). Prevalence of menopausal symptoms among women with a history of breast cancer and attitudes toward estrogen replacement therapy. *Journal of Clinical Oncology, 13*, 2737–2744.

Cox, K., & Avis, M. (1996). Psychosocial aspects of participation in early anticancer drug trials: report of a pilot study. *Cancer Nursing, 19*, 177–186.

Cox, K., & McGarry, J. (2003). Why patients don't take part in cancer clinical trials: an overview of the literature. *European Journal of Cancer Care, 12*, 114–122.

Critchfield, T. S., & Kollins, S. H. (2001). Temporal discounting: Basic research and the analysis of socially important behavior. *Journal of Applied Behavior Analysis, 34*(1), 101–122.

Cryder, C. E., Lerner, J. S., Gross, J. J., & Dahl, R. E. (2008). Misery is not miserly: Sad and self-focused individuals spend more. *Psychological Science, 19*, 525–530.

Damasio A. (1994/2003). *Descartes' error: Emotion, rationality, and the human brain.* New York, NY: Putnam.

Daugherty, C., Ratain, M. J., Grochowski, E., Stocking, C., Kodish, E., Mick, R., et al. (1995). Perceptions of cancer patients and their physicians involved in phase I trials. *Journal of Clinical Oncology, 13*, 1062–1072.

Davidson, J. R., MacLean, A. W., Brundage, M. D., & Schulze, K. (2002). Sleep disturbance in cancer patients. *Social Science and Medicine, 54*, 1309–1321.

Delanian, S., Lefaix, J. L., & Pradat, P. F. (2012). Radiation-induced neuropathy in cancer survivors. *Radiotherapy and Oncology, 105*, 273–282.

DeSteno, D., Gross, J. J., & Kubzansky, L. (2013). Affective science and health: The importance of emotion and emotion regulation. *Health Psychology, 32*, 474.

DeSteno, D., Petty, R. E., Rucker, D. D., Wegener, D. T., & Braverman, J. (2004). Discrete emotions and persuasion: The role of emotion-induced expectancies. *Journal of Personality and Social Psychology, 86*, 43–56.

Diefenbach, M. A., Miller, S. M., Porter, M., Peters, E., Stefanek, M., & Leventhal, H. (2008). Emotions and health behavior: A self-regulation perspective. In: M. Lewis, J. M. Haviland-Jones, & L. F. Barrett (Eds.), *Handbook of emotions* (3rd ed., pp. 645–660). New York, NY: Guilford.

Dillard, A. J., Fagerlin, A., Cin, S. D., Zikmund-Fisher, B. J., & Ubel, P. A. (2010). Narratives that address affective forecasting errors reduce perceived barriers to colorectal cancer screening. *Social Science and Medicine, 71*(1), 45–52.

DiMatteo, M. R., Lepper, H. S., & Croghan, T. W. (2000). Depression is a risk factor for noncompliance with medical treatment: Meta-analysis of the effects of anxiety and depression on patient adherence. *Archives of Internal Medicine, 160*, 2101–2107.

Dionne-Odom, J. N., Azuero, A., Lyons, K. D., Hull, J. G., Tosteson, T., Li, Z., . . . Bakitas, M. A. (2015). Benefits of early versus delayed palliative care to informal family caregivers of patients with advanced cancer: Outcomes from the ENABLE III randomized controlled trial. *Journal of Clinical Oncology, 33*, 1446–1452.

Dunn, J. R., & Schweitzer, M. E. (2005). Feeling and believing: The influence of emotion on trust. *Journal of Personality and Social Psychology, 88*, 736.

Earle, C. C., & Deevy, J. (2013). Cancer survivorship: Monitoring the long-term and late effects of treatment. In F. E. Johnson et al. (Eds.), *Patient surveillance after cancer treatment* (pp. 31–37). New York, NY: Humana Press.

El-Jawahri, A., Greer, J. A., & Temel, J. S. (2011). Does palliative care improve outcomes for patients with incurable illness? A review of the evidence. *Journal of Supportive Oncology, 9*, 87–94. http://dx.doi.org/10.1016/j.suponc.2011.03.003

Ellis, E. M., Homish, G. G., Parks, K. A., Collins, R. L., & Kiviniemi, M. T. (2015). Increasing condom use by changing people's feelings about them: An experimental study. *Health Psychology, 34*, 941.

Ellis, E. M., Kiviniemi, M. T., & Cook-Cottone, C. (2014). Implicit affective associations predict snack choice for those with low, but not high levels of eating disorder symptomatology. *Appetite, 77*, 124–132.

English, T., John, O. P., Srivastava, S., & Gross, J. J. (2012). Emotion regulation and peer-rated social functioning: A 4-year longitudinal study. *Journal of Research in Personality, 46*, 780–784.

Estrada, C. A., Isen, A. M., & Young, M. J. (1994). Positive affect improves creative problem solving and influences reported source of practice satisfaction in physicians. *Motivation and Emotion, 18*, 285–299.

Estrada, C. A., Isen, A. M., & Young, M. J. (1997). Positive affect facilitates integration of information and decreases anchoring in reasoning among physicians. *Organizational Behavior and Human Decision Processes, 72*, 117–135.

Fallowfield, L., & Jenkins, V. (2004). Communicating sad, bad, and difficult news in medicine. *Lancet, 363*, 312–319.

Ferrer, R. A., Green, P.A., & Barrett, L. F. (2015). Affective science and cancer control: Towards a mutually beneficial research agenda. *Perspectives on Psychological Science, 10*, 328–345.

Ferrer, R. A., & Klein, W. M. (2015). Risk perceptions and health behavior. *Current Opinion in Psychology, 5*, 85–89.

Ferrer, R. A., Klein, W. M. P., Lerner, J. S., Reyna, V., & Keltner, D. (2016). Emotions and health decision making: Extending the appraisal tendency framework to improve health and health care. In C. Roberto & I. Kawachi (Eds.), *Behavioral Economics and Public Health* (pp. 101–131). New York, NY: Oxford University Press.

Ferrer, R. A., Klein, W. M. P., Zajac, L., Land, S., & Ling, B. (2012). An affective booster moderates the relationship between message frame and behavioral intentions. *Journal of Behavioral Medicine, 4*, 452–461.

Ferrer, R. A., Maclay, A., Litvak, P. M., & Lerner, J. S. (2017). Revisiting the effects of anger on risk-taking: Empirical and meta-analytic evidence for differences between males and females. *Journal of Behavioral Decision Making, 30*, 516–526.

Ferrer, R. A., & Padgett, L. (2015). Leveraging affective science to maximize the effectiveness of palliative care. *Journal of Clinical Oncology*. Epub ahead of print.

Ferrer, R. A., Padgett, L., & Ellis, E. (2016). Extending emotion and decision-making beyond the laboratory: The promise of palliative care contexts. *Emotion*. Epub ahead of print.

Ferrer, R. A., Stanley, J., Graff, K., Goodman, N., Nelson, W., Salazar, S., & Klein, W. M. P. (2016). The influence of emotion on the informed consent process in cancer clinical trials. *Journal of Behavioral Decision-Making, 29*, 245–253.

Fredrickson, B. L., & Branigan, C. (2005). Positive emotions broaden the scope of attention and thought-action repertoires. *Cognition and Emotion, 19*, 313–332.

Fredrickson, B. L., Tugade, M. M., Waugh, C. E., & Larkin, G. R. (2003). What good are positive emotions in crises? A prospective study of resilience and emotions following the terrorist attacks on the United States on September 11th, 2001. *Journal of Personality and Social Psychology, 84*, 365–376.

Fried, T. R., Bradley, E. H., Towle, V. R., & Allore, H. (2002). Understanding the treatment preferences of seriously ill patients. *New England Journal of Medicine, 346*, 1061–1066.

Friese, C. R., Pini, T. M., Li, Y., Abrahamse, P. H., Graff, J. J., Hamilton, A. S., . . . Griggs, J. J. (2013). Adjuvant endocrine therapy initiation and persistence in a diverse sample of patients with breast cancer. *Breast Cancer Research and Treatment, 138*, 931–939.

Frijda, N. H. (1986). *The emotions: Studies in emotion and social interaction*. London, UK: Cambridge University Press.

Garg, N., Inman, J. J., & Mittal, V. (2005). Incidental and Task-Related Affect: A Re-Inquiry and Extension of the Influence of Affect on Choice. *Journal of Consumer Research, 32*, 154–159.

Gawande, A. (2014). *Being mortal: Medicine and what matters in the end*. New York, NY: Metropolitan Books.

Gottlieb, N. (2001). The age of breast cancer awareness: What is the effect of media coverage? *Journal of the National Cancer Institute, 93*, 1520–1522.

Gross, J. J. (2002). Emotion regulation: Affective, cognitive, and social consequences. *Psychophysiology, 39*, 281–291.

Gross, J. J., & Feldman Barrett, L. (2011). Emotion generation and emotion regulation: One or two depends on your point of view. *Emotion Review, 3*, 8–16.

Gross, J. J., & John, O. P. (2003). Individual differences in two emotion regulation processes: Implications for affect, relationships, and well-being. *Journal of Personality and Social Psychology, 85*, 348–362.

Grunberg, S. M., Deuson, R. R., Mavros, P., Geling, O., Hansen, M., Cruciani, G., & Daugaard, G. (2004). Incidence of chemotherapy-induced nausea and emesis after modern antiemetics. *Cancer, 100*, 2261–2668.

Han, S., Lerner, J. S. & Zeckhauser, R. J., Disgust Promotes Disposal: Souring the Status Quo (June 7, 2010). HKS Working Paper No. RWP10-021. Available at http://dx.doi.org/10.2139/ssrn.1624889

Han, P. K. J., Moser, R. P., & Klein, W. M. P. (2007). Perceived ambiguity about cancer prevention recommendations: Associations with cancer-related perceptions and behaviours in a US population survey. *Health Expectations, 10*, 321–336. http://doi.org/10.1111/j.1369-7625.2007.00456.x

Han, S., Lerner, J. S., & Keltner, D. (2007). Feelings and consumer decision making: The appraisal-tendency framework. *Journal of Consumer Psychology, 17*, 158–168.

Hay, J. L., Baser, R., & Weinstein, N. D. (2014). Examining intuitive risk perceptions for cancer in diverse populations. *Health, Risk, and Society, 16*, 227–242.

Hay, J., Shuk, E., Cruz, G., & Ostroff, J. (2005). Thinking through cancer risk: Characterizing smokers' process of risk determination. *Qualitative Health Research, 15*, 1074–1085.

Hoerger, M., Epstein, R. M., Winters, P. C., Fiscella, K., Duberstein, P. R., Gramling, R., . . . Kravitz, R. L. (2013). Values and Options in Cancer Care (VOICE): Study design and rationale for a patient-centered communication and decision-making intervention for physicians, patients with advanced cancer, and their caregivers. *BMC Cancer, 13*, 188.

Horneber, M., Fischer, I., Dimeo, F., Rüffer, J. U., & Weis, J. (2012). Cancer-related fatigue: Epidemiology, pathogenesis, diagnosis, and treatment. *Deutsches Ärzteblatt International, 109*, 161–172

Holland, J. C. (2003). Psychological care of patients: Psycho-oncology's contribution. *Journal of Clinical Oncology, 21*, 253s–265s.

Hoog, N. de, Stroebe, W., & Wit, J. B. de. (2007). The impact of vulnerability to and severity of a health risk on processing and acceptance of fear-arousing communications: A meta-analysis. *Review of General Psychology, 11*, 258–285. doi:10.1037/1089-2680.11.3.258

Hurria, A., Togawa, K., Mohile, S. G., Owusu, C., Klepin, H. D., Gross, C. P., & Tew, W. P. (2011). Predicting chemotherapy toxicity in older adults with cancer: A prospective multicenter study. *Journal of Clinical Oncology, 29*, 3457–3465.

Ifcher, J., & Zarghamee, H. (2016). Pricing competition: a new laboratory measure of gender differences in the willingness to compete. *Experimental Economics, 19*, 642–662.

Isen, A. M., & Means, B. (1983). The influence of positive affect on decision-making strategy. *Social Cognition, 2*, 18–31.

Jansen, L. A., Appelbaum, P. S., Klein, W. M., Weinstein, N. D., Cook, W., Fogel, J. S., & Sulmasy, D. P. (2011). Unrealistic optimism in early-phase oncology trials. *IRB, 33*, 1–8.

John, O. P., & Gross, J. J. (2004). Healthy and Unhealthy Emotion Regulation: Personality Processes, Individual Differences, and Life Span Development. *Journal of Personality, 72*, 1301–1334.

Keating, N. L., Landrum, M. B., Rogers, S. O., Jr., Baum, S. K., Virnig, B. A., Huskamp, H. A., . . . Kahn, K. L. (2010). Physician factors associated with discussions about end-of-life care. *Cancer, 116*, 998–1006.

Keller, P. A., Lipkus, I. M., & Rimer, B. K. (2003). Affect, framing, and persuasion. *Journal of Marketing Research, 40*(1), 54–64. doi:10.1509/jmkr.40.1.54.19133

Kelly, C., Ghazi, F., & Caldwell, K. (2002). Psychological distress of cancer and clinical trial participation: a review of the literature. *European Journal of Cancer Care, 11*, 6–15.

Keltner, D., & Gross, J. J. (1999). Functional accounts of emotions. *Cognition and Emotion, 13*, 467–480.

Kim, S. S., Kaplowitz, S., & Johnston, M. V. (2004). The effects of physician empathy on patient satisfaction and compliance. *Evaluation and the Health Professions, 27*, 237–251.

Kiviniemi, M. T., & Ellis, E. M. (2014). Worry about skin cancer mediates the relation of perceived cancer risk and sunscreen use. *Journal of Behavioral Medicine, 37*, 1069–1074.

Kiviniemi, M. T., Jandorf, L., & Erwin, D. O. (2014). Disgusted, embarrassed, annoyed: Affective associations relate to uptake of colonoscopy screening. *Annals of Behavioral Medicine, 48*(1), 112–119.

Kiviniemi, M. T., & Bevins, R. (2007). Affect-behavior associations in motivated behavioral choice: Potential transdisciplinary links. In P. R. Zelick (Ed.), *Issues in the psychology of motivation* (pp. 65–80). Hauppage, NY: Nova.

Kleef, G. A. van (2014). Understanding the positive and negative effects of emotional expressions in organizations: EASI does it. *Human Relations, 67*, 1145–1164.

Klein, W. M., Bloch, M., Hesse, B. W., McDonald, P. G., Nebeling, L., O'Connell, M. E., . . . Tesauro, G. (2014). Behavioral research in cancer prevention and control: a look to the future. *American Journal of Preventive Medicine, 46*, 303–311.

Kon, A. A. (2010). The shared decision-making continuum. *JAMA, 304*, 903–904.

Labott, S. M., Martin, R. B., Eason, P. S., & Berkey, E. Y. (1991). Social reactions to the expression of emotion. *Cognition and Emotion, 5*, 397–417.

Larsen, J. T., McGraw, A. P., Mellers, B. A., & Cacioppo, J. T. (2004). The agony of victory and thrill of defeat: Mixed emotional reactions to disappointing wins and relieving losses. *Psychological Science, 15*, 325–330.

Lazarus, R. S. (1991). Progress on a cognitive-motivational-relational theory of emotion. *American Psychologist, 46*, 819.

Lelorain, S., Brédart, A., Dolbeault, S., & Sultan, S. (2012). A systematic review of the associations between empathy measures and patient outcomes in cancer care. *Psycho-Oncology, 21*, 1255–1264.

Lerner, J. S., Han, S., & Keltner, D. (2007). Feelings and consumer decision making: Extending the appraisal-tendency framework. *Journal of Consumer Psychology, 17*, 181–187.

Lerner, J. S., & Keltner, D. (2000). Beyond valence: Toward a model of emotion-specific influences on judgement and choice. *Cognition and Emotion,14*, 473–493.

Lerner, J. S., & Keltner, D. (2001). Fear, anger, and risk. *Journal of Personality and Social Psychology, 81*, 146–159.

Lerner, J. S., Li, Y., Valdesolo, P., &Kassam, K. (2015). Emotion and decision making. *Annual Review of Psychology, 66*, 799–823.

Lerner, J. S., Li, Y., & Weber, E. U. (2013). The financial costs of sadness. *Psychological Science, 24*, 72–79.

Lerner, J. S., Small, D. A., & Loewenstein, G. (2004). Heart strings and purse strings carryover effects of emotions on economic decisions. *Psychological Science, 15*, 337–341.

Lerner, J. S., & Tiedens, L. Z. (2006). Portrait of the angry decision maker: How appraisal tendencies shape anger's influence on cognition. *Journal of Behavioral Decision Making, 19*, 115–137. doi:10.1002/bdm.515

Leroy, T., Christophe, V., Penel, N., Clisant, S., & Antoine, P. (2011). Participation in randomized clinical trials is linked to emotion regulation strategies. *Contemporary Clinical Trials, 32*, 32–35.

Leventhal, H., Diefenbach, M., & Leventhal, E. A. (1992). Illness cognition: Using common sense to understand treatment adherence and affect cognition interactions. *Cognitive Therapy and Research, 16*, 143–163.

Loewenstein G. (2005). Hot-cold empathy gaps and medical decision making. *Health Psychology, 24*, S49.

Loewenstein, G., & Lerner, J. S. The role of affect in decision making. In: R. J. Davidson, K. R. Scherer, H. H. Goldsmith (Eds.), *Handbook of affective sciences* (pp. 619–642). New York, NY: Oxford University Press, 2003.

Luce, M. F., Payne, J. W., & Bettman, J. R. (1999). Emotional trade-off difficulty and choice. *Journal of Marketing Research, 36*, 143–159.

Maglio, S., Gollwitzer, P. M., & Oettingen, G. (2013). Action control by implementation intentions. In A. Clark, J. Kiverstein & T. Vierkant (Eds.), *Decomposing the Will* (pp. 221–243). New York, NY: Oxford University Press.

McCahill, L. E., Smith, D. D., Borneman, T., Juarez, G., Cullinane, C., Chu, D. Z., et al. (2003). A prospective evaluation of palliative outcomes for surgery of advanced malignancies. *Annals of Surgical Oncology, 10*, 654–663.

Mellon, S., Kershaw, T. S., Northouse, L. L., & Freeman-Gibb, L. (2007). A family-based model to predict fear of recurrence for cancer survivors and their caregivers. *Psycho-Oncology, 16*, 214–223.

Mitchell, A. J. (2007). Reluctance to disclose difficult diagnoses: a narrative review comparing communication by psychiatrists and oncologists. *Supportive Care in Cancer, 15*, 819–828.

Monsuez, J. J., Charniot, J. C., Vignat, N., & Artigou, J. Y. (2010). Cardiac side-effects of cancer chemotherapy. *International Journal of Cardiology, 144*, 3–15.

Moskowitz, J. T. (2003). Positive Affect Predicts Lower Risk of AIDS Mortality. *Psychosom Med, 65*, 620–626.

Mullens, A. B., McCaul, K. D., Erickson, S. C., & Sandgren, A. K. (2004). Coping after cancer: Risk perceptions, worry, and health behaviors among colorectal cancer survivors. *Psycho-Oncology, 13*, 367–376.

Nelson, W. L., & Suls, J. (2013). New approaches to understand cognitive changes associated with chemotherapy for non-central nervous system tumors. *Journal of Pain and Symptom Management, 46*, 707–721.

Niederdeppe, J., Fowler, E. F., Goldstein, K., & Pribble, J. (2010). Does local television news coverage cultivate fatalistic beliefs about cancer prevention? *Journal of Communication, 60*, 230–253.

Ng, C. G., Boks, M. P., Zainal, N. Z., & de Wit, N. J. (2011). The prevalence and pharmacotherapy of depression in cancer patients. *Journal of Affective Disorders, 131*, 1–7.

Novak, S., Nemeth, W. C., & Lawson, K. A. (2004). Trends in medical use and abuse of sustained-release opioid analgesics: a revisit. *Pain Medicine, 5*(1), 59–65.

O'Connor, A. M. C., Boyd, N. F., Tritchler, D. L., Kriukov, Y., Sutherland, H., & Till, J. E. (1985). Eliciting Preferences for Alternative Cancer Drug Treatments: The Influence of Framing, Medium, and Rater Variables. *Medical Decision Making, 5*, 453–463.

Ofri, D. (2014). *What doctors feel: How emotions affect the practice of medicine*. Boston, MA: Beacon Press.

Pachur, T., Hertwig, R., & Wolkewitz, R. (2014). The affect gap in risky choice: Affect-rich outcomes attenuate attention to probability information. *Decision, 1*, 64–78.

Padgett, L., & Ferrer, R. A. (2015). Palliative care in cancer: Enhancing our view with the science of emotion and decision-making. *Journal of Palliative Medicine, 18*, 479.

Panagopoulou, E., Mintziori, G., Montgomery, A., Kapoukranidou, D., & Benos, A. (2008). Concealment of information in clinical practice: Is lying less stressful than telling the truth? *Journal of Clinical Oncology, 26*, 1175–1177.

Parker, S. M., Clayton, J. M., Hancock, K., Walder, S., Butow, P. N., Carrick, S., . . . Tattersall, M. H. (2007). A systematic review of prognostic/end-of-life communication with adults in the advanced stages of a life-limiting illness: Patient/caregiver preferences for the content, style, and timing of information. *Journal of Pain and Symptom Management, 34*, 81–93.

Parkes, C. M. (2000). Commentary: Prognoses should be based on proved indices not intuition [Peer commentary on the article "Extent and determinants of error in doctors' prognoses in terminally ill patients: Prospective cohort study," by N. A. Christakis & E. B. Lamont]. *BMJ: British Medical Journal, 320*, 469.

Parkinson, B., & Simons, G. (2009). Affecting Others: Social Appraisal and Emotion Contagion in Everyday Decision Making. *Personality and Social Psychology Bulletin, 35*, 1071–1084.

Parkinson, B., Simons, G., & Niven, K. (2016). Sharing concerns: Interpersonal worry regulation in romantic couples. *Emotion, 16*, 449.

Penman, D. T., Holland, J. C., Bahna, G. F., Morrow, G., Schmale, A. H., Derogatis, L. R., et al. (1984). Informed consent for investigational chemotherapy: patients' and physicians' perceptions. *Journal of Clinical Oncology, 2*, 849–855.

Persky, S., Ferrer, R. A., & Klein, W. M. (2016). Nonverbal and paraverbal behavior in (simulated) medical visits related to genomics and weight: A role for emotion and race. *Journal of Behavioral Medicine, 39*, 804–814.

Peters, E., Burraston, B., & Mertz, C. K. (2004). An emotion-based model of risk perception and stigma susceptibility: Cognitive appraisals of emotion, affective reactivity, worldviews, and risk perceptions in the generation of technological stigma. *Risk Analysis, 24*, 1349–1367.

Peters, E., Dieckmann, N. F., Västfjäll, D., Mertz, C. K., Slovic, P., & Hibbard, J. H. (2009). Bringing meaning to numbers: The impact of evaluative categories on decisions. *Journal of Experimental Psychology: Applied, 15*, 213–227.

Peters, E., Diefenbach, M. A., Hess, T. M., & Vastfjall, D. (2008). Age differences in dual information-processing modes. *Cancer, 113*, 3556–3567.

Peters, E., Hess, T. M., Vastfjall, D., & Auman, C. (2007). Adult age differences in dual information processes: Implications for the role of affective and deliberative processes in older adults' decision making. *Perspectives on Psychological Science, 2*(1), 1–23.

Peters, E., Lipkus, I., & Diefenbach, M. A. (2006). The functions of affect in health communications and in the construction of health preferences. *Journal of Communication, 56*, S140–S162.

Pirl, W. F., Lerner, J. S., Eusebio, J., Traeger, L., Fields, L., El-Jawahri, A., . . . Temel, J. (2015). Association between oncologists' dispositional affect and depressive symptoms in the patients with metastatic cancer. *Journal of Clinical Oncology, 33*, S9559.

Portnoy, D. B., Han, P. K., Ferrer, R. A., Klein, W. M., & Clauser, S. B. (2013). Physicians' attitudes about communicating and managing scientific uncertainty differ by perceived ambiguity aversion of their patients. *Health Expectations, 16*, 362–372.

Quinn, G. P., Koskan, A., Wells, K. J., Gonzalez, L. E., Meade, C. D., Pozo, C. L., & Jacobsen, P. B. (2012). Cancer patients' fears related to clinical trial participation: A qualitative study. *Journal of Cancer Education, 27*, 257–262.

Raghunathan, R., & Pham, M. T. (1999). All negative moods are not equal: Motivational influences of anxiety and sadness on decision making. *Organizational Behavior and Human Decision Processes, 79*(1), 56–77.

Reyna, V. F. (2008). Theories of Medical Decision Making and Health: An Evidence-Based Approach. *Medical Decision Making, 28*, 829–833.

Reyna, V. F. (2012). A new intuitionism: Meaning, memory, and development in fuzzy-trace theory. *Judgment and Decision Making, 7*, 332–359.

Reyna, V. F., Chick, C. F., Corbin, J. C., & Hsia, A. N. (2014). Developmental reversals in risky decision making: Intelligence agents show larger decision biases than college students. *Psychological Science, 25*, 76–84.

Richards, J. M., Butler, E. A., & Gross, J. J. (2003). Emotion regulation in romantic relationships: The cognitive consequences of concealing feelings. *Journal of Social and Personal Relationships, 20*, 599–620.

Robbins, M. L., Lopez, A. M., Weihs, K. L., & Mehl, M. (2014). Cancer conversations in context: Naturalistic observation of couples coping with breast cancer. *Journal of Family Psychology, 28*, 380–390.

Rodenhuis, S., Van Den Heuvel, W. J. A., Annyas, A. A., Schraffordt Koops, H., Sleijfer, D. T., & Mulder, N. H. (1984). Patient motivation and informed consent in a phase I study of an anticancer agent. *European Journal of Cancer and Clinical Oncology, 20*, 457–462.

Rottenstreich, Y., & Hsee, C. K. (2001). Money, kisses, and electric shocks: On the affective psychology of risk. *Psychological Science, 12*, 185–190.

Schuettler, D., & Kiviniemi, M. T. (2006). Does how I feel about it matter? The role of affect in cognitive and behavioral reactions to an illness diagnosis. *Journal of Applied Social Psychology, 36*, 2599–2618.

Smith, C. A., & Ellsworth, P. C. (1985). Patterns of cognitive appraisal in emotion. *Journal of Personality and Social Psychology, 48*, 813–838. doi:10.1037/0022-3514.48.4.813

Smith, J. L. (2000). Commentary: Why do doctors overestimate? [Peer commentary on the article "Extent and determinants of error in doctors' prognoses in terminally ill patients: Prospective cohort study," by N. A. Christakis & E. B. Lamont]. *BMJ: British Medical Journal, 320*, 469.

Srivastava, S., Tamir, M., McGonigal, K. M., John, O. P., & Gross, J. J. (2009). The social costs of emotional suppression: a prospective study of the transition to college. *Journal of Personality and Social Psychology, 96*, 883–897.

Stanton, A. L., Danoff-burg, S., & Huggins, M. E. (2002). The first year after breast cancer diagnosis: hope and coping strategies as predictors of adjustment. *Psycho-Oncology, 11*, 93–102.

Stanton, A. L., & Snider, P. R. (1993). Coping with a breast cancer diagnosis: A prospective study. *Health Psychology, 12*, 16–23.

Suter, R. S., Pachur, T., & Hertwig, R. (2015). How Affect Shapes Risky Choice: Distorted Probability Weighting Versus Probability Neglect. *Journal of Behavioral Decision Making, 29*, 437–449.

Tackman, A. M., & Srivastava, S. (2016). Social responses to expressive suppression: The role of personality judgments. *Journal of Personality and Social Psychology, 110*, 574–591.

Temel, J. S., Greer, J. A., Muzikansky, A., Gallagher, E. R., Admane, S., Jackson, V. A., . . . Lynch, T. J. (2010). Early palliative care for patients with metastatic non-small-cell lung cancer. *New England Journal of Medicine, 363*, 733–742.

Teno, J. M., Freedman, V. A., Kasper, J. D., Gozalo, P., & Mor, V. (2015). Is care for the dying improving in the United States? *Journal of Palliative Medicine, 18*, 662–666

Vahdaninia, M., Omidvari, S., & Montazeri, A. (2010). What do predict anxiety and depression in breast cancer patients? A follow-up study. *Social Psychiatry and Psychiatric Epidemiology, 45*, 355–361.

Vanneman, M., & Dranoff, G. (2012). Combining immunotherapy and targeted therapies in cancer treatment. *Nature Reviews Cancer, 12*, 237–251.

Vignemont, F. de, & Singer, T. (2006). The empathic brain: how, when and why? *Trends in Cognitive Sciences, 10*, 435–441.

Waters, E. A., Weinstein, N. D., Colditz, G. A., & Emmons, K. M. (2007a). Reducing aversion to side effects in preventive medical treatment decisions. *Journal of Experimental Psychology: Applied, 13*(1), 11.

Waters, E. A., Weinstein, N. D., Colditz, G. A., & Emmons, K. M. (2007b). Aversion to side effects in preventive medical treatment decisions. *British Journal of Health Psychology, 12*, 383–401.

Waters, E. A., Weinstein, N. D., Colditz, G. A., & Emmons, K. (2009). Explanations for side effect aversion in preventive medical treatment decisions. *Health Psychology, 28*, 201.

Wefel, J. S., Saleeba, A. K., Buzdar, A. U., & Meyers, C. A. (2010). Acute and late onset cognitive dysfunction associated with chemotherapy in women with breast cancer. *Cancer, 116*, 3348–3356.

Wegener, D. T., Petty, R. E., & Klein, D. J. (1994). Effects of mood on high elaboration attitude change: The mediating role of likelihood judgments. *European Journal of Social Psychology, 24*(1), 25–43. doi:10.1002/ejsp.2420240103

Willett, W. C. (2002). Balancing life-style and genomics research for disease prevention. *Science, 296*, 695–698.

Williams, D. M., & Evans, D. R. (2014). Current emotion research in health behavior science. *Emotion Review, 6*, 277–287.

Wilson, T. D., & Gilbert, D. T. (2003). Affective forecasting. *Advances in Experimental Social Psychology, 35*, 345–411.

Winterich, K. P., Han, S., & Lerner, J. S. (2010). Now that I'm sad, it's hard to be mad: The role of cognitive appraisals in emotional blunting. *Personality and Social Psychology Bulletin, 36*, 1467–1483.

Yang, Z. J., McComas, K. A., Gay, G. K., Leonard, J. P., Dannenberg, A. J., & Dillon, H. (2010). From information processing to behavioral intentions: Exploring cancer patients' motivations for clinical trial enrollment. *Patient Education and Counseling, 79*, 231–238.

PART 3

Conclusions and Future Directions

21

Affective Determinants of Health Behavior

Common Themes, Future Directions, and Implications for Health Behavior Change

RYAN E. RHODES, DAVID M. WILLIAMS, AND MARK T. CONNER

INTRODUCTION

In this concluding chapter we summarize common themes that cut across the preceding chapters, including different conceptualizations of affective concepts, dimensions of affect constructs, conceptual models of affect and behavior, behavior-specificity in affect–behavior relationships, and the relationship between affect, social processes, and behavior. Within each of these areas we highlight potential future directions. In the concluding section we discuss some immediate implications for health behavior intervention.

CONCEPTUALIZATIONS OF AFFECT IN THE CONTEXT OF HEALTH BEHAVIOR

There is some variability but also some emerging consensus regarding the conceptualization and labeling of affect concepts. First, many authors directly refer to or at least allude to a distinction between affect proper, which includes core affect, moods, and emotions, versus cognition about affect, which includes affective outcome expectancies, affective attitudes, and affective associations (Conner, this volume; Consedine, Reynolds, & Borg, this volume; Hall, Fong, & Lowe, this volume; Hansen, Gillman, Feldstein Ewing, & Bryan, this volume; Heyhoe & Lawton, this volume; Rhodes & Gray, this volume; Sheeran, Webb, Gollwitzer, & Oettingen, this volume; Wiers, Anderson, Van Backstaele, Salemink, & Hommel, this volume; Williams, this volume). However, the relationship between the two is not fully specified.

Within the affect proper domain, there is emerging consensus that core affect (i.e., pleasure versus displeasure and high versus low arousal) is more evolutionarily primitive and subcortically generated relative to more discrete emotions and moods (Hansen et al., this volume; Wiers et al., this volume; Williams, this volume). Likewise, consensus appears to be emerging regarding the distinction between "incidental affect" and "integral affect," with the latter term reserved for affect (proper) that is experienced in the context of the target behavior—that is, while thinking about or engaging in the target behavior (Rhodes & Gray, this volume; Sheeran et al., this volume). Moreover, within the integral affect domain there is a temporal distinction in the separations of anticipatory affect, immediate affective response, and postbehavior affect response, suggesting that temporality may be a defining dimension for affect constructs (Williams, Rhodes & Conner, this volume). There is, however, some disagreement regarding labeling of concepts within the affect proper category, including use of the labels "positive affect" and "negative affect" (Hagger & Protogerou, this volume; Williams et al., this volume).

Among concepts representing some type of cognition about affect, there is broad agreement regarding the distinction between instrumental and affective outcome expectancies and attitudes (Conner, this volume; Day & Coups, this volume; Hansen et al., this volume; Heyhoe & Lawton, this volume; Rhodes & Gray, this volume; Sheeran et al., this volume), representing an advance beyond the sociocognitive cost/benefit approach. A second distinction that is highlighted across the volume, but not necessarily within each chapter, is the level of conscious awareness attributed to cognition about affect. This is most prominent in chapters that feature dual process approaches (de Ridder & Evers, this volume; Ellis & Ferrer, this volume; Hall et al., this volume; Hansen et al., this volume; Heyhoe & Lawton, this volume; Reese, Yi, Bell, & Daughters, this volume; Rhodes & Gray, this volume; Sheeran et al., this volume; Wiers et al., this volume; Williams, this volume). The most noteworthy constructs in this distinction include affective associations and implicit attitudes, where affect is synonymous with type 1 determinants of health behavior (Evans & Stanovich, 2013). These are contrasted by affective attitude and anticipated affective reaction, which represent conscious mental representations of the affective experience.

The need for a taxonomy and discriminant validity among affect concepts is essential moving forward. Many authors highlight this issue directly, but this is also evident with the volume of labels employed across the chapters to describe various affect or affect-related constructs. Indeed, even the three coeditors use different labels for the broad category of cognition about affect, including "affect processing" (Williams et al., this volume), "affective judgements" (Rhodes & Gray, this volume), and "cognitively mediated affect" (Conner, this volume), although we all agree that these labels serve the same functional description. There is also some disagreement as to whether cognition about affect should even be considered as under the umbrella of research on affect and health behavior (Ekkekakis, Zenko, Ladwig, & Hartman, this volume). The present authors firmly believe that, given the interplay between affect, cognition, and behavior, the answer to the latter question is an unequivocal "yes," so long as one distinguishes between affect proper and cognition about affect.

Taken together, the distinctions referred to in the preceding paragraphs lay the groundwork for a preliminary taxonomy of affect constructs (Figure 21.1). In our preliminary taxonomy we distinguish between affect proper and affect processing. We include incidental affect, anticipatory affect, during-behavior affect, and postbehavior affect within the affect proper category. Although affect might be experienced above or below awareness (Lambie & Marcel, 2002), we do not try to make such a distinction, because definitions of affect usually include subjectively experienced feelings, so affect that is below awareness would not qualify (Davidson,

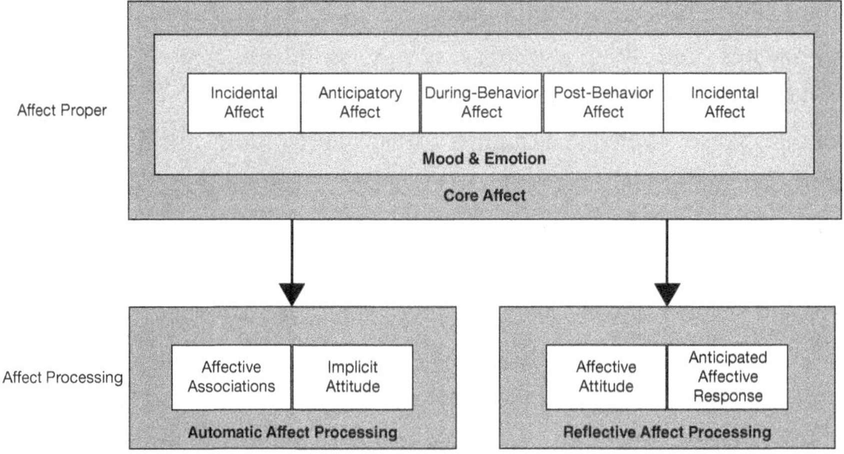

Figure 21.1. Proposed taxonomy of affect constructs.

Scherer, & Goldsmith, 2009; Ekkekakis, 2013; Kahneman, Diener, & Schwarz, 1999; Lewis, Haviland-Jones, & Barrett, 2008; Manstead, Frijda, & Fischer, 2004). Within affect processing we include a distinction between automatic affect processing (which includes affect associations and implicit affective attitudes) and reflective affect processing (which includes anticipated affective responses and affective attitudes).

While not included in our specific affect taxonomy, we view these constructs as antecedents of hedonic motivation and reflective motivation (see Williams, this volume). We see affect proper as mainly impacting on both types of motivation through affect processing. We also see affect processing as mainly impacting on behavior through hedonic and reflective motivation. Furthermore, we would also expect moderated relationships to be possible among affect constructs (e.g., affect proper moderating the impact of affective processing on motivation) and between affect and cognition constructs (e.g., affect processing moderating the impact of cognitive attitudes on motivation).

We concede this approach outlined previously and in Figure 21.1 as a mere starting point in order to classify key constructs. Whether these distinctions improve the conceptualization of affect in overarching health behavior models will be determined by future research. Furthermore, interventions designed with these distinctions will help determine whether they hold utility as an applied taxonomy for affect constructs.

CONCEPTUAL MODELS OF AFFECT AND BEHAVIOR

Nearly every chapter in the first part of this book (chapters 2–10) offers a conceptual framework for how affect influences behavior. Some chapters provide detailed and thorough focus on a particular affect concept (e.g., Baldwin & Sala, this volume; Kiviniemi & Klasko-Foster, this volume), whereas others emphasize multiple affective states and/or affect-related cognitive concepts and their interrelations (Conner, this volume; Hagger & Protogerou, this volume; Hall et al., this volume; Rhodes & Gray, this volume; Sheeran et al., this volume; Wiers et al., this volume; Williams, this volume). Frameworks include mediational pathways from affect proper to cognitively mediated affect processes to behavior (Conner, this volume; Rhodes & Gray, this volume), direct effects of affect on behavior (Baldwin & Sala, this volume; Kiviniemi & Klasko-Foster, this volume; Rhodes & Gray, this volume; Sheeran et al., this volume), affect as a moderator of the effects of cognition on behavior (Hall et al., this volume), or cognition as a moderator of the effects of affect on behavior (Sheeran et al., this volume). Additionally, some frameworks employ a dual-processing perspective, emphasizing the distinction between implicit and explicit affect and/or affect processing (Rhodes & Gray, this volume; Wiers et al., this volume; Williams, this volume). Another common theme is the interface between theories of affect regulation and theories of self-regulation that involve affect (Hagger & Protogerou, this volume; Rhodes & Gray, this volume; Sheeran et al., this volume). Whereas the former emphasizes how people use (health-related) behavior to manage their affect, the latter emphasizes the role of affect in managing behavior. Despite this difference in emphasis, there is room for integration across such affect-regulation and behavioral self-regulation models.

In general, more research is needed to test the conceptual models of affect and behavior that have been put forward in this volume and elsewhere. For example, more research is needed on the distinction between affect-related concepts. Is it possible to distinguish empirically (both in terms of measurement and manipulation) between affective associations and affective attitudes, and do these concepts have different relationships with behavior? Another area for future research is the effects of during-behavior versus postbehavior affective response on future behavior, and whether there are different mediators of these effects. These are exciting areas for the next decade of research.

BEHAVIOR-SPECIFICITY IN AFFECT–HEALTH BEHAVIOR RELATIONSHIPS

As we noted in chapter 1 (Williams et al., this volume) there does not appear to be any simple mapping between types of health behaviors and the relative importance of affect compared to other (e.g., cognitive) factors in determining behavior. For example, in the current book we have chapters that consider the role of affect for various preventive (e.g., physical activity: Hall et al., this volume; diet/eating: de Ridder & Evers, this volume; drinking alcohol: Reese et al., this volume; sexual behaviors: Hansen et al., this volume; smoking: McCarthy, Cook, Leyro, Minami, & Bold, this volume; suntanning: Day & Coups, this volume) and detective or curative (e.g., screening: Consedine et al., this volume; cancer-related behaviors: Ellis & Ferrer, this volume) health behaviors. Similarly, both approach (e.g., physical activity: Rhodes & Gray, this volume) or avoidance (e.g., drinking alcohol: Weirs et al., this volume; smoking: McCarthy et al., this volume; substance use: Reese et al., this volume; sun tanning: Day & Coups, this volume) health behaviors are addressed in the book. The book also contains chapters focusing on more (e.g., smoking: Weirs et al., this volume; physical activity: Hagger & Protogerou, this volume; diet/eating: Sheeran et al., this volume) or less (e.g., blood donation: Ferguson & Masser, this volume; health screening: Consedine et al., this volume) frequently performed health behaviors that might be considered to be more or less under habitual control (Ouellette & Wood, 1998). It is noteworthy that it is particularly in relation to more frequently performed behaviors that more automatic influences (that are normally tapped by more affective measures) have been studied.

Future research might usefully explore whether the different types of affect that are distinguishable (see Williams et al., this volume) show differential predictive power (i.e., effect size) for different health behaviors. For example, affect proper may be more predictive for some health behaviors and thus show only partial overlap with predictions from hedonic motivation or affect-processing variables (affective attitudes, regret, satisfaction, passion). Similar ideas about the power of cognitive determinants of intention and behavior have been reported in relation to tests of the theory of planned behavior in different groups of health behaviors (McEachan, Conner, Taylor, & Lawton, 2011). There has been limited work on this issue in relation to affective attitudes (Conner et al., in press; McEachan et al., 2016). McEachan et al. (2016) in a meta-analysis of the reasoned action approach (RAA) showed affective attitudes to be significantly stronger predictors of intentions and behavior for risk compared to protection behaviors, while in a multibehavior study testing the RAA, Conner et al. (in press) showed affective attitudes to be stronger predictors of behavior for risk compared to protection behaviors even when controlling for other RAA variables and past behavior.

Relatedly, the overlap between different types of affect as described in Figure 21.1 may vary across behaviors and this may have consequences for their relative power to predict behavior. For example, Conner, McEachan, Taylor, O'Hara, and Lawton (2015) showed that affective attitudes and anticipated regret were more strongly intercorrelated for risk compared to detection health behaviors (but not different from protection behaviors). Consistencies and inconsistencies between affective determinants and how this varies across behaviors may be an interesting area for further research on health behaviors. For example, in one individual physical activity might be performed only because of the positive affect experienced while performing the behavior, while in another individual it is performed only to avoid the anticipated regret of not taking physical activity, while in a third individual both types of affective determinant are important. The relationship of differing types of affect and how they vary across health behaviors could be an interesting avenue for future research. For example, work has considered affective ambivalence concerning differently valenced affective influences and cognitive-affective ambivalence where affective and cognitive influences are differently valenced (Conner & Sparks, 2002). Relatedly, the coherence of motivational influences including cognitive and affective factors as a moderator of intention–health behavior relationships has recently been examined (Sheeran & Conner, in press). Theory and applied comparisons in relation to various different individual or groups of health behaviors may yield interesting insights.

AFFECT, SOCIAL PROCESS, AND HEALTH BEHAVIOR

We noted a paucity of research and conceptualization on the role of social processes and affect constructs in health behavior across the chapters in this book. This may be deliberate, as affect proper is conceived as evolutionarily primitive (Wiers et al., this volume; Williams, this volume), yet emotions and moods are socioculturally moderated (Barrett, 2009) and affect-processing constructs have clear traditions in social learning (Bandura, 1986). Thus, social factors are likely critical in understanding the affect–health behavior relationship.

Eating behavior research appears to be the most advanced in this domain, with clear evidence that culture and social identity can influence perceptions of pleasure versus utility and subsequent behavior (see de Ridder & Evers, this volume). Relatedly, moral norms of health behavior have seen more advanced research in blood donation and health-screening behaviors, and research demonstrates the complex relationships between affect, societal expectations, and engagement with the behavior (see Consedine et al., this volume; Ferguson & Masser, this volume). The important relationship between the various affect constructs described in Figure 21.1 and social climate (e.g., caregivers, caregiving teams) is also highlighted in only a couple of chapters (see Ellis & Ferrer, this volume; Heyhoe & Lawton, this volume). Overall, the results of these chapters highlight the importance of social processes in understanding affect–health behavior relationship and underscore the importance of this issue for future basic and applied research in all health behaviors.

IMPLICATIONS FOR HEALTH BEHAVIOR CHANGE

Research on affect and health behavior can be placed on a continuum from more basic to more applied. A majority of the research represented in this volume, particularly Part 1 (chapters 2–10), is of a more basic variety, focusing on topics such as the conceptualization of affect, the interplay among different affect concepts and between affect and cognition, and the relationships between affect and health-related behavior. Moreover, much of the research discussed in Part 2 (chapters 11–20), while generally *more* applied than Part 1 (chapters 2–10), is still either laboratory based or involves field-based observational designs. As noted in the preceding sections, additional research of this kind is needed, particularly to the extent that it provides empirical tests of the multiple frameworks of affect and health behavior that have been forwarded in this volume and elsewhere.

Also sorely needed, however, is more applied research that translates theory and research on affective determinants of health behavior into behavior change interventions. Interventions on affect constructs may find contemporary theorizing of dual-process interventions as a useful template (e.g., Hoffman, Friese, & Wiers, 2008; Wiers et al., this volume; Williams, this volume; Williams & Evans, 2014). Specifically, it seems logical that behavioral interventions could focus on three routes: direct modification of other sources of behavioral influence (e.g., traditional social cognitive factors) in order to overcompensate for the affective constructs; direct modification of the affect constructs; or intervention on moderators of the affect–behavior link.

While much experimental research has accumulated on modifications of other cognitive sources of behavioral influence with mixed outcomes (Abraham & Michie, 2008; Prestwich et al., 2014), more research on modifications to affect constructs to potentially overcome the effects of other affect constructs may be useful. For example, a focus on anticipated affective reactions in order to lessen the effects of affective attitude on a given health behavior could be an effective means of intervention, when the experience of the behavior is less amenable to change (Conner et al., 2015). In a similar vein, interventions on satisfaction (Baldwin & Sala, this volume) or affective associations (Kiviniemi & Klasko-Foster, this volume) could also be useful in a similar capacity. More research is needed to examine how manipulations of one affect construct may improve health behavior by overriding the potency of other affect–behavior relationships.

A direct focus on affect constructs has seen limited attention. In this book, several chapters overview initial research that has focused on changing affect constructs to improve health behavior including affect-based games (Rhodes & Gray, this volume), messaging about affect (Conner, this volume; Day & Coups, this volume; Rhodes & Gray, this volume), and priming (Kiviniemi & Klasko-Foster, this volume; see also Hofmann, 2010). The state of this research suggests that some effects of health behavior change may be possible through directly targeting the affect construct as a putative mediator. Likewise, research is needed to test the malleability of hedonic motivation, as distinct from traditional emphases on socio-cognitive conceptualizations of motivation in terms of intentions or goals (Williams, this volume). For example, interventions might be designed to reduce hedonic desires for health-related stimuli such as calorically dense foods, cigarettes, and alcohol, or to reduce hedonic dread for behaviors such as vigorous exercise and cancer screenings. Still, these authors also note that this area of research is in its infancy, with only a handful of studies in any particular health behavior domain. We believe this route of affect–behavior intervention is an important area for sustained future research as it represents the most straightforward approach to intervention.

Intervention on moderators of the affect–behavior link, however, may be the most important future direction for affect science and health behavior (Sheeran et al., this volume). This route of intervention highlights affect regulation, with an overriding assumption that while affect constructs may be difficult to change (i.e., due to an evolutionary or primal foundation), we may be able to mitigate the impact of affect on behavior. Most of the chapters in this volume highlight the importance of affect regulation in some form, although it is clear that the research on this route of intervention is in its very early stages. For example, habit (Baldwin & Sala, this volume; Hall et al., this volume; McCarthy et al., this volume; Rhodes & Gray, this volume), identity (Rhodes & Gray, this volume), implementation intentions (Sheeran et al., this volume), mindfulness (Reese et al., this volume), and pharmaceuticals (Day & Coups, this volume; Reese et al., this volume) are all discussed as possible ways to alter the impact of affect-related constructs on health behavior. This pathway for health behavior intervention has seen the least amount of research and conceptual attention to date. We hope that burgeoning research in this area will provide for a more definitive understanding of interventions on of the affect–health behavior link in the next decade. Ideally, there is an ongoing feedback loop between basic and applied research, such that basic research provides a basis for intervention research and intervention research is used to further test and refine conceptual models (Head & Noar, 2014; Rothman & Salovey, 2007).

CONCLUSIONS

This book focuses on important and exciting ways in which researchers are exploring the impacts of various affect constructs and their pathways to determining health-related behaviors. Overall, the 21 chapters in this book highlight a range of thinking on affective determinants of health behavior and support research in a burgeoning field of study. Not all approaches are complementary, and this is helpful for future hypothesis testing and creative research (see Williams et al., this volume). Still, all the work compiled in this volume demonstrates a shift in the conceptualization of the determinants of health behavior from the historical emphasis on systematic processing of weighted expectancies and values to intentions and subsequent action (Edwards, 1954). We also noted several common themes across the chapters including conceptualizations of affective concepts that can be grouped by a limited number of distinctions (Figure 21.1). The growing interest in affect science and health behavior was also demonstrated by the variety of conceptual models across the chapters in this volume. Almost all of these models are slightly different, but they represent schematics to test in future research in order to further our understanding of the key pathways of affect on health and indeed other behaviors. We noted avenues that may require even more in-depth theorizing such as behavior-specificity in affect–behavior relationships and the interrelationship between affect, social processes, and behavior. Finally, we highlighted how affective determinants of health behavior may be intervened on using examples across various chapters within the volume. This interaction between basic science and applied behavior change intervention represents the purpose of public health research and the chapters within this book represent exciting future directions for new discoveries in affective determinants of health behaviors.

REFERENCES

Abraham, C., & Michie, S. (2008). A taxonomy of behavior change techniques used in interventions. *Health Psychology, 27*, 379–387.

Bandura, A. (1986). *Social foundations of thought and action: A social-cognitive theory.* Englewood Cliffs, NJ: Prentice-Hall.

Barrett, L. F. (2009). Variety is the spice of life: A psychological construction approach to understanding variability in emotion. *Cognition and Emotion, 23*, 1284–1306.

Conner, M., McEachan, R., Lawton, J., & Gardner, P. (in press). Applying the reasoned action approach to understanding health protection and health risk behaviors. *Social Science and Medicine.*

Conner, M., McEachan, R., Taylor, N., O'Hara, J., & Lawton, R. (2015). Role of affective attitudes and anticipated affective reactions in predicting health behaviors. *Health Psychology, 34*, 642–652.

Conner, M., & Sparks, P. (2002). Ambivalence and attitudes. *European Review of Social Psychology, 12*, 37–70.

Davidson, R. J., Scherer, K. R., & Goldsmith, H. H. (Eds.). (2009). *Handbook of affective sciences.* New York, NY: Oxford University.

Edwards, W. (1954). The theory of decision making. *Psychological Bulletin, 51*, 380–417. doi: 10.1037/h0053870

Ekkekakis, P. (2013). *The measurement of affect, mood, and emotion: A guide for health-behavioral research.* New York, NY: Cambridge.

Evans, J. S., & Stanovich, K. E. (2013). Dual-process theories of higher cognition: Advancing the debate. *Perspectives on Psychological Science, 8*, 223–241.

Head, K. J., & Noar, S. M. (2014). Facilitating progress in health behaviour theory development and modification: The reasoned action approach as a case study. *Health Psychology Review, 8*, 34–52.

Hoffman, W., Friese, M., & Wiers, R. W. (2008). Impulsive versus reflective influences on health behavior: a theoretical framework and empirical review. *Health Psychology Review, 2*, 111–137.

Hofmann, W. (2010). Evaluative conditioning in humans: A meta-analysis. *Psychological Bulletin, 136*, 390–421.

Hofmann, W., De Houwer, J., Perugini, M., Baeyens, F., & Crombez, F. (2010). Evaluative conditioning in humans: A meta-analysis. *Psychological Bulletin, 136*, 390–421.

Hoffman, W., Friese, M., & Wiers, R. W. (2008). Impulsive versus reflective influences on health behavior: A theoretical framework and empirical review. *Health Psychology Review, 2*, 111–137.

Kahneman, D., Diener, E., & Schwarz, N. (Eds.). (1999). *Well-being: The foundations of hedonic psychology*. New York, NY: Russell Sage.

Lambie, J. A., & Marcel, A. J. (2002). Consciousness and the varieties of emotion experience: A theoretical framework. *Psychological Review, 109*, 219–259.

Lewis, M., Haviland-Jones, J. M., & Barrett, L. F. (Eds.). (2008). *Handbook of emotions* (3rd ed.). New York, NY: Guilford.

Manstead, A. S. R., Frijda, N., & Fischer, A. (Eds.). (2004). *Feelings and emotions: The Amsterdam symposium*. New York, NY: Cambridge University.

McEachan, R., Taylor, N., Harrison, R., Lawton, R., Gardner, P., & Conner, M. (2016). Meta-analysis of the reasoned action approach (RAA) to understanding health behaviors. *Annals of Behavioral Medicine, 50*, 592–612.

McEachan, R. R. C., Conner, M., Taylor, N. J., & Lawton, R. J. (2011). Prospective prediction of health-related behaviors with the theory of planned behavior: A meta-analysis. *Health Psychology Review, 5*, 97–144.

Oullette, J. A., & Wood, W. (1998). Habit in every day life: The multiple processes by which past behavior predicts future behavior. *Psychological Bulletin, 124*, 54–74.

Prestwich, A., Sniehotta, F. F., Whittington, C., Dombrowski, S. U., Rogers, L., & Michie, S. (2014). Does theory influence the effectiveness of health behavior interventions? Meta-analysis. *Health Psychology, 33*, 465–474.

Rothman, A. J., & Salovey, P. (2007). The reciprocal relation between principles and practice: Social psychology and health behavior. In A. Kruglanski & E. T. Higgins (Eds.), *Social psychology: Handbook of basic principles* (pp. 826–849). New York, NY: Guilford Press.

Sheeran, P., & Conner, M. (2017). Improving the translation of intentions into health actions: The role of motivational coherence. *Health Psychology, 36*, 1065–1073.

Williams, D. M., & Evans, D. R. (2014). Current emotion research in health behavior science. *Emotion Review, 6*, 277–287.

INDEX

Page numbers followed by *f* refer to figures